Reproductive Rights in a Global Context

Reproductive Rights in a Global Context

South Africa, Uganda, Peru, Denmark, United States, Vietnam, Jordan

Lara M. Knudsen

Foreword by Betsy Hartmann

Vanderbilt University Press
NASHVILLE

© 2006 Vanderbilt University Press
All rights reserved
First Edition 2006

10 09 08 07 06   1 2 3 4 5

Printed on acid-free paper.
Manufactured in the United States of America
Design by Wendy McAnally

Library of Congress Cataloging-in-Publication Data

Knudsen, Lara M.
    Reproductive rights in a global context : South Africa,
Uganda, Peru, Denmark, United States, Vietnam, Jordan /
Lara M. Knudsen.– 1st ed.
        p. cm.
    Includes bibliographical references.
    ISBN 0-8265-1527-4 (cloth : alk. paper)
    ISBN 0-8265-1528-2 (pbk. : alk. paper)
    1. Birth control–Cross-cultural studies. 2. Contraception–
Cross-cultural studies. 3. Abortion–Cross-cultural studies.
4. Fertility, Human–Cross-cultural studies. 5. Sex instruction–
Cross-cultural studies. 6. Women's rights–Cross-cultural
studies. I. Title.
HQ766.K65 2006
363.9'6–dc22
                                            2005028191

Dedicated to the women who have suffered
needlessly from reproductive abuses,
to the women and men who help them,
and to my grandmother, Louise Dickson Morgan

Contents

Acknowledgments

I am particularly indebted to the eighty or so individuals in seven countries who so graciously offered their time and thoughtful opinions to me. I was between seventeen and twenty-one years old as I conducted this research, with little institutional affiliation or authority, yet these people were still kind enough to grant me personal interviews and to devote serious attention to my many questions. Without their willingness, this book would not have been possible. They are the following:

South Africa: Janet Cole, Tersia Cruywagen, Kim Dickson-Tetteh, Mandy Ewan, Ntuthu Manjezi, Claudia Mogale, Gloria Mokoena, Margaret Moss, Rachel Ramphora, Motsomi Senne, Khin San Tint.

Uganda: Jane Atergire, Florence A. O. Ebanyat, Joy Kyazike Kyeyune, Anthony Mbonye, Elly Mugumya, Jotham Musinguzi, Elizabeth Musisi, Stella Neema, Priscila Monica Nswemu, Josephine Othieno, Nestor Owomuhangi, Miriam Sentongo.

Peru: Susana Chávez, Daniel Gho Aspilcueta, Rossina Guerrero, Miguel Gutiérrez Ramos, Rocio Gutiérrez, Cecilia Olea Mauleon, Miguel Ramos, José Carlos Ugaz, Trixsi Vargas Vasquez, Tammy Quintanilla Zapata.

Denmark: Lau Sander Esbensen, Lisbeth Knudsen, Sniff Nexoe, Helle Samuelsen, Johan Seidenfaden, Charlotte Wilken-Jensen.

United States: Abbie Adams, Rachel Atkins, Brittney Camp, Terry Daley, Ann Osborne, Dorothy Roberts, Larry S. Rodick, Jane Ann White.

Vietnam: Sita Michael Bormann, Do Thi Thanh Nhan, Tine Gammeltoft,

Le Thi Nham Tuyet, Daniel Levitt, Nina McCoy, Lisa Messersmith, Nguyen Kim Cuc, Nguyen Thi Bich Hang, Nguyen Thi Hoai Duc, Quach Thu Trang, Tran Thi Phuong Mai, Vu Quy Nhan.

Jordan: Seifeldin Abbaro, Ayman Abdel-Mohsen, Zeinab Abu Al-Sha'ar, Basem Abu Ra'ad, Kholoud Abu Zaid, Issa Al-Masarweh, Nouf Al-Omari, Zuhair J. Al-Zu'bi, Michael Bernhart, Asma Bishara, Nisreen Haddadin Bitar, Leila Hamarneh, Basma Khraisat, Michel Laloge, Abdul Rahim Ma'ayta, Shatha Mahmoud, Dana Khan N. Malhas, Salwa Nasser, Lina Qardan, Salwa Bitar Qteit.

The Norcroft Women's Writing Retreat in Lutsen, Minnesota, provided me with a beautiful space to write a portion of the book, as did the Jones and Hermes-Roach families in Wisconsin. Thanks to my agent, Jodie Rhodes, for her belief in this project. Thank you to my editor at Vanderbilt University Press, Michael Ames, whose vision for this book I deeply appreciate.

I would also like to thank those individuals who gave comments on drafts of these chapters, though the usual caveats apply; all mistakes or misrepresentations are my own: Marie Adamo, Issa Almasarweh, Michael Bernhart, Janet Cole, Tersia Cruywagen, Florence A. O. Ebanyat, Tine Gammeltoft, Betsy Hartmann, Jane Hughes, Barbara Klugman, Lisbeth Knudsen, Le Thi Nham Tuyet, Daniel Levitt, Dana Khan Malhas, Margaret Moss, Jotham Musinguzi, Sniff Nexoe, Nguyen Thi Bich Hang, Nguyen Thi Hoai Duc, Ann Osborne, Lina Qardan, Salwa Bitar Qteit, Quach Thu Trang, Dorothy Roberts, Miguel Ramos, Larry Rodick, Vu Quy Nhan.

Special thanks to my two most dedicated editors, Sunny Daly and my sister, Jena Knudsen, for the many hours they poured into reading these chapters.

Dr. Elizabeth Newhall, medical director of the Downtown Women's Center in Portland, Oregon, introduced me to the reproductive rights movement; I have her to thank for helping me find this passion and encouraging me along my path. To the remarkable women and men who work at the Women's Center, I cannot adequately express my gratitude. They supported me as I grappled with issues familiar to most abortion clinic workers in the United States, such as security fears and ethical dilemmas. Perhaps most importantly, the women there showed me a model of health care delivery that, as I see it, approaches the ideal, complete with genuine respect for their patients and a desire to empower the women who walk through their doors. Additionally, the owners' flexibility allowed me to finance my travels by repeatedly returning to work after extended absences.

I would also like to thank the many devoted teachers and mentors who have inspired and challenged me, particularly Lynette Rummel, Bob Engel, Lisa Ann Richey, Agaryvette Rojas, Humberto Valdivia, and Riyard Mustafa. I owe everything to my family—parents Beth and Eric, sister Jena, and my extended family—for their unconditional support and encouragement. Thank you also to Christopher ML Jones, for his seemingly never-ending patience, love, and confidence in me. Thank you all.

Foreword

In *Reproductive Rights in a Global Context* author Lara Knudsen takes us on an inspiring yet sobering journey to seven countries—South Africa, Uganda, Peru, Denmark, the United States, Vietnam, and Jordan—where she introduces us to the multiple challenges women face in securing reproductive rights. The book combines both her personal passion for the subject, which began with her work in an abortion clinic in Portland, Oregon, and her ability to synthesize vast amounts of research and information. Ms. Knudsen is a skilled interviewer and in these pages we hear the voices of women's rights activists, health professionals, development workers, and government officials in each country who are committed, whether through the provision of direct services or policy advocacy, to advancing a full range of reproductive rights.

I first met Ms. Knudsen when she was an undergraduate student at Marlboro College, recently returned from fieldwork in Uganda. She told me about her plans for this book and I admired her then, as I do now, for her commitment to the project and her courage and ability to carry it through. She is a member of a new generation of reproductive rights activists and scholars with a holistic, transnational vision of the issues. She situates her analysis of the politics of population, contraception, abortion, HIV/AIDS, and sex education within a larger social, political, and economic framework. She does not hesitate to examine the powerful forces that constrain women's access to services whether they are patriarchal family structures, privatization of health services, the skewed priorities of national governments and international donors, racism, or right-wing assaults on reproductive freedom. At the same time she highlights the multiple forms of women's agency, from grassroots activism to policymaking, as women in all seven countries navigate and challenge these constraints.

Lara Knudsen also pays much needed attention to issues of access. Through the impressive work of women's health activists, South Africa's constitution, for example, guarantees women access to free and safe abortion, yet in some of the country's poorest regions abortion facilities remain few and far between, forcing many women to resort to illegal and unsafe abortions. In the United States too, many women lack access to services either because they do not have the money to pay for them or there are no nearby clinics or doctors to serve them. Population control programs meanwhile often target poor women with long-term, provider-controlled contraceptives like Depo Provera, Norplant, or the IUD without giving them access to a wider range of contraceptive choices. While Ms. Knudsen documents the achievements of the 1994 International Conference on Population and Development in Cairo in reaching a broad consensus in favor of women's empowerment and reproductive health, she also shows how wide a gap remains between rhetoric and reality.

This book is a major new contribution to the study of reproductive rights and Ms. Knudsen's clear exposition makes it particularly useful for undergraduate courses in women's studies, development studies, community health, and related disciplines. As a young woman who dared to journey around the world to find out first-hand about the status of reproductive rights, Lara Knudsen is also an important role model for students interested in these pressing and controversial issues.

—Betsy Hartmann,
Director, Population and Development Program,
Hampshire College

Preface

This book is the culmination of five years of traveling, interviewing, reading, and writing, all in the hope of gaining an understanding of women's sexual and reproductive rights in seven diverse countries. Although I am in the closing stages of this project, I feel that this book offers a beginning, for myself at least, in grasping a few fundamental concepts about reproductive rights, particularly as they relate to the countries highlighted.

My own work in reproductive rights started at home, in Portland, Oregon, when a local abortion clinic hired me part-time. I soon became interested in reading about issues such as abortion, contraception, and sex education in other countries, but a search at the bookstore revealed no such books. There were plenty of books written about reproductive rights in the United States, of course, and a few on global reproductive rights in general, but I failed to find a single one that gave a brief introduction to the topic in a variety of countries. From there grew the idea for this book. I wrote this book because I wanted to better understand how a reproductive health worker in, say, South Africa, deals with the challenges inherent to the work. Indeed, what *are* those challenges, in South Africa? Are they the same as those we face here in the United States? By listening to the stories of people involved in reproductive health work in a range of political, cultural, and economic contexts, my understanding of reproductive rights broadened considerably. I realized that what my coworkers and I do in Portland is only a small, though important, piece of the picture in securing reproductive freedom for women. I realized that, despite tremendous differences, common ground does in fact connect women in all of these countries; the challenges we face do contain similarities, though they may take distinct forms.

Between 2000 and 2004, I spent time in each country presented in this book, staying from just one month up to eight months in each place. I targeted a range of individuals for in-depth interviews; most of those with whom I spoke were women's rights activists, health professionals, development workers, and government officials. In each country, I tried to interview people with varying amounts of prestige and power, from top government officials to lay health workers who did not have medical credentials but worked with women in a reproductive health care setting every day. Approximately two-thirds of the respondents were women. I conducted about fifteen interviews per country, supplemented by every relevant publication I could find. All of the interviews for this book were conducted in English, with the following exceptions: The Peruvian interviews were all done in Spanish; two of the Ugandan interviews were done in Luganda; and two of the interviews in Vietnam were conducted in Vietnamese with the help of an interpreter. This book is based on these interviews and the literature.

I chose these seven countries—South Africa, Uganda, Peru, Denmark, the United States, Vietnam, and Jordan—for a number of reasons. I attempted to choose countries that differed from each other in geography, culture, religious influences, socioeconomic levels, and politics. Practical considerations were also taken into account concerning the feasibility of carrying out this type of research in each country, with attention paid to language barriers and safety issues, for example. Each country has unique characteristics that set it apart from all the others. South Africa, with its history of apartheid and coercive population control, now has one of the most liberal abortion laws to be found anywhere. Uganda, held up as an example of how to control a seemingly out-of-control HIV/AIDS epidemic, has some of the worst reproductive health indicators in the world. In Vietnam, where abortion has been used as birth control at the expense of other methods, the ethics of a strong, "successful" population policy are thrown into question. Denmark, praised for its exemplary health care system and progressive social culture, faces its own set of obstacles regarding the reproductive rights of a quickly growing immigrant population. Every one of these countries adds to the picture of what reproductive rights might look like from a global perspective.

These country studies are not meant to be representative of the region in which they are situated; the chapter about Peru, for example, should not be generalized to depict Latin America as a whole. In fact, these country studies are not even wholly representative of the countries they claim to describe. Although I have done my best to research as fully as possible, I will be the first to admit that a book about reproductive rights in seven countries, by one author, will not be comprehensive. Instead, each chapter offers a glimpse at the subject, with full awareness that it will not be all-encompassing or complete. The introductory chapter gives background information relevant to all of the country chapters, which may be read sequentially or individually. For those readers who desire a more in-depth look at a particular country described in this book, I have included a detailed bibliography at the end of the text, as well as a directory of reproductive rights contacts in each country.

As a young, white, middle-class American woman, my view of reproductive rights as I conducted this research was necessarily biased; each of us sees the world through our own particular lens. The authors of a similar cross-cultural study ask, "In attempting to transmit 'women's voices,' particularly in languages that are not their own, how can we avoid the risks of distortion and misinterpretation that come from multiple layers of translating, editing, rewriting, and decontextualizing?"[1] I have done my best to be true to the people who contributed to this project, soliciting their feedback throughout the writing process; however, the representations of each country in this book are undoubtedly filtered through my own lens, and thus are subjective.

This study is also limited by my decision to concentrate on a few key topics within the field of reproductive rights. Sexual and reproductive rights extend far beyond the confines of family planning; the field includes rights surrounding homosexuality (as well as bisexuality and transgender issues), infertility, STIs (sexually transmitted infections) and HIV/AIDS, domestic gender-based violence, harmful traditional practices, and the needs of women beyond their reproductive years, to name a few. I made this study more manageable by specifically focusing on fertility, contraception, abortion, and sex education. As is true for any reproductive rights issue, these topics are couched within larger political and economic structures that intimately affect women's reproductive freedom. As Dorothy Roberts articulates,

> Reproductive liberty must encompass more than the protection of an individual woman's choice to end her pregnancy. It must encompass the full range of procreative activities, including the ability to bear a child, and it must acknowledge that we make reproductive decisions within a social context, including inequalities of wealth and power. *Reproductive freedom is a matter of social justice*, not individual choice.[2]

Reproductive rights activism in the United States includes protecting women's right to refuse sterilization, as well as women's right to abortion. Working from Roberts's broadly defined concept of reproductive freedom, we can see that women's empowerment programs, such as income-generating projects in Vietnam, also influence the degree of reproductive autonomy women experience. Reproductive rights are inseparable from the larger economic and political structures under which we live; the more power women gain within those structures, the more say they will generally have over their bodies and their reproductive choices. Reproductive rights activism may take many different forms, then, and while there are very few people in Uganda openly advocating for the legalization of abortion, activism on girls' literacy or women's voter registration still contributes to wider reproductive freedom, if indirectly.

Devon Mihesuah quotes an American Indian woman who was present at the takeover at Wounded Knee: "In your culture you have lots of problems with men. Maybe we do too, but we don't have time to worry about sexism. We worry about survival."[3] Reading through these country studies, one finds that many of the women are doing just that—surviving. Poor women's resistance to patriarchal norms is usually less obvious than the loud protests and lobbying organized by largely middle-class activists, who have the luxury of being politically engaged. A common misconception persists that women, particularly poor women, are apathetic or ignorant about their own rights. While it is true that women are not very visible in public debates in a few of these countries, one must not underestimate the role of human agency. Even under difficult circumstances, women employ sophisticated ways of resisting and rebelling against unjust systems in their lives. However, even though they are invested in making independent decisions, it is far more difficult to do this successfully within a larger system that oppresses women and attempts to deny their power. Prevailing patriarchal ideology undermines women's efforts to claim control over their lives. Yet women are not rendered helpless as a result.

In this book I explore the intersections between reproductive rights in these seven countries and highlight commonalities found across borders, in spite of drastically different frameworks. As the literature on "global sisterhood" grows, so does the need for an understanding of global reproductive rights. This book sheds light on the concept of "universal reproductive rights" by considering the diverse contexts in which people strive for a more equitable society, with women claiming decision-making power over their bodies.

Reproductive Rights in a Global Context

Introduction

Reproductive Rights in a Global Context

Every year 530,000 women die during pregnancy and childbirth, and another twenty million become ill or permanently disabled during pregnancy.[1] These women, most of whom live in developing countries, have suffered the most from inadequate health care, poor reproductive health education, and lack of access to resources that may have saved their lives. Despite the large scale of tragedy associated with poor reproductive health, development programs addressing such issues face innumerable obstacles and controversy. Abortion, contraception, and sex education strike at the heart of the most intimate areas of life, challenging our perceptions of what it means to be human and what women's role in society should be. Worldwide, issues related to reproductive rights are some of the most vigorously contested, regardless of the population's socioeconomic level, religion, or culture.

What exactly is the concept of "reproductive rights"? The Program of Action from the 1994 International Conference on Population and Development (ICPD) includes one widely cited definition:

> [R]eproductive rights embrace certain human rights that are already
> recognized in national laws, international human rights documents
> and other consensus documents. These rights rest on the recognition
> of the basic right of all couples and individuals to decide freely and
> responsibly the number, spacing and timing of their children and to have
> the information and means to do so, and the right to attain the highest
> standard of sexual and reproductive health. It also includes their right to
> make decisions concerning reproduction free of discrimination, coercion
> and violence, as expressed in human rights documents.[2]

Unfortunately, in some countries, such as the United States, the term "reproductive rights" has become synonymous in many people's minds with "abor-

1

tion rights," and not surprisingly—of all sexual health topics, abortion is perhaps the most contentious. Despite long-standing taboos, abortion remains a common experience for women. Each year, thirty-five of every one thousand women of reproductive age in the world have an abortion—a number that adds up to roughly one abortion per woman over the course of her lifetime.[3] Twenty percent of all pregnancies worldwide end in abortion, and nearly half of those abortions are unsafe (and often illegal).[4] Access to safe abortion is clearly a crucial component of reproductive freedom, but it is only one of many related rights. Myriad forces influence a woman's reproductive autonomy, including her educational and job opportunities, her exposure to information about sexual and reproductive health, her power to negotiate the terms of sexual relationships, and her access not only to safe abortion but also to safe childbearing services.

Fears of overpopulation rather than a concern for women's reproductive rights have historically driven many reproductive health programs. The population control movement was effective throughout the latter half of the twentieth century in implementing family planning programs that frequently used coercion rather than a human rights–based approach in an attempt to reduce total fertility levels; this is true to a lesser extent today. For decades closely tied to contraceptive programs abroad, the population control movement must be acknowledged as a prime contributor to the reproductive health context one finds today. In the past few decades, tension has grown between feminist women's health activists who sought to expand women's reproductive rights for the sake of human rights and the population control advocates whose chief goal was to cut fertility levels as much as possible. To understand the state of reproductive health and rights today, a brief look at the population control movement is useful.

Roots of the Population Control Movement

Vivid imagery of a global population "bomb" or "explosion" has been invoked countless times in the three decades since Paul Ehrlich, an American biologist, claimed that humankind is breeding itself into oblivion.[5] Overpopulation has been blamed for everything from increased poverty, high unemployment rates, and overtaxed social services to degradation of the environment, famine, and genocide. In the past century, population control proponents have drawn from the insights of Thomas Malthus (1766–1834), a British clergyman-turned-economist who wrote *First Essay on Population*.[6] "Population, when unchecked, increases in a geometrical ratio. Subsistence increases only in an arithmetical ratio. A slight acquaintance with numbers will show the immensity of the first power in comparison of [*sic*] the second."[7] Malthus proceeded to claim that "preventive checks" on exponential population growth, such as poverty, famine, and war, will ultimately save humanity from itself. According to Malthus, human misery is, then, an "absolutely necessary consequence."[8] Today, the most extreme neo-Malthusians advocate cutting off famine relief to poor countries that are "overpopulated." They cite famine and epidemics like HIV/AIDS as the "natural" checks Malthus envisioned.

Ehrlich, the biologist and environmentalist mentioned above, published *The Population Bomb* in 1968, in which he advocated stringent population control policies that would even be compulsory if necessary.[9] His central argument about population is worth quoting at length:

> A cancer is an uncontrolled multiplication of cells; the population explosion is an uncontrolled multiplication of people. Treating only the symptoms of cancer may make the victim more comfortable at first, but eventually he dies—often horribly. A similar fate awaits a world with a population explosion if only the symptoms are treated. We must shift our efforts from treatment of the symptoms to the cutting out of the cancer. The operation will demand many apparently brutal and heartless decisions. The pain may be intense. But the disease is so far advanced that only with radical surgery does the patient have a chance of survival.[10]

Ehrlich referred to advances in modern medicine as "death control" and criticized the U.S. Department of Health, Education, and Welfare for being "much more concerned with death control than population control."[11] In his concluding chapter, Ehrlich offered a partial solution to the population "problem": "[We need] compulsory birth regulation . . . [through] the addition of temporary sterilants to water supplies or staple food. Doses of the antidote would be carefully rationed by the government to produce the desired family size."[12] Although Ehrlich's views have softened in recent years, his extreme views in the 1960s and 1970s were held by many population control advocates in the United States and Europe.

The Rise of Coercive Population Control Policies

In response to increasing concern about overpopulation, international agencies and governments around the world adopted policies, from the 1960s on, that were based on the rationale that population control for the sake of the nation takes precedence over individual human rights.[13] Developed countries poured substantial resources into controlling Third World population growth, garnering support for their campaigns through racist imagery that depicted the Western world being overrun by people from poor countries. Population policies that arose out of the alarmist debate on overpopulation were driven by demographic targets and contraceptive quotas created by governments and international donors. Working from the assumption that the U.S. model of the nuclear family is best, population policies became synonymous with family planning programs; they were often coercive and ignored the "user perspective."[14]

The most prominent actors in the international population arena are the United States Agency for International Development (USAID), the United Nations Population Fund (UNFPA), the International Planned Parenthood Federation (IPPF), and the Population Council—all of which fund reproductive health programs throughout the developing world. Although the World Bank is not generally associated with population control policies, it too has supported population activities since the 1970s. The World Bank even held loans for structural adjustment programs (SAPs) hostage in Egypt, Kenya, and possibly Tanzania until those governments agreed to implement a national population policy (NPP).[15] Today, the World Bank provides most of the funding for many of these NPPs. In many developing countries, the paltry government funds devoted to their NPP may signify a lack of political commitment, or it may be a strategic decision since donors are more willing to fund population policies than other policies.[16] The World Bank is one of the leading financers of what the bank calls "reproductive health/family planning information and services." As of 1994, the bank was releasing US$200 million per year in new loans for family planning, with another US$1 billion in credits and loans for population work.[17]

USAID is well-known for what Morsy calls its "protracted commitment to population control in the Third World."[18] Since the 1970s, the United States has been the single largest donor of population assistance (although it ranks last among donor countries in terms of the percentage of GNP spent on development aid).[19] Donors have historically viewed high population growth rates as the cause of underdevelopment rather than an outcome, and they insisted that the population "problem" be addressed before tackling development issues.[20] Richey reports results from a 2001 analysis, "If a country adopts a population policy, it is 12.5% more likely to receive USAID funding, and of those countries having received funding, adopting a policy increases the countries' expected assistance nearly threefold."[21]

The provision of family planning under such population policies is not purely in the interest of individual women, but rather is an instrument used to further demographic goals set by government officials working in conjunction with foreign aid agencies. In countless communities in developing countries, family planning came to be viewed with suspicion, as a Western intervention rooted in racist imperialism. In the past many developing countries have used vertical family planning programs, in which family planning is provided separately from any other health services; vertical programs are often characterized by poor counseling and inadequate follow-up care, and they sometimes contain an element of force.[22]

Despite an Indian delegate's comment at the 1974 UN World Population Conference in Bucharest that "development is the best contraceptive," the focus of fertility reduction programs remained the promotion of family planning.[23] By the 1984 UN World Population Conference in Mexico City, population control policies were under increasing attack from women's health advocates who argued that the policies' narrow focus led to coercion and decreased quality of care. These policies also ignored the varied social and cultural contexts in which family planning was provided in developing countries around the world.[24] Most family planning programs heavily relied on contraceptive methods like the IUD and Depo Provera, despite safety concerns in some instances, because they are provider-controlled, highly effective methods. Permanent methods, like female sterilization, have also been widely promoted.

Over the years, reproductive rights activists have become more effective at arguing the right of women to choose how many children they have, whether or not such a decision is in conflict with population control programs or antiabortion policies. As discussed, the international community's favoring population control policies that curb "unacceptable" fertility rates in the developing world has led to mistrust and suspicion from members of targeted populations.[25] Women's health activists in particular have become more organized and vocal in response to what many consider unethical population control policies. In addition, in the 1980s the HIV/AIDS epidemic forced a broader discussion of sex into public discourse in many countries, leading to more emphasis in development projects on reproductive health issues beyond access to contraception. This growing opposition to the narrow population control focus led to a significant departure in the early 1990s from past population policies.[26]

The 1994 ICPD in Cairo

The 1994 International Conference on Population and Development (ICPD) represents a major turning point in the international population movement. An incredible 179 nations (eleven thousand representatives from governments, NGOs, international agencies, and citizen activists) met in Cairo and adopted a twenty-year Program of Action that is credited with reframing the population discourse.[27] The new consensus shifts from a focus on slowing population growth to an emphasis on improving women's lives. Participants at the ICPD asserted that governments have a responsibility to meet individuals' reproductive needs, rather than demographic targets. Family planning should be provided in the context of other reproductive health services, including services for healthy and safe childbearing, care for sexually transmitted infections (STIs), and postabortion care (PAC). The ICPD cast more light on related issues like violence against women, sex trafficking, and adolescent health.

The Cairo Program of Action includes no demographic targets, and it is the first international policy document to define reproductive health: "Reproductive health is a state of complete physical, mental, and social well-being and not merely the absence of disease or infirmity, in all matters relating to the reproductive health system."[28] The document ventures, "Reproductive health [. . .] implies that people are able to have a satisfying and safe sex life and that they have the capability to reproduce and the freedom to decide if, when and how often to do so."[29] Including such a bold statement in the Program of Action, signed by 179 nations, signified a watershed moment in the reproductive rights movement.

Unlike previous population conferences, a wide range of interests from grassroots to government levels were represented in Cairo. Though feminist activists and neo-Malthusians have never been natural allies, they managed to form an alliance, albeit a tenuous one, at the ICPD, both agreeing on the necessity of widespread access to reproductive health information and services.[30] Since the conference, NGOs and citizen activists have taken on a larger role in scrutinizing government population policy; explicit population control policies are generally not accepted anymore.[31] The new language extols the centrality of women's empowerment in meeting broader development goals.

Controversy in the ICPD Program of Action (PoA)

Despite the gains won at the ICPD, many in the field argue that the Program of Action did not go far enough. Predictably, the issue of abortion was a contentious one, and the delegates eventually decided to omit any recommendation to legalize abortion, instead advising governments to provide proper postabortion care and to invest in programs that will decrease the number of unwanted pregnancies. Adolescent reproductive rights presented another controversy and source of dissension among more socially conservative countries; the Program of Action urges governments to "protect and promote the rights of adolescents to reproductive health education, information and care."[32] The ICPD did not adequately address the far-reaching implications of the HIV/AIDS epidemic, though this omission may reflect the lack of urgency felt about HIV/AIDS at the time.[33] By 1999, recommendations at the ICPD+5 were expanded to include commitment to AIDS education, research, and prevention of mother-to-child transmission, as well as to the development of vaccines and microbicides.[34]

Another criticism of the Cairo program is its acceptance of neoliberal economic policies, such as encouraging countries to adopt user fees for health services.[35] "Studies from Ghana, Swaziland, Zaire, and Uganda suggest that user fees result in decreased use of public health services, especially by poorer people and women. One outcome has been a rise in maternal and infant mortality rates."[36] Furthermore, the PoA did not recognize the devastating impact that structural adjustment programs (SAPs) and the transition to market economies had on health, especially for the poor.[37] Some groups, like the Corner House in England, highlight the need to link reproductive and sexual rights to broader human rights and macroeconomic reforms.[38]

Despite these limitations, the Cairo Program of Action represents a great step forward. Though some countries signed the PoA with noted reservations, the fact that delegates from 179 nations managed to reach a consensus on such emotive issues is an accomplishment in itself.

Implementing the Cairo Agenda

In many countries one finds evidence of post-ICPD tensions as a rights-based approach progresses from pure rhetoric to actual changes on the ground. The extent to which the Program of Action has been implemented varies considerably from one country to the next. Since the ICPD, many countries have broadened their reproductive health programs and attempted to integrate maternal and child health services with family planning. More attention is generally paid to adolescent health and the consequences of unsafe abortion than previously seen. The ICPD succeeded in getting feminist language into governments' and population agencies' literature; however, in many countries the underlying concepts are not yet widely put into practice.[39] In some instances, a superficial name change seems to be the extent of the ICPD's influence—for example, the former Population Crisis Committee is now known as Population Action International, though their working platform has not changed significantly.[40] Likewise, Richey points out that the Tanzania National Family Planning Program changed its name to the National Reproductive and Child Health Sector, but there had been few changes at the implementation level as of 2002.[41] Some countries have actually tightened their population control programs since the ICPD; an example may be found in the two-child policies implemented in many Indian states.[42]

Women's health organizations commonly argue that reproductive health programs still place disproportionate emphasis on family planning services, often at the expense of other services. Richey reports that many health centers in Tanzania have a constant supply of contraceptives, but they lack basic drugs like antibiotics.[43] Under the Cairo Plan, improving women's health includes both preventing unwanted pregnancy *and* ensuring safe delivery. A lack of antibiotics leads to increased maternal death from sepsis, yet the drugs are still not always considered essential supplies for reproductive health programs.[44] In Tanzania, USAID only funds health centers that are currently or soon will be family planning training centers. "In an ironic twist to the struggle in the 1970s to integrate family planning services into government primary care clinics, in the 1990s there is a failure to integrate any other services into what have become, in effect, family planning clinics."[45] The ICPD's holistic approach to women's health and empowerment is difficult to find on the ground in many countries. As Richey concludes, "We cannot expect that population policies will in fact improve women's health, choice, and empowerment, when women have no access to health care that is not contraceptives."[46]

Conservative Forces

In addition to the lingering influence of neo-Malthusian ideology and neoliberal economic policies, the surge of religious fundamentalism has also led, since the ICPD, to policies damaging to women's health.[47] At the same time that developed countries' fear of overpopulation shapes foreign aid, antiabortion political factions dictate the actions of many governments and nongovernmental organizations in regard to reproductive health. Written by the Reagan administration in 1984, the Mexico City policy (dubbed the "Global Gag Rule") forbids any foreign organization receiving population assistance from USAID to work on the topic of abortion. USAID-funded organizations may not provide abortion services, refer patients for abortions, or advocate the legalization of abortion, *even if they use separate funding for their abortion-related work.*[48] Ironically, such a rule would be unconstitutional if implemented within the United States; in the Supreme Court decision *Rust v. Sullivan,* the Court ruled that governmental restriction of an organization's legal activities violates that organization's free speech rights.[49] Furthermore, amid much confusion about the specifics of the rule, many organizations no longer carry out abortion-related research or provide postabortion care, even though these activities are technically allowed under the Gag Rule, because they are fearful of losing their U.S. funding. After a reprieve from the rule under President Clinton's administration, development workers worldwide had to contend with the Mexico City policy once again when President George W. Bush reinstated the rule his first day in office in January 2001. The impact has been far-reaching, effectively forcing organizations to choose between continuing to accept USAID funds and sticking to their full agenda of reproductive rights activism.

Along with the Global Gag Rule, the Bush administration and Congress withdrew U.S. funding for the United Nations Population Fund (UNFPA) and the International Planned Parenthood Federation (IPPF) in 2001. Since the beginning of Bush's first term as president, the U.S. government has been a difficult partner in international agreements like the one in Cairo. In two preparatory meetings for the ICPD+10 in Asia and Latin America, the United States was alone in opposing the ICPD's Program of Action. Additionally, the United States attempted, unsuccessfully, to derail passage of the reproductive health strategy at the WHO Executive Board meeting in January 2004.[50] As feminist activists in the United States and abroad have seen the diminution rather than expansion of women's rights in many areas, they have sought to organize against forces like the Bush administration to further advance the broad reproductive rights strategies outlined in Cairo. Hindering the success of feminist movements in some countries is their narrow focus on issues predominantly affecting privileged women.

Focus of Reproductive Rights Movements: Forging a New Conception of Reproductive Rights

Mainstream reproductive rights movements in many countries struggle to build an inclusive platform that includes women from all socioeconomic backgrounds. In the United States, for example, the best-known reproductive rights organizations historically focused almost exclusively on issues that were most important to white, upper- and middle-class American women rather than addressing matters that more directly affected the less privileged. Narrowly concentrating on a woman's legal right to abortion, for example, American feminists until recently have largely neglected other reproductive rights issues that greatly affect women of color and poor women, such as sterilization abuses and inadequate access to health services, not to mention access to information and contraception. While the issue of abortion clearly has a tremendous impact on all women, the greatest obstacle to procuring a safe abortion for poor women and women of color in the United States is usually a matter of *access* and not one of legality. The legalization of abortion may ensure that a wealthy white woman can obtain an abortion from her private physician, but legalization by itself does not ensure that a poor, black woman in a rural area will have the financial resources or physical access to get an abortion. Likewise, interviewees in Peru took note of the concentration of the Peruvian women's movement in the capital city of Lima and its limited strength in more remote areas of the country. Kholoud AbuZaid in Jordan opined that feminist activists there are disconnected from the average woman and have a difficult time translating abstract feminist theories into practical, on the ground assistance. To maximize their strength and effectiveness, women's movements throughout the world must include in their agendas the needs of poor women in particular, all the while attempting to carve out a new definition of reproductive rights—one that takes into account the broader socioeconomic structures that influence women's autonomy.

The Changing State of Women's Reproductive Health and Rights

Although the seven countries highlighted in this book are each unique, they fit into larger, global patterns. In each of the countries, one can easily find a vibrant core of people dedicating their time, energy, and resources to furthering the cause of women's reproductive freedom. What form that freedom takes varies drastically from country to country and is specific to each cultural, religious, and ethnic background. Though confronted with myriad obstacles, ranging from depressing economic conditions to a devastating HIV/AIDS epidemic to fundamentalist political forces, women in each of these countries attempt to gain control over their health, their bodies, and their lives. Only in recent years have feminists become more effective at clearly defining the values behind reproductive rights and separating those values from the motivations of population control proponents. As today's reproductive rights movements grow, so do their abilities to clearly articulate a vision of reproductive rights that is far-reaching in both its definition and appeal.

1

South Africa

Background

South Africa is a country of extremes in regard to reproductive rights. On one hand, the country's experience with apartheid has left a legacy of deep-rooted inequities between segments of the population; South Africa's history is fraught with racist population control policies. The raging HIV/AIDS epidemic has largely sabotaged advances in reproductive health, as has the challenge of severe poverty in most areas of the country. Yet South Africa boasts what is perhaps the most progressive legislation in the world concerning abortion, and the country is widely commended for its successful integration of reproductive health services in line with the sentiments of the International Conference on Population and Development in Cairo.

With eleven official languages, South Africa's people are diverse; of 44.8 million people, 79 percent are African (black), 9 percent white, 9 percent "Colored," and 3 percent Indian.[1*] Grave health inequities persist along racial lines after decades of oppressive rule by the apartheid government. Historically, whites have enjoyed the best access to education and health care, followed by Indians, "Colored" people, and, lastly, blacks. South Africa's overall fertility rate is one of the lowest on the continent; in a study of over eleven thousand women, the fertility rate from 1995 to 1998 was 2.9—a decrease of 1.0 from the figure twenty years before. Fertility rates are lowest in the wealthiest and most urban provinces (Gauteng, Western Cape, and the Free State) and

---

* The term "Colored," first used by the apartheid government, refers to anyone of mixed racial heritage. During apartheid, data were gathered according to the labels White, Black, Colored, and Indian. The current government continues to use this system for data disaggregation. The small percentage of "Colored" people is partly due to the strict prohibition against interracial marriage during apartheid.

11

highest in the impoverished Northern Province, Eastern Cape, and Kwa-Zulu Natal. The total fertility rate masks substantial differences in fertility among various sections of the population; women with no education have an average of 4.5 children, compared to 1.9 for women with some university-level education. Broken down by race, the fertility rates are 3.1 for Africans, 2.5 for "Coloreds," and 1.9 for whites.[2] Several historical, cultural, and socioeconomic factors contribute to the varying fertility rates of South Africa's racial groups, as discussed below.

South African Reproductive Rights History: From Precolonial Traditional Societies to Apartheid

Despite the devastating effects of colonialism and apartheid on South Africa's native people, traditional lifestyles and values remain strong in parts of the country and continue to influence South Africans' morals and actions today. Traditional African societies that occupied present-day South Africa did not view sex as taboo or dirty; adults expected young people to enjoy sex, though within a tightly controlled framework. People made use of traditional methods of family planning, such as the rhythm method, withdrawal, and postpartum abstinence. As long as a woman continued to breastfeed, her husband would ejaculate outside the vagina to protect the infant from semen, thought to seep into the rest of the woman's body, contaminating her breast milk and harming the baby (hence, the widespread practice of *ukusoma*—"thigh sex"). Most of these traditional societies believed that a woman should not become pregnant again until her child is weaned and able to stand or walk. For hundreds of years, midwives and traditional healers aided women in using local herbs for both contraception and abortion.[3]

By the nineteenth century, abortion was not uncommon among Xhosa, Afrikaner, and "Colored" women, despite the increasing presence of missionaries who preached the evils of abortion.* The practice was not widely accepted, however. Myths circulated about abortion; for example, rural Pedi and Tsonga men believed that if a woman had an abortion, the rains would not come. Women who had abortions were labeled abnormal and thought to be witches.[4] In the early 1900s, white doctors claimed that abortion for white women was a threat to white supremacy. The South African judicial system concurred, and abortion became a "crime against the state."[5]

---

* Afrikaners are descendants of Dutch settlers, who first came to South Africa in the 1600s.

The apartheid government formally came into power in 1948 and later claimed that the black population was draining the country's resources. In order to control black population growth and hold onto white minority rule, the Afrikaner government implemented a vertical family planning program in 1974.[6] Under this program, patients paid fees for all health services except contraceptives, sterilization, and medical exams for victims of rape or assault.[7] In most rural areas, long-term methods such as injectables served as the sole contraceptive option. Hundreds if not thousands of black women were unwilling recipients of Depo Provera when health professionals gave them a shot immediately following childbirth without consent or even knowledge. Such postdelivery shots were so common that health workers dubbed this practice the "fourth stage of labor."[8]** Similarly, some doctors have been charged with performing tubal ligations after a cesarean section without the woman's knowledge or consent.[9] Testimony before the Truth and Reconciliation Commission in 1998 revealed an extreme example of the apartheid government's determination to control black fertility: The Chemical and Biological Warfare Program of the South African Defense Force undertook research for an infertility vaccine intended for use among black women.[10]***

While black and "Colored" women faced the government's attempts to stifle their reproduction, at the same time the authorities denied women the option of legal abortion. In 1975, the 99 percent male, all-white South African Parliament passed the Abortion and Sterilization Act, which made abortion illegal except for the very few women who met the stringent requirements. A woman was eligible for a legal termination of pregnancy only if she met one of the following criteria: the pregnancy seriously threatened her physical health or life; continuing the pregnancy would result in permanent damage to her mental health (usually defined as brain damage only); the fetus could be proven "irreparably" seriously handicapped (for example, if it had no brain); the woman was legally classified as an "imbecile"; or the woman could prove the pregnancy was a result of rape or incest.[11] Two doctors had to swear that the woman met one of these conditions before she would be granted a termination.[12] Inequities of race and class are obvious upon consideration of who managed to secure a legal termination; access to safe and legal abortions was almost

---

** Labor and delivery is typically broken down into three stages: contractions leading to full cervical dilation (stage one), delivery of the baby (stage two), and delivery of the placenta (stage three).

*** The postapartheid government established the Truth and Reconciliation Commission (TRC) in an effort to hear victims' and perpetrators' accounts of abuses that occurred during apartheid.

exclusively limited to wealthy, white women who could pay for a gynecologist to guide them through the bureaucracy. Of 868 legal abortions performed in 1988, 69 percent of the patients were white, though whites only comprised 12 percent of the general population at the time.[13] Likewise, in 1990 white women accounted for 800 of the 1,200 legal terminations performed.[14]

Refused the right to abortion, black women facing an unwanted pregnancy also dealt with pressure from within the black population to carry the pregnancy to term. Responding to the oppression and murder of blacks under the apartheid system, coupled with black women's forced contraceptive use and sterilization, a loud voice among the black "freedom fighters" from 1976 on urged women to have more children to aid the struggle.[15] In the midst of pressure from part of the black community to procreate and pressure from the government to be sterilized, women's own desires often went unmet.

The End of Apartheid and the Arrival of the African National Congress

After nearly a half century under an oppressive apartheid system, the anti-apartheid movement was successful in ousting the white government and replacing it with the African National Congress (ANC), led by Nelson Mandela. In 1994, for the first time since colonialists arrived in South Africa in the 1600s, the African population gained control over the state government, and the ANC introduced far-reaching changes. The 1994 Constitution includes a Bill of Rights that prohibits discrimination based on race, sex, gender, pregnancy, marital status, or sexual orientation.[16] The new government also ratified international human rights treaties, such as the Convention on the Rights of the Child and the Convention on the Elimination of All Forms of Discrimination against Women (CEDAW) (the latter of which the United States still refuses to sign).[17] In late 1996, the ANC legalized abortion in one of the most sweeping abortion reforms in the world.

During apartheid, the government repressed and denied expression of many progressive ideas; activists working for development faced being labeled "counter-revolutionary" or charged with treason. When the ANC came into power, a space suddenly opened for dialogue on issues like racism, sexism, and classism. Almost overnight, people with energy and creativity gained the freedom to work to improve their communities without fear of retaliation from government forces. South Africans did not waste time taking advantage of their newly won freedom. A crucial subject for reform was health care.

When the apartheid government finally fell apart and the ANC came into power, health services in South Africa were "fragmented, vertical, and over-lapped between provincial and local government authorities," though they were still of a relatively high standard.[18] The public health system was oriented toward tertiary care (the most sophisticated and expensive, curative procedures), while primary care remained underfunded. Divided into separate institutions on the basis of race, geographical area, and government authority, the health system's structure encouraged a severely unequal distribution of resources. Fallout from decades of racial discrimination was perhaps most obvious in the national health indicators; at the time of the government change in 1994, the infant mortality rate for blacks was ten times higher than the rate for whites, and the maternal mortality rate for blacks was sevenfold that for whites.[19]

The ANC sought to establish accountability and respect between the government and the health sector, but it encountered an atmosphere of mistrust and skepticism among health professionals. Historically, doctors and government officials never enjoyed a friendly relationship, partly due to many doctors' perception of government officials as overly authoritarian and bureaucratic.[20] Mistrust of the government extended to the general black population as well; whites have always had greater access to health care and health information than others, and black South Africans have often met anything perceived as "white" with suspicion. Furthermore, contraception was seen as "population control" for so long that this idea is only gradually dissolving.[21] A greater element of trust in the government exists today, and people are less suspicious about contraceptives. The new Patient Charter aims to protect patients from coercive contraception use and forced sterilization.[22] The Sterilization Act of 1998, in addition to affirming the right to sterilization, details the conditions under which it may be performed.[23]

Acting in accordance with the ANC's socialist, human rights roots, Dr. Nkosazana Zuma, the minister of health, declared free health care for pregnant women and children under the age of six in 1994. Two years later, under her leadership, the Ministry of Health extended universal primary health care to everyone—a particularly admirable accomplishment considering the shortage of outside funding for health care in South Africa. During apartheid, sanctions on the country resulted in scant international funding for health care. Even today only 1 percent of South Africa's total health budget comes from donors; the system is financed mainly by taxes.[24] The ANC has demonstrated its commitment to health by allotting a generous budget; in 1996–1997, the government spent US\$3.62 billion on health care—nearly 10 percent of its total budget.[25] Exactly how to spend that money, and how to strike a balance between preventive and curative services, remains a contentious issue.

Sex Education

Despite extensive reforms after apartheid in a number of sectors, sex education for young South Africans remains limited in scope and availability, though the situation appears to be improving. Beginning in the 1980s, a contingent of nurses entered the public school system to talk to children about sex.[26] The Planned Parenthood Association of South Africa (PPASA), contracted by the National Department of Health, now has a program to train teachers in sex education, and the subject has recently become compulsory and included in examination.[27]

Dr. Janet Cole, a gynecologist at Groote Schuur Hospital in Cape Town, explains parents' resistance to sex education: "Their children are now getting better educated than [the parents] are and that's causing all sorts of family tensions. It's got to do with linguistic things as well, learning a language which is not your ancestral home language and becoming alienated in your parents' eyes from your own culture, and taking up all these new sort of 'foreign affairs,' so to speak."[28] Many South Africans view sex education, contraception, and abortion as "Western" ideas that have been imported to their communities. In a country suffering from a devastating HIV/AIDS epidemic, the inadequacy of current sex education programs directly contributes to deaths. Mandy Ewan, a clinic worker in Cape Town, believes, "South Africans are not being practical because we don't want to educate our youngsters. There's too much fear and shyness."[29] Exacerbating the problem, most reproductive health information has traditionally been disseminated to girls and women only, ignoring men's role in reproductive health.

In some areas, information related to sexual and reproductive health is withheld from the schools by conservative community leaders.[30] Dr. Margaret Moss, head of Contraceptive Services at Groote Schuur Hospital, explains, "[T]here have always been the very vocal antagonists who believe that if you teach children about sex they're going to go out and do it, instead of recognizing that giving them information allows them to make responsible choices." Dr. Moss acknowledges, "[T]here's been a great divide between education levels and different groups of the population. But even in the very privileged schools, sex education has been at best very erratic."[31] It is often left to the individual principal to decide; consequently, sex education programs usually fall short of the ideal.[32]

Parts of South Africa have a strikingly high teenage pregnancy rate; nationally, by the age of nineteen, 35 percent of all teenage girls have been pregnant, though that figure is as low as 15 percent in the Western Cape.[33] Not surprisingly, teen pregnancy is higher among women of color and rural Africans, women with little or no education, and those living in Mpumalanga, Northern Cape, and Eastern Cape provinces.[34] Over half of all live births by black women are to women under twenty years old.[35] Legally, pregnant girls can remain in school, but they are often ostracized and forced to drop out (though there are no consequences for the father of the baby, frequently a fellow pupil or even a teacher).[36] Many people believe that the presence of a pregnant girl in class causes drowsiness in other students.[37]

Several of the health professionals interviewed point out the need to address broader socioeconomic structures that impede adolescents' ability to avoid both unwanted pregnancy and HIV infection, including economic barriers and the high levels of coercion, rape, incest, and domestic violence in South Africa. The Planned Parenthood Association of South Africa (PPASA) is one of many organizations working on a more integrated approach to youth services. PPASA's Youth Project provides training on leadership, self-esteem, assertiveness, responsible decision making, negotiation for safer sex, and facilitation (youth are trained to teach the program to their peers). The organization's CEO, Motsomi Senne, is a certified nurse-midwife who first became involved with the organization as a volunteer in 1989. He emphasizes that PPASA's youth services "recognize the fact that HIV/AIDS and teenage pregnancy hit the most underprivileged communities. No matter how many contraceptives, how much education you could give, it is very difficult for you if you don't look at the broader indicators like social-economic problems."[38] The youth services that PPASA runs include career development programs (such as computer literacy and business courses), as well as recreation facilities.

An incredible 37 percent of South Africa's population is under fifteen years old, and most adolescent-centered services are now run by nongovernmental organizations (NGOs) like Planned Parenthood rather than the government.[39] The National Adolescent Friendly Clinic Initiative (NAFCI), the service arm of loveLife, which started in 1998, is a collaborative program between the national and provincial governments, the Reproductive Health Research Unit (RHRU), Health Systems Trust, and PPASA.[40] Clinics managed by the NAFCI attempt to be hip and trendy, with popular music, colorful walls, and a specially designed "chill room." LoveLife has also trained a group of volunteers who are eighteen to twenty-five years old to carry out peer education about reproductive and sexual health issues, both in the clinics and surrounding communities.[41] The program so far appears successful in drawing more young people into reproductive health centers.

Referring to PPASA's youth centers, Motsomi Senne explains, "We put those there so the young person recognizes that the prevention of HIV or the deference of pregnancy makes sense if you look at it within the development context. 'If I want to accomplish these things, I cannot continue to work hard, study hard, and at the same time put my life at risk of HIV/AIDS.' "[42] Organizations like PPASA and loveLife desperately try to meet the reproductive and sexual health needs of today's youth, needs that the public school system fails to adequately address; however, NGOs are small in scope and cannot replace the role of public education and health services.

Access to Health Services and Family Planning

Poverty may be the single largest barrier South Africans, and women in particular, face in their attempt to access health care. In 1995, nearly half (49%) of all female-headed households were poor, compared to 31 percent of male-headed households. Women earn 72 to 85 percent of what men with identical education levels earn, and among farmers in the Northwest, women earn only 57 percent of men's wages.[43] Even the simplest health care visit incurs hidden costs, like transportation, time away from work, and medications—costs that most women cannot afford.

Public hospitals in South Africa only charge fees for their services if the patient earns above a designated income level or if he or she has private health insurance.[44] Although health care is free, many employers provide private health insurance and, as in the United States, those companies decide what they will and will not cover. (Abortion, IUD removal, and, to a lesser extent, contraception, are frequently not covered.) Dr. Moss explains, "The vast majority of the population doesn't have the resources to access private services, so they rely on the state."[45] Those who can afford a private clinic usually choose to obtain services there and most likely obtain better quality health care than that available in the public sector.

In addition to women's concerns about the quality of care provided at public health facilities, physical access is poor, especially in rural areas. Twenty-two percent of the black population must travel more than an hour to access hospital care. Eighteen percent must do so to reach a primary care facility (compared to 3% of whites).[46] Although more than half the population lives in rural areas, only 12 percent of doctors practice there.[47] The mere cost of transportation places health care out of reach for many underprivileged South Africans. The public clinics that do exist in rural areas work on rigid schedules of mornings and afternoons only, and they are usually closed on the weekends. This poses a dilemma for women who are in school or have to work and for working men who want to accompany their partners, not to mention men who have reproductive health needs themselves.[48] In some provinces, such as the Western Cape, mobile clinics providing primary health care travel to small settlements and farms to increase access to services.[49]

Many patients have concerns about confidentiality in public health clinics, which is particularly crucial when accessing sensitive services like abortion. In many public hospitals, all pregnant women are held together in one waiting room, regardless of whether they are there for an abortion, antenatal care, or treatment after a miscarriage. The lack of privacy and sensitivity deters many; others complain that the public hospitals are understaffed and that, due to lengthy waiting lists, a woman may easily become too far along in her pregnancy to have an abortion by the time she is seen.[50] Women may also feel uncomfortable or embarrassed to be seen by male providers, and in Kwa-Zulu Natal's public hospitals, for instance, 74 percent of all physicians are male (a fact that contributes to the popularity of midwives, most of whom are women).[51] Of those clinics with adequate facilities, some have reputations for being rude to patients desiring terminations. Clinic worker Mandy Ewan points out, "Women are afraid they will be judged at the public hospitals—that the sisters [nurses] will say to them, 'Why do you need this pill? You are so young,' or 'Why are you here again?' "[52]*

Dr. Cole believes the largest obstacle to reproductive health services is the lack of knowledge in the community, particularly in regard to contraceptive usage.[53] A 2000 study found that only 47 percent of women knew a missed period could signify pregnancy, and only 47 percent knew that early symptoms of pregnancy can include vomiting, weight gain, facial changes, moodiness, change in appetite, or breast changes. Six percent could not identify any signs of pregnancy at all.[54] In another study (of 537 women *already visiting* a reproductive health clinic) only 18 percent could offer a definition of a Pap smear.[55] The lack of knowledge pertaining to reproductive health partially stems from illiteracy and the challenge of disseminating materials in the country's eleven official languages.[56] Those suffering most from high illiteracy rates and, consequently, less access to reproductive health information are undoubtedly black

---

* Note that the term "sisters" in this context refers to nurses and has no religious connotation.

and "Colored" South Africans. Educational levels vary depending on one's race; just before the change of government, in 1993, 99 percent of white South Africans were literate, compared to 84 percent of Indians, 66 percent of "Coloreds," and a mere 54 percent of Africans.[57] A moving population—particularly an influx to cities from rural areas—also creates gaps where the message fails to get through.[58]

Dr. Tersia Cruywagen, owner of the Reproductive Choices clinic located near Johannesburg, recalls the ignorance of one patient: "I had one woman the other week who came in and she was taking the birth control pill, her partner was using condoms, and she still took the Morning-After Pill every other day!"[59]* Ignorance about emergency contraception (EC, or the "Morning-After Pill"), is particularly common. Dr. Cole laments, "There is almost no public knowledge about [emergency contraception] in this country, and unfortunately the majority of clinicians and pharmacists do not even know about it."[60] A 2000 study in Gauteng province demonstrated that only 1 percent of clients had ever heard of EC, though another study in Western Cape reported more encouraging results, with 17 percent of the population being aware of the drug.[61] Even for women who do know about EC, it is problematic to obtain the medication from a doctor in the evening or on the weekend. Emergency contraception is available free of charge at any public hospital or at Planned Parenthood and may be obtained directly from a pharmacy without a prescription, but it is highly underutilized.[62] In another study, 83 percent of women were completely unaware of EC, and of the remaining 17 percent not one could provide an adequate description.[63] To rectify the situation, the University of Stellenbosch, in collaboration with the Western Cape Provincial Health Department, launched an emergency contraceptive hotline for youth in October 2003, which is being extended to other provinces (for example, to Kwa-Zulu Natal in June 2005).[64]

While lack of knowledge is a problem, so is the presence of misinformation or rumors; the persistence of myths surrounding family planning heavily discourages women from seeking services. Gloria Mokoena, a nurse-midwife at the Hillcare Women's Clinic in Hillbrow, Johannesburg, says that her patients believe all sorts of myths about sex and contraceptives, like "injectables will make me fat."[65] Common rumors about contraception include that they cause infertility and decreased sexual libido. Some people believe that a woman cannot get pregnant if she has sex while standing up; has sex with more than one man; drinks twenty glasses of water before and after intercourse; jumps up

---

* The Morning-After Pill, also known as emergency contraception (EC), may be taken within seventy-two hours of unprotected intercourse to prevent pregnancy.

and down fifty times after sex; urinates after sex; or inserts a cloth soaked in Coca-Cola into the vagina before and after sex.[66]

Even though the prevalence of misinformation concerning contraception is well-known, there is no government-sponsored mass media campaign to educate people about contraception; most public education campaigns are the work of various NGOs, like Planned Parenthood.[67] PPASA had a program in the past in which they sent trained community members door-to-door, providing birth control pills and condoms and giving informative talks on reproductive anatomy and correct condom use. Differences in acceptance of contraception and abortion are less linked to cultural differences among various ethnic groups (Xhosa vs. Zulu) and more directly related to geographical region: urban or rural.[68]

Despite the paucity of accurate family planning information and high fertility rates, contraceptives are generally accessible and widely used in South Africa. According to the law, anyone at least fifteen years old may obtain contraception without parental consent. South Africa's 1998 Demographic and Health Survey found universal knowledge of at least one family planning method. Of the women questioned, three quarters had used family planning before. Nationally, injectables were the most common method, at 57 percent; 38 percent had used the Pill, and 18 percent had used condoms.[69] Although injectables are the most common method used by Africans, their use is decreasing as more contraceptive choices are made available. The Pill is the most widely used method for other racial groups.[70]

Injectable use has historically been very high among black women for a number of reasons, perhaps the foremost being lack of choice. Prescriber bias toward injectables has played a key role in their use among black women; even today, many service providers present the Pill in a negative light because they believe women are incapable of remembering to take it every day.[71] Health workers often do not properly counsel patients about how to take the Pill correctly or about the effects that other drugs (like antibiotics) can have on the Pill's efficacy.[72] In the past ten years, South Africa has seen an increased rate of women starting contraceptive use but a decreased rate of continued use, which reflects more on the services than on the women themselves.[73] As Dr. Kim Dickson-Tetteh, formerly of the Reproductive Health Research Unit, states, "South Africa has one of the highest rates of contraceptive use in the world, and certainly in the African region—around 60 percent. The problem lies in the high rates of discontinued use and the lack of choice of contraceptive methods. People are not counseled about the effects of contraception and there are all sorts of myths and misconceptions."[74] It is no surprise that women who believe the common myths about contraception are quick to abandon their method of choice.

Other, nonhormonal contraceptives, such as condoms or sterilization, do not even approach injectables or the Pill in popularity. Condoms have not been well received by South African men for a number of reasons, ranging from insufficient access and information to myths and distaste for them. The 1998 Demographic and Health Survey reveals that just 2 percent of women report their partners using condoms, though this number is increasing in light of the HIV/AIDS epidemic.[75] Female sterilization is not widely accessible, due to long waiting lists at hospitals, though 16 percent of currently married women have been sterilized. Male sterilization is much less common and is unacceptable in the majority of communities; it is mostly used by white couples in urban areas.[76]

The Influence of Men and Traditional Cultural Values on Women's Family Planning Use

Many respondents cited men's attitudes as another major obstacle for women trying to use family planning. Dr. Margaret Moss believes that many women discontinue using contraceptives because of their partners. "We've ignored men far too long as far as giving [. . .] effective information, and men don't like to be ignorant. They hate to admit that their female partner knows more than they do, so they tend to sort of dig in their heels and [. . .] be rather negative."[77] Poor communication between partners often leads women to use contraception in secret.[78] This contributes to the popularity of injectables, which are easy to conceal from a partner.

One study of eighty providers and 436 community members in the Northern Cape reveals that the power imbalance between men and women is the most frequently mentioned factor contributing to an unwanted pregnancy.[79] Both sexes view a woman's request for safe sex as an admission that she has a sexually transmitted infection (STI) or is promiscuous. Among younger women, the financial support they receive from older men may deter them from negotiating protected sex.[80] Such "sugar-daddy" relationships between young women and financially stable, older men are quite common in South Africa, particularly in urban areas.

While more recent social phenomena like "sugar-daddy" relationships abound in urban areas, women in rural areas face stronger traditional beliefs that influence their reproductive health. Deeply entrenched cultural beliefs shape, to a large degree, the power dynamics between the sexes. In a customary union, *lobola* was given for the bride by the groom or his family. The ensuing sense of ownership made it difficult for women to make their own decisions about fertility.[81] Motsomi Senne points out, "If you walk into a village and ask the chief of that particular tribe if you can bring contraceptives into the community, you are likely to be met with a 'no' answer. [. . .] I think that empowering women to stand up and make a decision, to be assertive, is all talk unless the men see it as well, because at the end of the day [. . .] women end up in the villages where men make the decisions about sexuality."[82]

The high traditional value placed on fertility undoubtedly affects women's and men's reproductive decisions. Dr. Moss notes that men commonly measure their wealth and manhood by the number of children they produce, and although these beliefs are strongest in rural areas, they are felt by urbanites as well.[83] Motsomi Senne describes the desire of traditional men to have many children—at least one boy to carry on the family name and then many girls to increase the family's wealth from their dowries. Women who choose to not have children are often considered selfish and unnatural. Dr. Cole explains,

> In some of the cultures in this country, it is incumbent on a young woman to show that she's fertile before she's really accepted as a decent member of the community. Before she's considered marriageable, she needs to have had a baby first. [. . .] There's a very strong push on people, particularly in rural communities, to do just that. [. . .] Perhaps in a bygone era, when the rural communities were strong and there was good family matrix and lots of support, that was entirely appropriate— culturally, that was the thing. But these days, that has been so fractured, and there is such a lot of poverty in rural communities that we see a lot of problems as a result of it.[84]

Many young, single mothers find themselves without an adequate support network now that the traditional extended family system has been partly dismantled by poverty and urbanization. Some women are in a difficult position in which they must produce many children to fit traditional norms, but they have little help supporting those children.

Some people continue to view family planning as a Western construct that is in direct opposition to traditional values. In order to adapt family planning to local cultures, Senne suggests, "What we need to do as a solution is use traditional practices. For instance, a lot of tribes believe in initiation rites of girls and boys, where they go to the mountain and get educated. [. . .] All [that the boys] are taught is that now they are men—they should have sex, they should have babies—but there is no link between that and other issues beyond the mountain, when they move out of rural areas into metropolitan areas and universities and so forth." Young men who have undergone the traditional initiation rites are ill-equipped to deal with such complex issues as STIs and unwanted pregnancy. Senne argues that community leaders need to incorporate training on proper child spacing and obligations to women in the initiation rites.[85]

Finally, a major obstacle to women obtaining health services is violence. Though present in most countries of the world, violence against women in South Africa has certainly been exacerbated by the country's turbulent history. During apartheid, the South African government denied black men their dignity while constantly employing the use of force to control them. According to one perspective, in this context violence against women thrived, as some men took out their anger on the only people they could: their wives. Today, under the ANC, women fare little better. An estimated one thousand women are raped daily in South Africa; the country has a higher rate of rape than any other country that is not currently at war. One woman is killed by her partner every six days in Gauteng province alone, and one study of all-male city council members in Gauteng revealed that one-third admitted to beating their wives. [86] An estimated quarter of all young women in South Africa are currently in relationships with abusive men.[87] Violence keeps women in a compromised state and affects their self-esteem, preventing them from asserting their full reproductive rights and exposing them to STIs and unwanted pregnancy.

Abortion

South Africa's abortion history is a conservative one; until 1997, abortions were illegal except in extreme cases. Although the government kept no official statistics of illegal abortions and estimates are difficult to calculate, health professionals approximate that forty-two thousand to three hundred thousand illegal abortions occurred each year throughout the 1980s and early 1990s.[88] More than fourteen thousand women ended up in a hospital every year for complications from illegal abortions, and a 1994 study by the Medical Research Council found that an average of 425 women died annually from unsafe abortions before its legalization.[89] Yet today, the country boasts one of the most liberal abortion laws in the world, and abortion-related morbidity and mortality have greatly diminished. The South African story is one that offers myriad lessons to reproductive rights activists worldwide.

When President Nelson Mandela signed the Choice on Termination of

Pregnancy Act into law in November 1996, it became one of the most progressive pieces of abortion-related legislation in the world.[90] The law allows for abortion on demand through the twelfth week of pregnancy, and from thirteen to twenty weeks under broad medical, socioeconomic, ethical, and eugenic indications (such as with a fetal diagnosis of Down's Syndrome). No parental or spousal consent is required. One of the most radical elements of the law is that trained midwives are allowed to provide first trimester abortions. The act even has a clause stating that anyone who tries to prevent a lawful termination or obstructs access to a facility will be guilty of an offense and liable to a fine and/or imprisonment.[91]

South Africa's Choice on Termination of Pregnancy Act is worth quoting at length. The act reads:

> Recognising the values of human dignity, the achievement of equality, security of the person, non-racialism and non-sexism, and the advancement of human rights and freedoms which underlie a democratic South Africa;

> Recognising that the Constitution protects the right of persons to make decisions concerning reproduction and to security in and control over their bodies;

> Recognising that both women and men have the right to be informed of and to have access to safe, effective, affordable, and acceptable methods of fertility regulation of their choice and that women have the right of access to appropriate health care services to ensure safe pregnancy and childbirth;

> Recognising that the decision to have children is fundamental to women's physical, psychological, and social health and that universal access to reproductive healthcare services includes family planning and contraception, termination of pregnancy, as well as sexuality education and counseling programmes and services;

> Recognising that the State has the responsibility to provide reproductive health to all, and also to provide safe conditions under which the right of choice can be exercised without fear or harm;

> Believing that termination of pregnancy is not a form of contraception or population control;

This Act . . . promotes reproductive rights and extends freedom of choice by affording every woman the right to choose whether to have an early, safe and legal termination of pregnancy according to her individual beliefs.[92]

The act went into effect on February 1, 1997, and in the first year alone 31,312 legal terminations were performed.[93] That number increased to more than 100,000 by August 1999.[94] The number of abortions performed in public health facilities in the first six months of the act was double that of legally conducted abortions in the seven-year period of 1984 to 1991.[95] In the first year of the law's implementation, doctors at the Kalafong Academic Hospital in Pretoria witnessed a significant decrease in the number of patients admitted with complications from abortion, from a 50.7 percent complication rate in 1996 to just 29.4 percent in 1997.[96] Even though many barriers to safe and legal abortions persist in South Africa today, the situation now is far superior to what it was prior to 1997. Claudia Mogale, a labor and delivery nurse in Johannesburg, says that the number of women arriving with complications from abortion decreased dramatically after 1997.[97] One midwife who worked in a public hospital before the Choices Act describes the scene:

> There were a lot of women who came and they were willing to pay you for an abortion, and you didn't have the means to do a safe abortion. You did your best to help because [. . .] if you didn't help the woman, [she] would go and buy something [to self-abort]. [. . .] When I was dealing with a woman once in a hospital, I found a wire inside the vagina and the pregnancy was far advanced. [. . .] This woman had hoped that if this child was going to come out the vagina, then she must put a wire in there to kill if before it came out. [. . .] I've seen many things inserted in vaginas [in an attempt to self-abort]. Women will insert such horrible chemicals into their vaginas, and then come to me to help. So there was a huge demand for it.[98]

Abortion-related mortality has decreased significantly in South Africa since the new law went into effect. The number of legal abortions is increasing each year, but health officials expect it will plateau in the next few years, as has been the case in other countries.[99]

Despite South Africa's liberal legislation, illegal abortions persist in great numbers due to poor access to legal services. Although, on paper, South African women are entitled to free and safe abortions, in reality, their access to termination services has been extremely limited in some areas of the country. Three years after the law went into effect, a report released by the Department of Health in April 2000 revealed that out of 299 government-designated abortion facilities, only 59 were fully functional.[100] In Kwa-Zulu Natal, one of the country's poorest provinces and the one with the largest female population, only 6 of 49 designated facilities performed terminations at that time. Furthermore, the vast majority of those facilities are located in urban areas. In the first three months following implementation of the Choices Act, 60 percent of all legal terminations were done in Gauteng, South Africa's most heavily populated province, which includes the cities of Johannesburg and Pretoria.[101] Almost all of these terminations were performed in tertiary centers, at a far greater cost to the government than if they were done at the primary-care level.[102] On average, women in the year 2000 lived 100 kilometers away from a public facility providing abortions, despite Department of Health guidelines that call for a maximum distance of 10 to 16 kilometers.[103] The long distances translate into later term abortions; a discouraging 34 percent of abortions are done in the second trimester.[104] In the very poor Eastern Cape province, most people have no electricity or running water, and women must travel long distances on foot to reach a clinic, sometimes only to be told that they are too advanced in their pregnancies to receive a termination.[105]

The private sector stepped in to help fill the gap in accessibility to abortion services; as of 1999, there were 138 private facilities in South Africa offering terminations.[106] Private clinics, though they charge fees, usually have more flexible hours of operation than the public clinics. Marie Stopes International has opened eleven clinics in South Africa since 1993, with plans to expand even more.[107] Another clinic, Reproductive Choices, is trying to carve out a middle path in South Africa's dichotomous health care system—between the underfunded, inadequate (but free) public services and the outrageously expensive, elitist private clinics. Some private clinics charge up to R4000 (US$450) for an abortion, according to Dr. Cruywagen, compared to the R800 (US$120) that Reproductive Choices charges.[108] Yet even the reasonable rates found at Dr. Cruywagen's clinic are far out of reach for most South Africans; in 2000, the average annual household income was only US$7,500.[109]

Given the high percentage of abortions done in the second trimester, a crucial factor affecting access is how those abortions are performed. In the United States, a second-trimester abortion can be done (usually under general anesthesia) in less than ten minutes by a skilled surgeon. The patient is only asleep for fifteen to twenty minutes, and she remains under observation in the recovery room for forty-five minutes to an hour. Until recently, however, there were no doctors in South Africa trained to do late second-trimester abortions surgically. As of early 2000, Dr. Tersia Cruywagen, owner of Reproductive Choices, was the only doctor in South Africa trained to do surgical terminations up to sixteen weeks.[110] Dr. Cruywagen received her training from a Dutch physician, Dr. Marijke Alblas, who since 2001 has trained additional physicians in the Western Cape to do the procedure.[111] Dr. Cruywagen now travels to Cape Town, Pretoria, and Mpumalanga province to train other physicians how to conduct first-trimester abortions. She explains how frightening it was for her when she first started doing sixteen-week terminations, because she knew that there is not a single doctor in South Africa—or in all of Southern Africa, for that matter—whom she could consult if she encountered any difficulty.[112]

The vast majority of second-trimester abortions in South Africa are performed with medication rather than instruments. Unlike surgical abortions, medical abortions use a drug called misoprostol to soften the cervix and induce a miscarriage, therefore requiring a prolonged hospital stay. Especially because many women do not have a telephone at home or reliable transportation in case of an emergency, medical providers require them to stay under observation in the hospital for the duration of their miscarriage, which can be as long as twenty-four hours. Dr. Janet Cole, formerly of Groote Schuur Hospital in Cape Town, explains that in 2000, each of the three hospitals in Cape Town that perform second-trimester abortions were capable of handling four patients per week, which meant only twelve women per week could have a second-trimester abortion in Cape Town. Starting in 1999, the hospital introduced a "first come, first served" policy instead of making appointments. They had found that a large number of the women who made appointments were already too far along, and that wasted the spot someone else could have used. But the "first come, first served" system also has its flaws, as Dr. Cole illustrates,

> Every Monday morning, we would take the first fifteen people to be
> assessed by the doctor. [. . .] I'm sure you can picture the scene. [. . .]
> People would come here, try and sleep overnight to be closest to the
> door early in the morning. There were physical fights breaking out.
> [. . .] A security guard had to be obtained. [. . .] The staff would—still
> are—being threatened both verbally and physically and are subjected to
> an enormous amount of abuse and stress. Now we're trying to see if we
> can go back to the booking system and force providers to make a proper
> assessment on first contact, at the primary-care level, to try and reduce
> the load here. Some of the women that I have been admitting have been
> already four or five times to try and get to be one of the first numbers

and it's just a mess. By the time they get here they are often turned away because their pregnancy is too advanced. [. . .] Many of these women are hysterically anxious that they're not going to be done and for them the consequences then are really dire, usually financial. Then they get here and just can't believe they got up at four in the morning and are being turned away. We are pushed absolutely to the limits.[113]

If more South African doctors received training in surgical second-trimester abortions, all of those desperate women could be seen in one day. Yet few doctors are willing to be involved in abortion care; as Dr. Cole laments, "Most South African doctors have been taught for years that this is a very dangerous procedure and the risks are too great."[114]

In 2000, a tertiary abortion clinic in Johannesburg Hospital provided second-trimester abortions to eight patients a day, and the waiting list was over two weeks long. Rachel Ramphora, head nurse at the clinic, reports that her staff saw two to three patients a day who were past twenty weeks—the cut-off—and had to be referred for prenatal care.[115] A sign posted on the front door of the clinic reads:

TO ALL PATIENTS OF THIS CLINIC:
This clinic will attend to your problem, but procedures will not be performed immediately as the daily requests outnumber our available facilities. The sisters [nurses] will help you to the best of their ability and will give you the earliest date possible for your procedure. Please do not abuse or argue with the sisters as I have instructed them to adhere to departmental policy. Should you be uncooperative and/or abuse our system, you will not be attended to until you see the Superintendent of the hospital.
    Professor F. Guidozzi
    Department of Obstetrics & Gynaecology

The tone of this notice reflects the high tension that health professionals working in abortion care experience. And for patients who are beyond the cut-off for abortion, few choices remain.

Even once a woman manages to be seen at a health facility that performs abortions, she may face an imposing barrier to quality service—the negative attitudes of health workers. Although retraining programs are helpful, Dr. Moss points out that it is much easier to transfer information and knowledge than it is to change attitudes and behavior patterns.[116] Legally, there are no restrictions on young women getting abortions or contraception, but some biased service providers make the patients feel "wicked or sinful."[117] Motsomi Senne acknowledges, "Access is about friendliness. It's about knowing that you can approach someone for help, without being prejudiced. That is still not there."[118] In one study, nurses interviewed in a public hospital reported that they do not identify with women seeking abortions. They feel the abortion patients are irresponsible and uncaring, or denying their womanhood by choosing to terminate their unwanted pregnancies. Most of the nurses do not expect men to take responsibility for preventing pregnancy—that is considered the woman's domain.[119] Although the law requires health workers to tell patients about their rights, it does not oblige them to refer patients to abortion providers.[120]

Some women have reported that health workers denied them the results of a pregnancy test or a referral letter when they sought an abortion. Some are told that abortion is immoral and sinful; others are given inaccurate information about the procedure or their eligibility to get one.[121] In one extreme example, complaints received by the officer at the Commission on Gender Equality held that "women in rural areas who go to abortion clinics are sometimes forced into signing consent forms for sterilization."[122] One study found that less than 8 percent of nurses and social work students supported the availability of abortions "on-request," without any forthcoming reason to justify the abortion. Even of those individuals involved in abortion services, only 56 percent believe abortions should be available on request.[123] In one study conducted by Reproductive Choices, 22 percent of community members and 7 percent of providers felt abortion should not be provided under *any* circumstances.[124] Out of eighteen patients who confided in a partner, family member, or friend about their decision to have an abortion, twelve received an unsupportive response, including desertion (six), abuse (three), and forcefully preventing the abortion (one).[125] Loveday Penn-Kekana, spokesperson for the Reproductive Rights Alliance, states, "Many women feel that if you go to [the] hospital with an incomplete abortion you will get better treatment than if you go there to request an abortion."[126] In some hospitals, the radiation department refuses to do ultrasounds for patients considering termination.[127] One respondent claimed that, as of early 2000, the gynecology wing of Pretoria Hospital refused to do abortions at all.[128]

Medical students are not required to learn how to do terminations, though this may change in time as it eventually becomes harder for obstetricians who ethically object to abortion to find a job.[129] The Choices Act states that doctors must have enough basic knowledge about the procedure to be able to refer patients to another provider and to deal with complications; a physician may refuse any training beyond that on ethical grounds.[130]

To address the widespread negative attitudes of health providers toward abortion, Ipas, an international NGO experienced in abortion training and care, collaborated with the Women's Health Directorate of the Limpopo Department of Health and Welfare to conduct "values clarification workshops" for both health providers and community members. These workshops were quite successful: "Most participants reported increased empathy, support and comfort regarding TOP service delivery."[131] By including in their workshops individuals who are community leaders, Ipas hopes to sway public opinion in favor of a more accepting, nonjudgmental view of abortion.

Beyond attitudinal problems, many health workers have been slow to learn of the new abortion law. Two years after the abortion law went into effect, a study in the Free State found that only 78 percent of physicians *already providing abortions* demonstrated fair knowledge of the Choices Act, and only 67 percent of those referring cases to other providers gave correct answers to basic questions about the act.[132] Of course, ignorance about abortion extends to the public as well. Dr. Khin San Tint of the Women's Health Project in Johannesburg conducted a study of knowledge about abortions among the general population in 2000: "We found that the community doesn't know anything about terminations! Some said that they knew one can get an abortion, you don't have to go to jail, but the majority did not even know that much."[133] Studies conducted in 1999 and 2000 revealed poor knowledge of the new abortion law; one by the Reproductive Health Research Unit (RHRU) reported that just 53 percent of the people questioned felt they could explain the new abortion law to others.[134] In another study, only 44 percent of people were aware that abortion is available on request, 22 percent knew that consent from the partner is not required, and just 20 percent knew that parental consent is not required.[135] Dr. Janet Cole, speaking in early 2005, believes the situation has not changed much since 2000: "The average woman still has no idea of the law about abortion in this country, and how liberal it actually is."[136] Given the general lack of knowledge about the new abortion law, it is not surprising that the number of illegal abortions remains high.

Health professionals who choose to involve themselves in abortion care feel unsupported by others in their profession, and they often bear the brunt of colleagues' antagonistic views of abortion.[137] When Dr. Tersia Cruywagen opened Reproductive Choices in 1998, she had to work to establish credibility with her colleagues by doing research trials and strengthening her relationships with doctors for referrals. Beyond her own profession, she struggled to get the support of the community. In the beginning, it was a tremendous financial challenge to continue her work when the bank withdrew all loans upon discovering that Reproductive Choices is an abortion clinic.[138] Although such discrimination may be prohibited by law, it would be difficult and costly to bring a case to court against the bank. As a result of both negative attitudes toward abortion and the marginalization of providers, relatively few people, despite the great need, are willing to provide this service or even participate in the process. The law states that no one may prevent a woman from obtaining an abortion, but the same result is often achieved when the majority of practitioners refuse to provide abortions.[139]

A clause of the Choice on Termination of Pregnancy Act makes it a criminal offense for anyone who is not qualified to perform abortions to do them.[140] Nevertheless, many women pay for illegal providers. The quality of these backstreet abortions varies considerably, and, according to Dr. Cruywagen, some providers tell women on the phone that they go up to twenty-four or twenty-seven weeks in gestation. These providers then send women home with drugs to "miscarry," but, as Dr. Cruywagen points out, "What will they do with that fetus? It must be a horrible experience, but they're desperate."[141] According to the law, abortions may not be performed beyond twenty weeks into the pregnancy except in cases of fetal malformation or risk to the woman's life, but this gestational limit is not yet strictly enforced.[142]

Despite encouraging preliminary statistics of falling mortality and morbidity rates for abortion recipients, health providers know that the number of legal abortions performed constitute only a fraction of all abortions done in South Africa each year. As outlined in the Choices Act, the government implemented the Midwifery Abortion Care Training Program to counteract some of the barriers to accessing a legal abortion. In coalition with the Maternal, Child and Women's Health Directorate of the Department of Health and the international NGO Ipas, the Reproductive Health Research Unit developed a 160-hour training course in abortion, including theory and practical instruction.[143] The South African Nursing Council certifies midwives once they have completed their abortion training.[144] In October 1998, the revised training manual was ready; an impressive 148 requests for training poured in during the first six months of the training.[145] The program trains midwives in all nine provinces in manual vacuum aspiration (MVA), treatment of postabortion complications, and family planning counseling.[146] Training in MVA is particularly advantageous because its use does not require electricity, and it may therefore be used in even the most rural parts of the country. A 2000 evaluation of midwives performing abortions in all nine provinces found that they provided high-quality medical care and were competent providers.[147]

Organized nongovernmental opposition to abortion services has become an increasingly visible obstacle. Six months after the Choices on Termination of Pregnancy Act became law, three antichoice groups challenged its constitutionality in court on the grounds that a fetus is entitled to human rights. In July 1998, the High Court ruled in favor of the act, though additional legal challenges related to minors and second-trimester abortions are currently pending.[148] When clinics first started providing abortions in 1997, there were some protests, though not many. One sizable protest outside the Cape Town Marie Stopes clinic drew attention in 1999, but it was nonviolent.[149] Today, most harassment of "abortion sisters" (abortion clinic workers) comes from desperate patients stuck on a waiting list, not from fanatical antichoice activists.[150] South Africa has no history of abortion-related violence or intimidation, unlike some other countries, including the United States.[151] Doctors for Life and the Christian Lawyers Association, two groups opposed to the abortion law, are perhaps the most visible opposition to the new law.[152] Prochoice groups have little political power, as it is difficult to rally around an issue already considered by most a won battle.[153]

South African women still face myriad obstacles to obtaining a safe abortion, but the legal framework is in place to protect their right to this service, even if legal challenges are underway. South Africa has succeeded in passing a law that not only advances women's reproductive rights in South Africa, but also provides a model for other countries to emulate. Attention must now be paid to increasing *access* to abortion and other reproductive health services, as well as attempting to diminish health inequities in South Africa, which are so clearly carved out along lines of race, class, and sex. Though activists have made great progress in recent years, numerous barriers remain. The burgeoning HIV/AIDS epidemic has stalled progress on nearly every reproductive health issue.

The HIV/AIDS Epidemic

While entire texts have been devoted to the issue of AIDS in South Africa, this section will give only a brief introduction to the topic. South Africa has the fastest growing AIDS epidemic on the continent, with an estimated fifteen hundred people newly infected with HIV each day. Average life expectancy is expected to fall from sixty to forty years between 1998 and 2008 due to AIDS.[154] An incredible 15 to 18 percent of South Africans aged twenty to forty years are infected with HIV, with crippling effects on the country's economy, health care, and education systems.[155] Progression of the epidemic has been rapid; national prevalence of HIV/AIDS jumped from 2.4 percent of women testing positive in prenatal clinics in 1992 to 27.9 percent in 2003.[156] Among the poorest populations in South Africa, that figure is even higher, as in Kwa-Zulu Natal (33%) or Mpumalanga (30%).[157] Of the total population, an estimated 12.9 percent (5.6 million people) have HIV/AIDS.[158] Women are more vulnerable to the HIV/AIDS epidemic than men; two-thirds of HIV-positive individuals in South Africa are women.[159]

The South African government's early handling of the HIV/AIDS epidemic was inadequate and lacked political leadership, according to many in the field. Although a governmental AIDS program was written in 1994, it was criticized for being disorganized and poorly planned; a 1997 national review of South Africa's response to the AIDS epidemic found that there was little political leadership.[160] At the International Conference on AIDS in Durban in 2000, President Thabo Mbeki made the statement that AIDS is caused by poverty, not HIV.[161] In establishing a group to help solve South Africa's AIDS problems, Mbeki appointed "AIDS dissidents" like Peter Duesberg, who believe that treatment drugs like AZT actually *cause* AIDS, despite strong evidence from numerous international research studies showing the drug's efficacy.[162] As late as 2001, President Mbeki expressed doubts about both the link between HIV and AIDS, and the extent to which the disease had spread in the country.[163] A leaked document in September 2001 from the Ministry of Health claimed that the government's policies for coping with AIDS were unacceptable from a human rights perspective.[164] Dr. Cole comments, "The majority of my colleagues in the private sector, where I now work, feel that the government's response to the HIV epidemic is hopelessly inadequate and at times positively dangerous."[165]

In 1998 a pressure group called the Treatment Action Campaign (TAC) was established to advocate for the rights of people living with HIV/AIDS and particularly to fight for access to antiretroviral medications (ARVs).[166] TAC sued the Ministry of Health in 2002, claiming that the government was not reducing the risk of mother-to-child-transmission of HIV because it failed to provide prophylactic anti-retrovirals, such as Nevirapine, in the public health sector.[167] The South Africa High Court ordered the government to offer Nevirapine to pregnant HIV-positive women.[168] TAC campaigners have remobilized civil society, continuing their protests and civil disobedience in an attempt to shame the government into offering antiretrovirals for HIV-positive individuals. In November 2003, the government reversed its position on ARV treatment and agreed to administer the drugs; Glaxo SmithKline and other pharmaceutical companies granted permission for the production of low-cost generic versions of their drugs.[169] The national Comprehensive HIV/AIDS Care, Management, and Treatment Plan went into effect in 2004 and by the end of the year, sixty-five thousand South Africans were on antiretroviral treatment in public and private clinics. Voluntary counseling and testing (VCT) uptake more than doubled in the first year of the program.[170]

South Africa has made great strides in the provision of services for sexually transmitted infections (STIs); such services are a central component of a solid HIV/AIDS program. In one study, 40 percent of people with a history of an STI were HIV-positive; on average, half of patients coming to clinics with a current STI are HIV-positive.[171] The National Department of Health has initiated a program intended to strengthen the training and referral practices of traditional healers for STI care.[172] STI service at the primary health care level is one of the main entry points for HIV-positive people into health care system; all efforts to encourage voluntary counseling and testing should be promoted at this level.[173] Increasing the availability of VCT sites is crucial to both prevention and treatment, as individuals who learn of their positive status can not only receive treatment, but also modify their behavior to avoid infecting others.

Despite all the media attention on HIV/AIDS in South Africa, some respondents insist that the message is not getting through to people, that young people still exhibit a blasé attitude in regard to protecting themselves from HIV. According to the South African Demographic and Health Survey, only 8 percent of all women report using a condom during their last sexual encounter—only 6 percent of married women and 16 percent who had sex with a boyfriend or casual partner.[174] Additional research is needed to determine if the low use of condoms is due to lack of information, denial, or something else entirely. In one study, 95 percent of teenage girls knew about AIDS, citing television, radio, friends, and health workers as their most common sources of information. Yet more than half did not know that a healthy-looking person can have AIDS, and only 13 percent said they knew someone with HIV/AIDS, an unlikely reality in a country with such a high infection rate.[175] Ntuthu Manjezi of Planned Parenthood asserts that people are aware of HIV/AIDS but many myths still abound. One—perhaps the most dangerous—is that sleeping with a virgin can cure someone who is HIV-positive.[176] Another is that only whites (or only blacks) can get AIDS, or that only gay men, prostitutes, or promiscuous people get AIDS. Some people believe that anyone who uses a condom has

AIDS, and others believe that "AIDS is a myth put out by the Western nations to trick developing countries into reducing their population."[177]

The stigma of AIDS remains; Dr. Cole believes HIV patients are often mistreated by medical workers and by members of their greater community. HIV-positive women may be encouraged to get abortions if they become pregnant, even up to twenty-four weeks and often unnecessarily, given the availability of Nevirapine to significantly reduce the chance of mother-to-child-transmission.[178] The stigma seems to be lessening, however, as the epidemic grows. Former president Nelson Mandela lost his son to AIDS in early 2005 and has been a vocal advocate of AIDS work.

Perhaps the only positive outcome of the AIDS epidemic is the serious attention now paid to reproductive health issues. More people recognize the need to expand sexual health awareness in general and to introduce "life skills" education in primary and secondary schools.[179] The number of programs targeting men, as well as those targeting youth, has also increased substantially.[180] Subjects that were formerly taboo to discuss have now been forced into public dialogue given the immensity of the AIDS epidemic.

Influence of the ICPD

The 1994 International Conference on Population and Development (ICPD) in Cairo took place just five months after the change in government in South Africa; it was the first major international conference in which South Africa participated under a democratic government. Even before the ICPD's preparatory process, South Africa's National Health Plan included basic components of sexual and reproductive health.[181] In the formation of its population policy, the South African government solicited opinions from the population through community-based workshops, public radio, and newspaper ads.[182] The population policy today treats high fertility as an indicator rather than a cause of poverty and poor quality of life.[183] Since the ICPD, South Africa has shown considerable success in integrating sexual and reproductive health care into primary care.[184] Several major developments have taken place: The government has introduced a cervical screening policy, improved STI services, and focused more attention on supporting victims of domestic violence.[185] The Department of Health has also better incorporated the issue of gender into its policies and official documents.[186]

South Africa's constitution lays out women's right to make decisions concerning their reproduction and reproductive health, as outlined in Cairo. Section 12(2) includes, "Everyone has the right to bodily and psychological integrity, which includes the right (a) to make decisions concerning reproduction." Likewise, Section 27(1) states, "Everyone has the right to have access to (a) health care services, including reproductive health care."[187] Both the Choice on Termination of Pregnancy Act in 1996 and the Sterilization Act in 1998 further entrench women's reproductive rights on a legislative level. South Africa's turbulent history with coercive population control programs may be a contributing factor to the new government's willingness to actively improve women's reproductive health.

International Influences on Reproductive Rights in South Africa

South Africa is unique in that donor countries have not historically had the same degree of influence over the government as is found in most developing countries. Because of South Africa's history with apartheid, the majority of Western nations imposed sanctions on the country and refused to take part in many development efforts. Even today, only 1 percent of current expenditure on public health comes from donors.[188] Though large amounts of development assistance have poured into the country in recent years in light of the HIV/AIDS epidemic, South Africa still has a tradition of being more financially independent than most other African nations. Nonetheless, the country is undoubtedly influenced by the international discourse on reproductive health and by the policies and politics of donor countries. As seen in other countries highlighted in this book, the Global Gag Rule has had a particularly noticeable effect.

The Planned Parenthood Association of South Africa prides itself on being "a model of efficient, quality services for the government to copy," as CEO Motsomi Senne describes it. When abortion became legal in 1997, Planned Parenthood—an international organization with decades of experience—was eager to assist the government in setting up quality abortion services. Yet PPASA has been forbidden from participating directly in abortion services because a portion of its funding comes from the U.S. government. The United States' so-called Mexico City Policy, also known as the Global Gag Rule, prohibits the use of any federal funds by an organization involved in abortion services, even if the abortion component of the organization's work is funded separately. Senne explains, "It's sad because foundations in the U.S. receive funds from the government and then they turn around and give aid to us, but we are punished by the politics in that country and we are affected by their law."[189]

Setbacks and Gains: A Look to the Future

In a land of scant economic resources, a major ethical dilemma presents itself: What portion of the limited funds should go to prevention, and what portion should be spent on curative services? Should patients with AIDS get the best possible medications on the market, or should teenagers receive comprehensive sex education and free condoms? Should women have easy access to safe and legal abortions, or should contraceptives be widely disbursed and promoted? It is tragic when a health system is so overtaxed that these decisions must be "either/or." As Dr. Moss explains, "Unfortunately, one of our greatest concerns is that other reproductive health services are suffering, and contraceptive services have taken a backseat with focus not only on termination of pregnancy, but also on the rising epidemic of STDs and HIV infection."[190]

How does one deal with such a situation? First, Motsomi Senne argues, South Africans need to integrate their two health systems—the expensive private sector and the overcrowded, inadequate public sector-in order to make more equitable services accessible to the population. Today, abortions are often provided in a costly manner, later in the pregnancy than ideal and at the tertiary level. Abortion provides just one example of how the government could save valuable funds as access to services increases, as women have abortions earlier in their pregnancies and at a primary health clinic.

Also crucial to the future of South African women's reproductive health is the availability of physicians who are well trained in a range of abortion procedures. For decades during the apartheid era, South Africa was almost completely shut off from the outside world, ineligible for international aid. Now, with a democratic government firmly in place, many health-related NGOs are turning to foreign donors for help. South African universities and medical schools, long considered among the best in the world, should be at the forefront of additional abortion training for physicians.

Asked where South Africa is headed in the area of reproductive health, Ntuthu Manjezi insists, "We need to continue a holistic approach—all aspects, sexual and reproductive health issues, for a healthier person. It starts with an individual and then it spreads until the whole community becomes healthier."[191] As Dr. Dickson-Tetteh elaborates, "We really need to educate our girls in particular, to try and empower them so they have more control over their lives. We need to educate men to transform their thinking about women's bodies and women's health care."[192] Such fundamental shifts in cultural and societal thinking, however, will require focused activism and time to transpire.

Emerging from one of the most turbulent periods in its history, South Africa is a newly democratic country attempting to catch up from years lost to an oppressive regime. With a solid human rights foundation embedded in the nation's constitution and legislation, South African activists have reason to be optimistic for the future. The country's leaders express a commitment to social justice that few countries can boast. Yet the obstacles South Africa faces are indeed massive: intense poverty, an AIDS epidemic that affects every citizen, and rampant violence against women, to name a few. Gross economic inequities, and their attendant social unrest, will not disappear overnight; until these broader issues are addressed, women will not enjoy the reproductive freedom they deserve.

2

Uganda

Background

Bordered by Kenya, Tanzania, Rwanda, the Democratic Republic of Congo, and Sudan, Uganda sits in East Africa on the shores of Lake Victoria. Of the countries highlighted in this book, Uganda presents one of the most challenging environments for reproductive rights activists. The country suffers from extreme poverty, devastating maternal and infant mortality rates, and a serious HIV/AIDS epidemic. Uganda's human development index (HDI) falls below the average not only for sub-Saharan Africa, but also for the category of "least developed countries in the world."[1] Just one out of four households in Uganda has safe drinking water, and 5 percent have electricity for lighting.[2] The gross domestic product per capita is $1,390 per year, and life expectancy at birth is only 46.2 years.[3]

With an average of 6.9 children per woman, Uganda has one of the highest fertility rates in the world.[4] Though women have about seven children on average, they only want an average of five children; nearly half of all births are unwanted or mistimed.[5] Largely influenced by the international population movement, the Ministry of Health in Uganda (as in many other developing countries) has concentrated a disproportionate amount of resources on provider-controlled, long-term contraceptives in an effort to reduce fertility levels. Family planning programs are often treated as the end-all solution to women's high morbidity and high fertility, despite the myriad factors that play equally, or even more, crucial roles in women's state of health.[6] Notwithstanding the attention paid to family planning, only 23 percent of married women use contraception, according to the 2000 Demographic and Health Survey, though this does represent a fivefold increase since 1988.[7] Women's reproductive health remains poor in Uganda, and complications from unsafe abortion are a leading cause of maternal morbidity and mortality.[8] Multiple barriers impede women's ability to care for their health in this East African nation.

Cultural Views of Fertility

Uganda's fertility rate has not changed significantly in the past thirty years, hovering around seven children per woman, though total fertility rates mask the changes that are occurring in different subsets of the population.[9] As Richey points out, "When fertility rates were analyzed according to socio-economic rankings, it was shown that fertility levels increased by nearly one child per woman for the poorest two quintiles over the past five years and decreased by around one child for the richest 40 percent."[10] Poor women in Uganda are in fact having more children now than in the past due to a number of factors, including limited access to quality health services, ignorance about contraceptive methods, women's inability to negotiate contraceptive use, and cultural views of fertility. Though Uganda has a diverse population of nine major ethnic groups and many other smaller groups, a fairly consistent value across these cultures is the importance placed on fertility.[11]

Asked how a community would view an older woman who chose to remain single and childless, Dr. Florence Ebanyat answered, "It is very rare for women to choose to be single or not to have a child!"[12] Dr. Ebanyat points out that those couples who have no children usually suffer from infertility. Another physician, Dr. Joy Kyeyune, believes that "They wouldn't understand her. [. . .] You are sort of a different person if you don't aspire to get married."[13] Several respondents echoed similar sentiments.[14] Interestingly, more than one respondent pointed out that even if a woman chose to refrain from getting married, her community would likely still expect her to have a child. Stella Neema, an anthropologist, relates, "In fact they say, 'Why don't you—even if you don't get married—get yourself a child!' "[15] Social worker Elly Mugumya explains that in many Ugandan cultures, if an adult dies without having children, it is considered a bad omen and requires special rituals.[16]

Most men in Uganda expect to have many children, and many see family planning as a Western construct. Nurse-midwife Priscila Nswemu explains, "The community may say, 'That one is a *mzungu* [white person]—he only has two or three children.' "[17] The strong preference for sons also leads to high fertility, since families often continue having children until they have the number of boys desired.[18] The prevalence of polygamous unions (one-third of all marriages) also leads to higher fertility, due to competition among co-wives: "One wife wants to have more than the other to get the love of the husband or to build the clan."[19] Still, this desire is gradually changing, particularly as the cost of living and school expenses increase.[20] One of the reasons for Uganda's high fertility is the early age at which women begin childbearing, which is influenced not only by cultural traditions but also by poor sex education.

Sex Education in Uganda

The vast majority of Ugandan youth receive very little instruction in reproductive and sexual health matters from either their school curricula or at home. Even if a comprehensive sex education program were introduced into the school system, the challenge of reaching adolescents who are not in school would be great; only 43 percent of fifteen-year-olds have completed primary school, and even fewer continue on to secondary school.[21] The literacy rate in the country is just 61 percent for women and 76 percent for men.[22] Uganda recently implemented universal primary education (UPE), in which children are entitled to free primary education, but Dr. Jotham Musinguzi insists that universal secondary education is what is truly needed to make a measurable impact on the health of adolescents and young adults.[23]

In some traditional Ugandan cultures, youth receive most of their information about sexual matters from a paternal aunt, called a *ssenga* among the Baganda people. In many cultures, however, there is no such provision.[24] Despite the Buganda Kingdom's attempts to revive this tradition as a way to transmit reproductive health information, the system has weakened and adolescents increasingly turn to churches, school groups, the media, and nongovernmental organizations (NGOs) for their reproductive health–related information.[25] The importance of more attention to adolescent reproductive health is underlined by the prevalence of early marriage and childbearing. Nearly half of all eighteen- to nineteen-year-old women have had a baby, and another 16 percent are pregnant at any given time.[26] The median age at first marriage for women is just 17.7 years, and for men, 21.9 years, though Ugandans marry later today than in the past.[27]

Increasing awareness of sexual violence should be a central component of any sex education program, given the prevalence of sexual violence against adolescents. A study of secondary-school students in Kabale found that 31 percent of girls and 15 percent of boys reported being coerced into having sex.[28] Likewise, a study of fifteen- to nineteen-year-old sexually experienced girls reported that 14 percent were coerced into having sex the first time. Those girls who reported coerced sex were less likely to be currently using contraception or to have used a condom with their last sexual encounter, and they were more likely to have experienced an unwanted pregnancy and a sexually transmitted infection (STI).[29] Protecting youth from sexual violence is crucial to their future reproductive health, even beyond the immediate impact of the abuse.

Equally important to comprehensive sex education is access to an adequate health care system, which is not currently the case for the majority of the Ugandan population.

Uganda's Health Care System—Recent History

Since colonial times, Uganda's health sector has been composed of government providers, NGOs (often missionaries), "modern" private practitioners, and traditional healers (bone setters, herbalists, psychotherapists, and traditional birth attendants [TBAs]). These different systems were never integrated nor coordinated. Religious organizations—namely, the Roman Catholic Church, the Church of Uganda (affiliated with the Church of England), and the Seventh-Day Adventists—ran the most efficient health units, but the traditional sector remained the most widely utilized of all. In rural areas especially, people turned to traditional healers as a first option for treating everything from malaria, burns, and respiratory infections to diarrhea, infertility, and "bad luck."[30] The private sector and nongovernmental organizations (NGOs) filled some gaps in the system by offering more accessible, speedy, and flexible services; however, these services were prohibitively expensive for the vast majority of the population.[31]

Despite its faults, Uganda's health care system was consistently rated one of the best in sub-Saharan Africa throughout the 1960s and 1970s, but the system collapsed under the weight of such widespread instability and destruction as witnessed in the 1970s and 1980s.[32] The political tyranny and instability of the Amin and Obote II regimes (1971–1985) shattered Uganda's health care system. Between 1971 and 1986, gross domestic product (GDP) per capita halved, and many Western donors fled.[33] "Rural physical and social infrastructure degenerated to the point of helplessness and despair."[34] Both the Amin and Obote II regimes largely ignored rural health services; health centers lacked basic equipment, running water, and electricity. Beyond the scant resources, morale among staff was low—rooms were left unclean and grass uncut, and people felt no sense of community ownership for the government-installed health units.[35]

In January 1986, the National Resistance Army/Movement (NRA/M) came into power with Yoweri Kaguta Museveni as its president. Although criticism of Museveni mounts today as he refuses to relinquish power, most agree that

Museveni has done more for the country than his predecessors. With the relatively stable political history of the past twenty years, the health care system has gradually improved and, though grossly underfunded, all public health services are currently available to the population free of cost.[36]

Access to Health Services and Family Planning

In Uganda, 46 percent of the population lives below the absolute poverty line, and the Uganda Participatory Poverty Assessment Project (UPPAP) in 1998 found ill health to be the most frequent cause of poverty.[37] Multiple barriers impede women's ability to care for their health, not the least of which is the dilapidated state of the public health care system.[38] Eighty-eight percent of the country's 24.4 million inhabitants live in rural areas, where health services are least accessible.[39] Perhaps the most visible and devastating obstacle to accessing health care in Uganda lies in the general lack of transportation and communication infrastructure across the country.[40] Uganda's road system, particularly in the countryside, is extremely limited. Small dirt roads often become impassable during the two rainy seasons of the year, and the near-total lack of street names in rural areas further impedes emergency services.[41] Outside of the major cities, the most common mode of transportation to a health clinic is a bicycle—clearly not the ideal for someone who is already in a physically compromised state, not to mention someone in need of emergency care. A 1995 Safe Motherhood Needs Assessment revealed that, in most areas, the local "ambulance" was a bicycle pulling a trolley, or a stretcher that could be carried to the nearest health center. Most rural areas are without phone lines, and in some isolated parts of the country even mobile phones do not function. Indeed, the Safe Motherhood assessment found that lack of transport and communication were the two largest barriers to obtaining health services, particularly for emergency obstetric care.[42]

Communication lines are key in transmitting crucial health-related messages and information about the value and use of available health services to the community. Rural women are the most disadvantaged in this regard, since they often have no access to newspapers, radio, or television, and they are more likely than men to be illiterate. Elly Mugumya, a social worker, points out the difficulty in spreading reproductive health information in Uganda's dozens of languages to a geographically scattered population.[43] Further compounding the communication dilemma is the fact that health promotional materials are often written in English, which few people in rural areas can read or understand.[44]

The disproportionate number of government health centers located in urban areas exacerbates transportation and communication difficulties that many women face. Over 50 percent of hospitals are located in urban areas, where only 12 percent of the population resides, and in 1992 urban areas housed 76 percent of all doctors, 80 percent of midwives, and 70 percent of nurses in Uganda.[45] When one considers the dearth of medical professionals to begin with—the doctor to population ratio in Uganda is 1:28,000—this unequal distribution is even more alarming.[46] Service provision favors hospitals, which consume over 45 percent of the Ministry of Health's total budget.[47] The Ministry of Planning and Economic Development estimates that less than half of Ugandans (49.0%) have access to static health units and the average Ugandan woman lives 19 kilometers from the nearest family planning facility.[48] Dr. Musinguzi argues that a community-based approach, in which services are taken directly to people who live in rural areas, would be most effective in providing needed care to the population, particularly when coupled with anti-poverty programs so people can afford the costs attendant to obtaining health services.[49]

One approach to improving access to health providers is to invest in midwives. Jane Atergire of the Uganda Private Midwives Association (UPMA) emphasizes that midwives are in a unique position to provide quality, affordable services at the grassroots level. The UPMA, established in 1948 as a member of the International Confederation of Midwives, boasts five hundred members throughout the country. Though, in the past, midwives were only qualified to deliver babies and provide prenatal care, recent policy changes and updated training have expanded the abilities of Uganda's midwives to include postnatal services, immunizations, HIV treatment, STI management, and family planning provision.[50] Atergire points out that the government is weak in regulating unqualified health providers who carry out maternal services; UPMA attempts to standardize the training midwives in the country receive.[51]

Elly Mugumya, executive director of the Family Planning Association of Uganda (FPAU), explains that access to services includes not only physical ability to reach a clinic, but also the availability of competent and trained staff, the necessary medical supplies, and a private and confidential environment for delivery of care.[52] If a woman is able to overcome the numerous barriers to reaching a government health unit, she often finds upon arrival a limited range of services offered. In 1997, only 60 percent of health units countrywide offered family planning services.[53] Ministry of Health statistics from the following year show that only two-thirds of health units provided antenatal care (67%), fewer than half offered maternity services (48%), and only 39 percent had the capacity for inpatient care. Most health centers have an irregular supply of contraceptives and only offer one or two methods of contraception, even when they are in stock.[54] The public hospitals in Uganda are grossly underfunded and often run out of such basic supplies as latex gloves and essential drugs, not to mention emergency blood supplies.[55] According to reports from Kiboga, one of the country's most impoverished districts, the hospital there often runs out of antibiotics by midweek; it is not uncommon for women who have a cesarean section later in the week to go without the antibiotics necessary to prevent sepsis.[56] Patients are expected to compensate for the hospital's shortages by purchasing their own gloves and drugs at local pharmacies; this financial burden places health care out of reach for a great number of people living in rural areas.

Nearly all government health centers are understaffed; poor living and working conditions make it difficult to attract doctors and other trained professionals to rural areas. Keeping medical professionals in the country in general is a challenge, in fact; like most developing countries, Uganda suffers from the "brain drain" phenomenon, in which highly trained professionals seek employment in wealthier countries. Compounding the problem is the fact that medical professionals in Uganda are paid poorly and irregularly. A general practitioner makes about US$3,000 per year, which, even in the context of Uganda's low cost of living, is inadequate considering the amount of schooling doctors have to complete and the long hours they work. Nurses make just half that figure. Health workers frequently take up second jobs in order to pay their bills; a 1997 study found that, for added income, some doctors were involved in agriculture and livestock rearing, operating drug and medical supply stores, teaching, baking pancakes to sell, providing abortions, and prostitution.[57] Although the government has improved the regularity with which staff are paid since decentralization in the mid-1990s, pay is still often erratic, with workers going weeks, or sometimes even months, at a time with no income.[58] Strikes are uncommon, though, perhaps because staff know that their refusal to work would result in lost lives of people who have no control over pay schedules. It is not surprising, then, that many drugs and supplies intended for public hospitals mysteriously end up in the private practices of physicians and nurses alike. Low morale among hospital staff also adversely affects provider attitudes and encourages the reputation of nurses and doctors as being rude or judgmental, and often truant. This further discourages the general population from accessing health care.

Health services are particularly inaccessible in the parts of northern and western Uganda that currently experience civil strife and insurgency. Hundreds of girls and young women have been raped and forced into marriages with soldiers as a result of these conflicts.[59] Conservative estimates place the number of children abducted by the Lord's Resistance Army (LRA) in the north to be twenty thousand; one study found that 85 percent of abducted children contract at least one sexually transmitted infection while in captivity.[60] Adolescents affected by the twenty-year war have little power to protect their health.

The Ministry of Health estimates that, nationally, only 38 percent of women are attended by a trained health worker during childbirth.[61] The majority of women deliver at home, with the assistance of female relatives, older children, and sometimes a traditional birth attendant (TBA).[62] A study Stella Neema conducted found that many women who do not deliver at a health clinic explain that they do not attend partly because of financial barriers, but also because of their perception of the hospital. "They were saying that 'Pregnancy is not sickness, why do I go to the hospital?' "[63] The hospital is seen as the place to go for health problems, but most people view pregnancy and delivery as a natural occurrence rather than a disease requiring care from medical professionals. A large percentage of pregnant women (around 80%) in the study went to the hospital for antenatal care, but only 30 percent returned to the hospital for delivery. Neema discovered that women considered the antenatal card they receive as a kind of insurance, "because if you don't have that card [when you deliver], the health workers are going to chase you out. So some of these mothers would go, get the card, and keep it there, in case of a problem—they could go back to the hospital."[64]

Several sociocultural factors place women at greater risk than men, both for becoming ill in the first place and for delaying, or never receiving, health care. Uganda's female morbidity rate is staggering; studies show that, at any one time, over 70 percent of the country's women are sick.[65] Yet these women have little opportunity to improve their health. Cultural preferences dictate that men eat the best food, so women already living in malnourished communities have the worst nutrition of all. Dr. Kyeyune notes, "When there is little meat, the boy eats the meat and the girl doesn't eat the meat. The girls don't eat the eggs."[66] This inequality persists despite the fact that pregnant and lactating women are most in need of balanced diets; they are also more likely to develop anemia—an especially dangerous condition for pregnant women.[67]

Once women do fall ill, restoring their health is usually a low priority in the family's budget. Women seek health care often solely in relation to their reproductive health, partly because their societal value is closely linked with

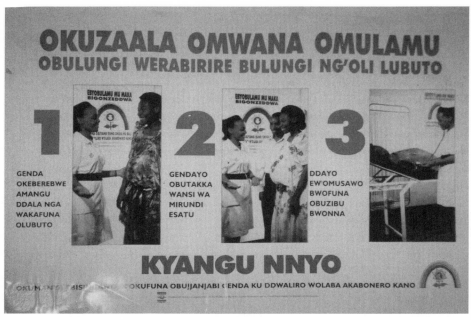

This poster reads, "To give birth to a healthy child, take care of yourself when you are pregnant. Go quickly to get examined when you become pregnant. Go to the doctor a minimum of three times while you are pregnant. Return to the doctor if you have any problems. It's very easy!" As discussed in this chapter, obtaining prenatal care, or any other health services, is far from easy for the majority of Ugandan women. Poster produced by Uganda Delivery of Improved Services for Health (DISH).

their fertility and partly because these are the services offered to them, often at the expense of other services. Since most women have very little or no independent income, the decision of whether or not they will seek health services rests largely with the woman's husband. Women account for 70 to 80 percent of Uganda's agricultural work force, yet only 7 percent of them own land and 30 percent have access to or control over the proceeds of their work.[68] Nationally, only 15 percent of women are self-employed or employed in the formal sector, and nearly all of these women live in urban areas.[69] Women work an average of fifteen to eighteen hours each day, compared to the eight to ten hours that men work.[70] They often cannot afford to leave their domestic duties for a day to seek health care. Even though public health care is free, transportation to the health unit, and sometimes additional needed drugs, can cost women money they do not have, requiring the notification and consent of the husband. This lack of financial autonomy becomes especially crucial in relation to family planning services.

Men's Involvement in Family Planning

Men's reluctance to support family planning use presents another barrier to many women. As Nestor Owomuhangi of the United Nations Population Fund (UNFPA) explains, "The husband is normally the king of the home," the decision-maker and breadwinner, who chooses how many children to have and which children go to school.[71] Men's own ignorance about reproductive health and family planning likely contributes to their resistance to its use. Dr. Ebanyat notes, "Very rarely do you find men coming up with their spouses for [family planning] services, although we try to encourage that."[72] Dr. Kyeyune relates that men sometimes come with their wives to the family planning clinics on their bicycles but then wait under a tree for her to finish the appointment. "So we are encouraging them, 'No! You can come and sit with your wife, and you all learn together.' "[73] Though today more reproductive health clinics recognize the need to involve men in their services, most men believe that family planning is purely the woman's domain and do not want to be associated with it. Even men who work in the field of reproductive health, with the Ministry of Health, will often say, "No, I don't want to go on radio for that!"[74] Dr. Kyeyune explains her strategy of starting with men who are working in reproductive health offices, encouraging them to be public advocates for reproductive health so that other men will follow.

Men's reluctance to learn more about family planning, coupled with their resistance to their wives using it, has led to a great number of women using contraception without their husbands' knowledge.[75] There is considerable demand for methods like Depo Provera (a hormonal injection whose effects last three months) and Norplant (hormonal implants that work for five years), since those are two methods that a woman can use relatively easily, without leaving evidence around the house of her family planning use.[76] "They will use the excuse of coming to bring a sick child to the hospital, or coming to the market," and then stop by the family planning clinic to receive their shot or implants.[77] Elly Mugumya of the Family Planning Association of Uganda relates that many women ask clinic staff to hold onto their appointment cards so their husbands will not discover them.[78] Women's secret use of contraception underlines the importance of involving men in family planning services. Hiding contraceptive use and procuring funds for transportation can be a burden for many women.

"Men are the decision-makers, and they are the people who control finances in the home," believes Josephine Othieno.[79]

Dr. Jotham Musinguzi, while recognizing the presence of cultural obstacles to family planning use, explains, "To me, a lot of what is called cultural barriers is more ignorance, rather than these other things."[80] Once the population is well informed of the benefits of family planning, Musinguzi insists, use will increase.

Religious beliefs likely prevent some women from using contraception, considering the fact that 42 percent of the population is Catholic, 36 percent Protestant, and 12 percent Muslim.[81] Yet Dr. Musinguzi believes religious barriers are not a major influence; studies have shown that even Catholic Ugandans use family planning services in great numbers.[82]

The consequences of the lack of access to services may be partially seen in high mortality rates: The infant mortality rate in Uganda is 88 deaths per 1,000 live births, compared to a rate of 7 deaths per 1,000 live births in the United States (and mortality rates in the United States are among the highest of all developed countries).[83] The maternal mortality rate is equally staggering, at 505 deaths per 100,000 live births, compared to 7.5 deaths per 100,000 live births in the United States.[84] Elly Mugumya points out the need for improving emergency obstetric care, which has a tremendous impact on maternal mortality.[85]

Contraception

Family planning has been in Uganda since 1957, but before Idi Amin came into power in 1971, the government scarcely mentioned the issue of population.[86] Birth control was a contentious issue because of ethnic tensions, as different groups were vying for power in the country. "The politics of population growth has therefore been played out in terms of the power-sharing potentials of regional, ethnic, religious, and interest groups rather than in terms of the overall impact of population growth on national development."[87] The 1971/1972–1975/1976 Health Sector Strategic Plan (HSSP) supported family planning, but many government policies remained pronatalist. For example, eligibility for government housing was based on the number of children in the family, and it was difficult for families with only a few children to obtain it. In 1976, the Ugandan government first expressed the view that the country's population was too high, but a population policy was not incorporated in national development plans until 1987.[88] For years, civil strife inhibited the government's attempts to reduce fertility rates.[89] In 1990, the government finally eliminated some restrictive policies that were inhibitory to women using family planning, such as the requirement for spousal consent.[90] In 1993, the Ugandan government recognized access to family planning as a basic human right.[91]

Available family planning services often fall short of the ideal, partly explaining Uganda's low contraceptive prevalence rate (CPR); just 23 percent of currently married women use contraception.[92] Though this represents a noticeable increase from 5 percent in the early 1990s, it is still low by regional standards; Dr. Musinguzi points to Kenya, with a CPR of 38 percent, and Zimbabwe, with a CPR of 54 percent, as examples of comparable countries that have managed to make family planning more accessible than Uganda, where use remains low.[93] Among sexually active fifteen- to nineteen-year-olds in Uganda, one study found, only 19 percent of young women and 42 percent of young men currently use a modern contraceptive method.[94]

Those who do enjoy access to family planning may not receive adequate counseling, follow-up care, or access to the full range of contraceptives they deserve. Hardon et al. argue that access to contraceptives requires, minimally, a range including methods for both men and women, temporary and permanent methods, hormonal and nonhormonal methods, user-controlled methods (i.e., the Pill and barrier methods), and methods that are safe for breastfeeding women. They also call for postcoital methods, such as emergency contraception and abortion (the latter is illegal in Uganda and the former is practically nonexistent).[95] In many hospitals in Uganda, only two or three contraceptive methods are available, the most common of which are the Pill and Depo Provera.[96]

The most popular contraceptive methods in Uganda are injectables, exclusive breastfeeding after delivery, and the Pill, followed by the rhythm method.[97] Just 3.8 percent of women report using male condoms.[98] Dr. Neema notes that the female condom has been introduced in Uganda, but it is prohibitively expensive compared to the male condom. She laments, "Yet the female condom would have been the best because it is a woman's technology—the woman is the one to handle it—the woman knows when to put it on or when not to put it on, but that problem of the expense will hinder people [from using] it."[99]

Beyond the government-run family planning clinics, women who can afford it have the option of attending clinics in the private and nongovernmental sectors. The Family Planning Association of Uganda (FPAU), a private nongovernmental organization, provided a large portion of contraceptive services to Ugandans from the late 1950s until 1990, when the government fully developed its family planning policy and trained service providers.[100] A survey done in 1988–1989 found that 33 percent of people using family planning in Uganda obtained services from FPAU, while 42 percent used government health services. Since then, FPAU's share of the market has declined to between 20 and 25 percent, as more private clinics and NGOs offer family planning services.[101]

Most private and NGO clinics, including those of FPAU, charge fees for their services, though not at full cost recovery. Elly Mugumya, executive director of FPAU, outlines the benefits of their fee-for-service policy as threefold: "One, it contributes to the resources that we get from the donors; two, it prepares our communities for paying for services and attaching value to the services they receive; and three, it gives us accuracy—we can talk with confidence about [our] services" because the fact that someone has committed his or her money to purchasing the Pill, for example, likely means that they intend to use it.[102] Likewise, clinics run by Marie Stopes Uganda charge nominal fees for their services; a three-month supply of the Pill costs just over $1, as does an injection of Depo Provera, and an IUD insertion costs $6. Male and female sterilization cost $12 apiece.[103] Still, for the great number of Ugandans who have no money to spare, visiting a private clinic for family planning services is an impossibility; they must rely on the government-run clinics.

Beyond the logistical barriers outlined above that women face when attempting to access a family planning clinic, a number of cultural barriers are also present. Women may be hesitant to suggest family planning use to their husbands for fear of being thought of as promiscuous. Dr. Florence Ebanyat describes the stigma attached to family planning, "Most men think that when a woman uses contraceptives she is likely to move around with other men because she knows that she will not get an unwanted pregnancy."[104]

The perception of family planning as a means of birth control rather than birth spacing discourages many from its use. Josephine Othieno explains this belief: "[When] somebody comes and talks to you about family planning, that's what they are advocating for you—never to deliver [again]."[105] Stella Neema, an anthropologist and women's health expert, believes that the way donors and the government have marketed family planning is problematic. She believes family planning has been packaged as a method of birth control, when a more effective message may be to emphasize the importance of birth spacing.[106] Nestor Owomuhangi agrees: "The main message of family planning has been to reduce the number of children you have—people don't want that."[107] Owomuhangi continues, "If someone gets the message that family planning improves your health—maybe you live longer, you increase your income because these numbers of children will cut down—those messages have not been sent. It is

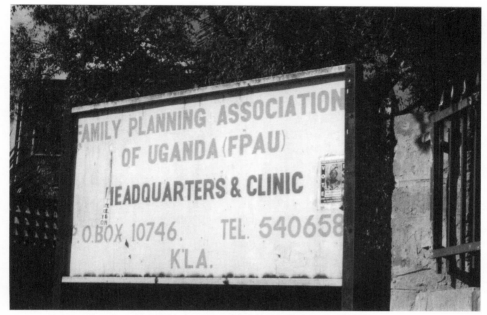

The Family Planning Association of Uganda (FPAU) is one of the primary providers of family planning in Uganda; its headquarters is announced by this rather dilapidated sign.

more like 'Use this thing and it will reduce on children.' So people know this thing but they do not realize it improves their health. Until the moment that people link this thing to their own well-being, they will still know about it and leave it there."[108]

Overall awareness of family planning is high, but Elly Mugumya points to the gap between information and use. "All they know is awareness, and that awareness has not been developed further to creating sufficient knowledge and understanding."[109] Though most Ugandans can name various contraceptive methods, few can explain how they work. "So the level of awareness needs to be transformed into knowledge and motivation. You can get awareness creation on the radio, but the motivation for use calls for programs that are really person-to-person counseling, to let people ask those questions and gain deeper understanding of what you are talking about. Such programs really would be more intense than awareness."[110]

The lack of basic knowledge about contraception leaves the population vulnerable to myths and misconceptions. Myths about contraception remain a substantial barrier to women's use, even among educated women; common is the belief that certain contraceptives make women infertile or diminish her sexual libido.[111] Inadequate counseling at most family planning clinics contributes to the existence of myths. Women's fear of side effects is the most commonly cited barrier to using modern contraceptives.[112] Though many women's concerns about contraceptive side effects are well-grounded, this particular obstacle to family planning use could be tackled by counseling women about common side effects of the various contraceptive methods, including the fact that many side effects disappear after several weeks of use.

Considering the dearth of sex education that adolescents receive, the relatively inaccessible health services, and the numerous social and cultural barriers to family planning use, it is not surprising that thousands of women in Uganda face unwanted pregnancies each year. A number of those women choose to illegally end their pregnancies in abortion.

Abortion

Abortion is illegal in Uganda except to save the mother's life, yet many respondents felt that abortion is not uncommon, and a study in Mbarara reports that 78 percent of teenage girls know someone who had an abortion.[113] The government rarely enforces the law that criminalizes abortion; few women are prosecuted, even when a woman's illegal abortion is well-known in her community. Elly Mugumya explains, "For example, on the hospital card it is written 'illegal abortion' and that card will be attached to the patient and she is treated and goes to surgery and at the end of day there will be no police officer calling or a government official asking for all those who have been treated for this illegal abortion."[114]

Though few women are in prison for having illegal abortions, the law is effective in deterring the establishment of safe, easily accessible abortion services for women. An estimated 22 percent of all maternal deaths are caused by unsafe, illegal abortions, according to the Ministry of Health.[115] Admissions at hospitals due to incomplete abortions account for close to 30 percent of pregnancy-related admissions—a statistic that has changed little in many years.[116] An abortion provided by a private sector physician, nurse, or midwife costs approximately $64—far out of reach for most Ugandans—but drugs for inducing abortion can be obtained for just $7 from a pharmacist.[117] For those women who cannot afford even that much, many rely on traditional healers or self-induce an abortion, often with dangerous consequences.[118]

Confronted with an unwanted pregnancy, most women end up carrying the pregnancy to term; as Nestor Owomuhangi of UNFPA puts it, "Most people really don't do anything, once they find they are pregnant, they say, 'What can we do? It's God.' They say, 'We are pregnant—too bad. I can't go [to get an abortion] because you know someone died—the other one went and she died.' "[119] Though there has been little research done on abortion in Uganda, several respondents felt that young women, and students in particular, are most likely to have abortions. A Ugandan school policy forbids pregnant students from remaining in classes or resuming school after the delivery; therefore, young female students may be more likely to seek an abortion in order to continue studying.[120] A recent policy review allows girls to return to school after delivery, but they may not return to the same school.[121] Married women seem less likely to have abortions, though women with young babies at home may be an exception.[122] Respondents generally have the impression that abortion is more common in urban areas than rural areas.[123] Jane Atergire points out that girls and young women in urban areas who have greater educational opportunities may have more goals that are not compatible with childbearing than their rural counterparts.[124] Also, when a man impregnates a woman in a rural area, "he is forced to marry her so she does not need to have an abortion."[125] Still, Dr. Musinguzi wonders if this perception of abortion as an urban phenomenon is simply because "in urban areas we are likely to capture it—that's where the doctors are, or rather the health services."[126] He believes abortion is a major problem in rural areas as well. More than one respondent felt that abortions in rural areas tend to have higher complication rates than those found in urban areas.[127]

Women who have an abortion face tremendous stigma from their community if people discover what she has done.[128] Dr. Joy Kyeyune describes the stigma attached to abortion, "It's almost equivalent to prostitution."[129] Stella Neema recalls, "It is really negative, very negative. In fact, I got surprised when I was in Denmark, a friend of mine—a student, a girl, told me that she aborted and she was talking about it normally, like it's a normal thing. I said, 'What?!' Here, they don't talk about it, they don't want to hear about it, and they think you are a murderer."[130] Dr. Miriam Sentongo describes a recent incident, "Just yesterday there was a case of a woman who had twins, and I think she got pregnant when the twins were too young. [. . .] She aborted, then threw the fetus on the rubbish pit. So they found the fetus, and the whole village was mobilized to check every woman, until they got this woman and they took her right down to the police. [. . .] You are condemned right away. Some are even beaten."[131]

Although this societal problem could partly be addressed on the policy level by legalizing abortion, the number of deaths from clandestine abortions could be significantly reduced if proper postabortion care (PAC) were available; today, only 30 percent of health units offer such care, needed for both induced abortion and spontaneous abortion (miscarriage).[132] Dr. Anthony Mbonye believes women are not yet confident about seeking postabortion services from the hospital: "They only come when it is too late and this quite often leads to high deaths."[133]

Elly Mugumya of FPAU states that his organization offers postabortion treatment and counseling when needed, though they refer patients with incomplete abortions to the hospital.[134] Dr. Kyeyune explains that, after the abortion has occurred, a woman can relatively easily find a medical professional who will complete the evacuation of her uterus; initiating the abortion is the difficult, and most dangerous, part.[135] Dr. Florence Ebanyat of the Ministry of Health (MOH) describes the postabortion care program in place at the MOH, which calls for managing emergency complications, including the removal of products of conception using dilatation and curettage (D&C) or the manual vacuum aspirator (MVA—the safest method available); counseling for family planning to reduce a repeat of unwanted pregnancy; and referral for other reproductive health services as necessary.[136] The Ministry of Health policy is that the provision of PAC services should exist regardless of whether the abortion was induced or spontaneous.[137] Counselors at Marie Stopes intentionally ask their patients whether the abortion was induced or spontaneous in order to better provide postabortion counseling and contraceptive counseling, if necessary. Josephine Othieno, of Marie Stopes Uganda, emphasizes that MSU clinics provide postabortion care in the most empathetic manner possible and have never reported a patient for an illegal abortion.[138] Still, a nurse-midwife at one of MSU's clinics insists, "No, we don't want to handle those patients because we don't want to be associated with that. It would taint our name if everyone knew they could come to Marie Stopes after an abortion."[139] Women commonly rely on traditional healers not only for the abortion but also for treatment of postabortion complications, due to fear of mistreatment in the health clinics, as well as the distance and economic cost of attending a clinic.[140]

A recent survey of health facilities managers throughout Uganda found that 90 percent agree that better PAC services are needed.[141] The managers called for better stocks of basic supplies in the health centers, more advanced medical equipment (such as manual vacuum aspirators), transportation services for referrals, a campaign to educate the public about the risks of unsafe abortion, and an expanded capacity for midwives and other providers to treat abortion complications. To this end, the Uganda Private Midwives Association, with technical support from the international reproductive rights group

Ipas, trains midwives to provide PAC services, including the use of manual vacuum aspirators.[142] The United Nations Population Fund (UNFPA) has also been involved in training midwives in PAC, as well as assisting the government in training staff to provide abortions.[143] Dr. Anthony Mbonye laments that the government's policy on the management of abortion complications has not yet been widely disseminated and implemented. The policy calls for extensive training of health workers in managing complications like sepsis, evacuation of the placenta, and blood transfusion. A shortage of antibiotics, blood, and other basic supplies in most health units hampers the management of abortion complications.[144]

Most health professionals interviewed were not optimistic about the future of legalizing abortion in Uganda. The experience of trying to make emergency contraception available has adequately squelched the immediate ambitions many had to push for legalization of abortion. In 2001, a mass media campaign by Commercial Market Strategies to raise awareness about emergency contraception was met with a very negative response, including a letter from Uganda's Catholic cardinal to officials at USAID and to the Minister of Health, who tactfully withdrew from the project.[145] Commercial Market Strategies had to make implementation of their project "low-key."[146] Today, emergency contraception is available in Uganda, but Dr. Ebanyat explains that few providers will direct patients where to obtain it or how to use it; "[I]t's not something you can get easily."[147]

There is essentially no debate in Uganda today about legalizing abortion, and several respondents felt that the reaction to the topic is so extreme that it will be years before any progress is made in liberalizing the abortion law.[148] Uganda is primarily a conservative Christian country in which most people believe abortion to be murder.[149] Owomuhangi points out that Uganda has historically been divided along religious lines—Protestant, Catholic, and Muslim— as well as ethnic lines. "I can't see the president, coming from a Protestant background, coming out in favor of abortion and cutting off the Catholics. At least now, they are trying to heal political wounds, not divide them more."[150]

Dr. Ebanyat points out that even if abortion were legalized, the facilities and supplies needed to provide abortions are not forthcoming. "We still have a lot of room where we can do a lot without getting in anyone's way."[151] Dr. Kyeyune concurs, "When we are thinking of having an advocacy issue in a network we say legalizing abortion and everybody says, 'No, let us start with things which can be achieved!' "[152] Yet Kyeyune is optimistic that someday the law will change. She points to the AIDS epidemic as an example; when AIDS first became a problem in Uganda, "it wasn't okay to talk to children about sex.

[. . .] It was a moral issue," but as the problem came to affect more families, the silence was broken.[153]

The dearth of research conducted on abortion complicates the matter. Dr. Jotham Musinguzi, a doctor in support of liberalizing the abortion law, explains, "The reason why some of us have not gone out to explode on it is basically because we think we need to collect some more information about what unsafe abortion is doing to our maternal mortality, and once we have the data then we can go out and talk to all these people and work with civil society."[154] Musinguzi argues that, given pressure from civil society to change the abortion law, the government may be willing to at least engage in an informed debate on the topic. A study of fifty-three abortion experts in Uganda found that two-thirds support liberalizing the current law.[155] Nevertheless, serious consideration of the issue among the general public appears to be in the distance.

The HIV/AIDS Epidemic

Uganda reported the highest HIV infection rates in the world in the early 1990s.[156] Like many other sub-Saharan African countries, Uganda had many characteristics that would make it the perfect environment in which AIDS could flourish, yet the country managed to stem the tide of the epidemic and has since been lauded as an example of how other nations should tackle the problem. In 1986, the Ugandan government launched a multisectoral approach to AIDS, including many partners in their programs and adopting a comprehensive behavior-change approach focusing simultaneously on abstinence, partner reduction, and condom use, as well as reducing stigma and improving access to testing and treatment.[157] President Museveni was a public figure in the fight against AIDS, and he insisted that the epidemic's reach went far beyond the work of the Ministry of Health. The government designed a new curriculum to ensure that STI/HIV/AIDS information was integrated into reproductive health programs.[158] The country also implemented a major policy change for midwives, allowing them to diagnose and treat HIV-positive patients, even prescribing medications for them.[159] As a result of their efforts, in 1995 Uganda became the first country to register a decrease in the number of new cases each year, and the HIV/AIDS prevalence declined from 18 percent of the total population in 1992 to just 5 percent in 2001.[160] In 1998, Uganda became one of the first African countries to distribute antiretroviral medications (ARVs), at a reduced cost, to HIV-positive people. Since June 2004 ARVs have been available free of charge to the population, though not everyone in need of ARVs has access to the life-prolonging drugs.[161] Today,

Uganda is home to the Joint Clinical Research Center, one of the largest AIDS care centers in sub-Saharan Africa.[162]

Despite Uganda's great success in controlling this deadly epidemic, much work remains to be done. The consequences of the epidemic are far-reaching and will have an impact on the country for decades to come, particularly since the epidemic disproportionately affects young people. Ten- to twenty-four-year-olds make up 33 percent of Uganda's population, for example, yet they account for half of all new HIV cases. Girls and young women in this age group are four times more likely than boys to be infected.[163] Additionally, a troubling fact unearthed by a recent study is that only 10 percent of teenage girls and 40 percent of teenage boys aged fifteen to nineteen report using condoms.[164] Knowledge of HIV/AIDS is high in Uganda, but that knowledge does not necessarily translate into action.[165] More than one respondent mentioned the stigma associated with condom use; many people consider them suitable only for nonregular partners. Married couples and even unmarried individuals in serious relationships may consider the nonuse of condoms as demonstrating trust and love.[166] The stigma attached to AIDS itself is also significant; in one recent study, over half of teenagers reported that they do not believe HIV-positive teachers should be allowed to keep their jobs.[167]

The effect that the HIV/AIDS epidemic has had on the nation's fertility remains unclear. Anecdotally, some respondents mentioned that people may choose to have more children as a way of repopulating the country after seeing so much death around them. Stella Neema continues, "But then there are those who say 'Oh, what if in the course of our life, we get the disease and then we have given birth to so many children? How are they going to survive?' So there is that balancing."[168] There are an estimated 1.7 million orphans in Uganda (out of a population of 24 million), many of them orphaned by AIDS.[169]

Beyond the obvious human and economic costs of such an epidemic, some respondents pointed out the negative impact of the disease on reproductive health work. Pregnancy endangers the health of a woman with HIV/AIDS more significantly than an HIV-negative woman, and children who contract HIV from their mothers during delivery are less likely to survive. Nestor Owomuhangi of UNFPA notes, "The gains made in the area of, for instance, reducing maternal mortality and infant mortality are being jeopardized by the problem of HIV/AIDS."[170] Owomuhangi also mentions that HIV/AIDS has inevitably diverted funds from other reproductive health issues in general.[171] While President Museveni frequently talks about AIDS in public, Owomuhangi believes equal attention should be paid to safe motherhood issues. "Imagine if the level of attention given to HIV/AIDS is given to a number of other issues related to reproductive health, for example, changing people's attitudes towards health care. 'All mothers should go for five antenatal care visits.' "[172]

For all the pain and suffering that has resulted from the AIDS epidemic, some reproductive health workers pointed out that the epidemic has helped people talk more openly about sexual and reproductive health issues, particularly for adolescents.[173] The International Conference on Population and Development (ICPD) in Cairo has also bolstered recent emphasis on adolescent reproductive health.

Influence of the ICPD

Kirumira argues that historically in Uganda there has been a "general failure to see family planning as a component of a comprehensive population policy, rather than as its equivalent. The two have been assumed to be synonymous."[174] The government's reluctance to wholeheartedly support population policies led to increased donor funding and control of the issue; global definitions and interpretations of population policy had a correspondingly substantial influence on Ugandan policy.[175] Needless to say, the ICPD had a tremendous impact on population and family planning issues in Uganda. A national population policy (NPP) had been drafted in 1994 prior to the ICPD, but when it went into effect in January 1995 it included revisions that incorporated principles from the Cairo Program of Action.[176] The Population Secretariat, housed in the Ministry of Finance and Economic Planning, was also established in 1994. In reference to the NPP, the Population Secretariat states, "A major aspect of the implementation strategy is that the policy is not coercive; rather the broad aim is to create a population that is cognizant of the interrelationships among population and development."[177] The emphasis at the ICPD on the need for *voluntary* family planning services is heard in this statement.

Much of the language used in government policy documents reflects principles developed at the ICPD. In the Sexual and Reproductive Health and Rights section of the Ministry of Health's annual report, a list of twelve main objectives includes "advocate for sexual and reproductive rights" (listed first) and "reduce fertility rate" (listed last).[178] In the same section of the most recent health sector strategic plan, the ministry outlines its specific goals for reducing maternal mortality, increasing the contraceptive prevalence rate (CPR), and increasing the percentage of deliveries supervised by a trained health worker. Absent from the list, however, are any demographic targets or mention of fertility reduction.[179]

Since the ICPD, the Ugandan government has drafted the Uganda National Plan of Action on Women, the National Gender Policy, the Children's Statute, the Local Government Act, and the Decentralization Policy, all of which incorporate principles outlined in the Program of Action.[180] The Ministry of Health's Maternal and Child Health Department was renamed (and demoted to) the Reproductive Health Division, housed within the Department of Community Health.[181] Uganda also adopted a Reproductive Health Minimum Package, which emphasizes safe motherhood and child survival, family planning, prevention and management of STI/HIV/AIDS, adolescent health, infrastructure, and information, education, and communication (IEC).[182] According to Dr. Florence Ebanyat, assistant commissioner of reproductive health at the Ministry of Health, the government has adopted a more integrated approach to reproductive health services, and certain issues that were previously on the periphery, such as adolescent health, abortion, and female genital mutilation (FGM), are now given more attention.[183] Midwives are now allowed to diagnose and treat STIs, offer family planning, immunize, provide postabortion care, and manage HIV patients, when previously their duties were confined to antenatal care and deliveries.[184] Dr. Jotham Musinguzi, director of the Population Secretariat, describes the post-Cairo shift as one of "less emphasis on family planning alone as a panacea for solving the population problem."[185] Rather, family planning is one of many strategies in the context of working for women's equality, equity, and empowerment. Musinguzi also cites improved coordination among NGOs, donors, the government, and civil society as a positive outcome of the ICPD.

Still, the degree to which the sentiments of the ICPD as reflected in national documents are felt by government officials and health care workers remains unclear. Uganda has effectively incorporated the language of the ICPD into its national policies, but changing the mentality of reproductive health and population workers may take more time. When asked how important fertility reduction is compared to the other goals of the national population policy, Dr. Musinguzi replies, "It is a *very* high priority—in fact, one of our highest priorities, as far as we are concerned, that we may reduce fertility."[186]

Influence of Donors

Contributing over 60 percent of Uganda's health budget, international donors undoubtedly wield significant influence in the health sector.[187] The largest contributors are the World Bank, USAID, DFID (U.K.), the World Health Organization (WHO), UNICEF, and World Vision.[188] Like the Ugandan government, donors are changing their methods and strategies as a result of the ICPD. The

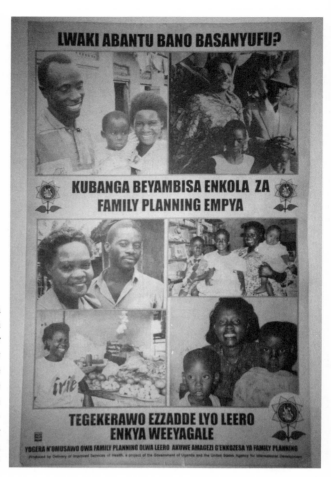

Produced by a USAID program in Uganda, this poster proclaims, "Why are these people happy? Because they chose the new family planning. Plan for your family today for a better tomorrow."

associate program officer of reproductive health in UNFPA, Nestor Owomu-hangi, reports a dramatic shift in the organization since 1994. Moving away from vertical family planning programs, UNFPA has adopted a more integrated approach to reproductive health, which focuses less on reducing fertility and more on child spacing.[189] Its programs are developed within the human rights framework outlined in the ICPD.[190] Similarly, USAID was unwilling to put resources into any non–family planning programs when it first came to Uganda; now, with increased domestic and international pressure, the agency is slowly widening its focus to related issues, like safe motherhood, though "the support has been diluted."[191]

Despite gains made since the ICPD, donors still place disproportionate emphasis on promoting family planning rather than supporting the general infrastructure of the health care system. Traditionally, a large portion of resources went to the physical rehabilitation of health centers; "there was a strong tendency to focus on generating measurable outputs, rather than supporting the underlying processes which support health systems and health development."[192] Donors are less willing to fund health workers' salaries, staff recruitment, or basic supplies and equipment, like gloves and drugs—other than contraceptives—at health centers, even though such support has the potential to dramatically increase the quality of services offered, lowering mortality rates.[193] Dr. Sentongo notes that the Reproductive Health Division's program to train more midwives is difficult to secure funding for, but "they support us in terms of procuring contraceptives."[194] Dr. Ebanyat points out other areas in which it is difficult to get donor support, such as infertility, reproductive health cancers, and men's involvement programs.[195] Donor-funded programs are disbursed unevenly, both geographically and in terms of subject area. Grants from outside sources are often earmarked for specific projects that may be inconsistent with local needs.[196] The United States' recent dramatic drop in foreign aid for reproductive health has also had an influence on Ugandan women's health, as both the government and NGOs, including UNFPA, grapple with a greatly reduced budget.[197]

Gender Equality in Uganda

Uganda has long boasted one of the strongest women's movements in Africa. The country was the first in Africa to have a female vice president, and women have held ministry posts as well.[198] An impressive one-quarter of parliamentarians are women. The women's movement has not made reproductive health and rights a priority issue, however, perhaps partly because of the need to follow the socially conservative agenda that the government embraces—one that is popular with the churches. Uganda's "no-party" political system does not encourage advocacy of political interests by NGOs, leaving them to focus on public education campaigns and community programs to raise awareness in the population at large about gender-related issues. Dr. Joy Kyeyune emphasizes the importance of gender equality taking place in the home when children are young. "Boys and girls should be treated equally, and then even when they start going to school—take both to school. Don't take only the boy, because once the girl misses out on education, then she will miss out on job opportunity, she will become poor—she will be a poor woman and suffer in whatever marriage. If she's in a bad marriage, she can't walk out because of economic reasons."[199]

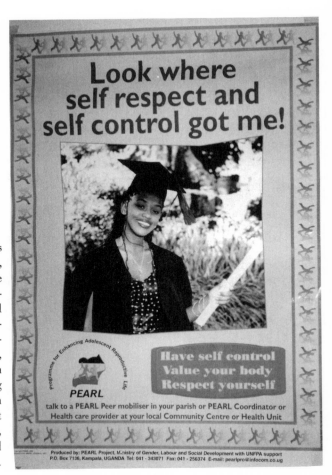

Look where
self respect and
self control got me!

**Have self control
Value your body
Respect yourself**

programme for Enhancing Adolescent Reproductive Life

PEARL

talk to a PEARL Peer mobiliser in your parish or PEARL Coordinator or
Health care provider at your local Community Centre or Health Unit

Produced by: PEARL Project, Ministry of Gender, Labour and Social Development with UNFPA support
P.O. Box 7136, Kampala, UGANDA Tel: 041 - 343071 Fax: 041 - 256374 E-mail: pearlpro@infocom.co.ug

The posters on this page and the next, produced by the Ugandan government and a local NGO with funding from international donors, target 'hip' urban youth, spreading reproductive health messages that promote abstinence, monogamy, and condoms.

More than one respondent mentioned the need to empower women economically in order to improve their health. Stella Neema notes that when women start earning their own income, "their health will also improve because when they are sick they won't wait for the husband, they will just go use the money from their earnings. But the problem has been that the man is the one in control of the money because he is the one who brings the money."[200] Several NGOs have implemented microfinance and revolving fund programs to help women in this regard.

Further involving men in women's reproductive rights would be beneficial to all concerned, but the task is not an easy one. Dr. Sentongo explains that even in planning meetings at the Reproductive Health Division, few men are

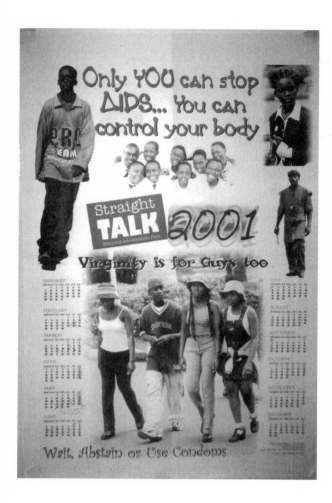

willing to talk about women's rights. "The minute you bring in gender issues, they shut off. They think maybe this is women's empowerment and we want to overshadow them—things like that."[201] Finding allies among men to further the cause of reproductive rights is a challenge in Uganda, though one that has the potential to help the movement tremendously.

Conclusion

Like other countries that endorsed the Program of Action, Uganda adopted the feminist language of the ICPD in its relevant government documents. Concrete changes have been realized at the implementation level, particularly in regard to integration of services, but much work remains to be done. Experience demonstrates that policies often fail to translate into action; the feminist ideals expressed in select Ministry of Health documents are likely not felt on the ground where service delivery occurs. Access and quality of care for reproductive health services in Uganda remain low, and donors continue to weigh family planning as a disproportionately higher priority than other equally essential areas. Frequent evaluation of existing programs and sensitization of service providers and communities alike is needed if the idealist principles outlined in the ICPD ever translate into reality in Uganda.

The aims of Uganda's health care system are admirable—to provide universal coverage of quality services free of cost. Yet the reality is far from this ideal, and over half of Ugandans have no access to a health care clinic at all. The main culprit for the wide gap between policy and practice is the most obvious one: poverty. But it is not only a lack of resources that creates weaknesses in the health care system; the uneven distribution of resources (favoring tertiary urban hospitals) is directly responsible for inadequate facilities in rural areas, where health care is needed most. When most health units are far from an individual woman's home, the burden of paying for transport and taking time away from her domestic duties is often sufficient to prevent access. Both of these factors also hinder a woman's ability to seek family planning services without the knowledge or consent of her husband. Approaching family planning from the more holistic view espoused in the ICPD's Program of Action, reproductive health services should be expanded in scope and breadth to reach a broader segment of the population.

Taking care of their reproductive health is a struggle for most Ugandan women, who face multiple barriers throughout their lifetime that greatly restrict their ability to exercise reproductive freedom. Beginning with the dearth of sex education as children, women later face pressure to be in sexual relationships though they may not be well equipped to protect themselves against sexually transmitted infections, HIV/AIDS, or an unwanted pregnancy. Lacking easy access to contraception, or any other health services for that matter, millions of Ugandan women have little power to control their bodies and their fertility. In the attempt to do so, many die from illegal, unsafe abortions. Until women enjoy access to a wide range of health services not limited to family planning, until they gain economic independence and share equal educational and job opportunities with men, until Uganda's abortion law is liberalized for both public health and human rights reasons, women in this country will have difficulty achieving the reproductive autonomy they deserve.

3

Peru

Background

Nestled in the western crook of South America between Ecuador and Chile, Peru is a country with a history of diverse cultural influences. Many of the indigenous people in Peru are descendents of the Incas and continue to live in the Andes Mountains, speaking Quechua or Aymara, while others inhabit the low-lying Amazon rainforest in the north and speak dozens of different languages. African influence from Peru's history with slavery is most prevalent on the coast, as are the traces of Japanese and Chinese culture that came along with mass migrations.[1] Peru's peoples are diverse in their ethnicity, language, religion, and lifestyle, and wide economic disparities persist. As in many countries, one can see the vast differences in access to reproductive health services between the rural poor and the urban elite, though urbanization has led to a booming population of urban poor. In the slums surrounding Lima, the country's sprawling capital city on the coast, living conditions are comparable to, or even worse than, those found in rural areas.

Reproductive rights activists in Peru face many difficulties. The majority of the population receives scant sex education and limited access to reproductive health services, including family planning. Around 60 percent of all pregnancies in Peru are unplanned—one of the highest figures in the world.[2] Not surprisingly, unsafe abortions are commonplace in this predominantly Catholic country where abortion is illegal except to save the woman's life. Peru's recent history includes a coercive population control program that targeted the nation's indigenous women. Yet Peru is also a country with a vibrant and growing feminist movement and a core of health professionals committed to improving women's reproductive freedom. Feminist activists are responsible for many gains in reproductive rights, including better access to contraception and increased public debate about abortion. Although the conservative sector is well financed and powerful, the overall direction of Peru's reproductive rights movement is a positive one.

Sex Education

Peru's generally abysmal sex education lays the groundwork for the country's high proportion of unwanted pregnancies. Sex education within the home is practically nonexistent; rumors and misconceptions abound. Strongly influenced by the Catholic Church, the Ministry of Education's commitment to comprehensive sex education has been lacking. In the mid-1990s, the ministry implemented a new sex education program, but after the irate reaction of a Catholic cardinal upon review of the curriculum, dissemination stopped. Ministry officials drew up a second curriculum, which was acceptable to the Catholic Church yet lacked the most crucial health messages adolescents need concerning contraception and the prevention of sexually transmitted infections (STIs).[3] Even when individual schools decide to adopt progressive sex education programs, the curricula eventually fall by the wayside in most cases, when the authorities in that particular school change. Students are aware of family planning methods in general but are usually unable to describe even one method in detail—how the method works and how to use it.

Despite progress on other fronts in reproductive health, Peru's teenage pregnancy rate has not changed since studies first measured the indicator in the early 1970s. Nationally, 12 to 13 percent of teenage women are pregnant at any given time, though this figure rises to as high as 25 to 35 percent in some rural areas.[4] Given the intense efforts activists have directed toward increasing access to contraception and advocating for a more liberal abortion law, one wonders why the topic of sex education has not received similar attention. Perhaps most fundamental to a woman's ability to take care of her sexual and reproductive health is the availability of complete and accurate information about subjects like anatomy, pregnancy, family planning, abortion, and protection from STIs and HIV/AIDS. Without such basic knowledge, women must rely on the numerous myths and misconceptions that circulate in nearly every community. The near absence of sex education that many Peruvians experience today endangers women's health and impinges on women's ability to exercise their reproductive rights.

Barriers to Using Family Planning

Although early childbearing has remained a dominant feature of Peru's demographic picture, overall fertility rates have dropped in the past fifty years. However, women still have an average of one or two more children than they desire, indicating a need for greater access, in the broadest sense of the word, to family planning services.[5] Peru's total fertility rate (TFR) stands at 2.9 children per woman, though the national figure masks gaping inequities within the population, according to socioeconomic level, residence, and education. Women with no formal education, for example, have an average of 5.1 children per woman, while women with higher education have only 1.8 children.[6] As in many countries, rural women tend to be the most disadvantaged, with the least amount of formal education, employment opportunities, and negotiating power with their husbands.

The Ministry of Health has provided contraceptives since 1983 and in 1994 began offering contraceptives in public health clinics free of charge, yet numerous barriers impede women's access to reproductive health services.[7] Women in Peru report a high level of awareness and acceptance of family planning methods, yet contraceptive prevalence remains low for a number of reasons. Perhaps the most obvious barrier for women attempting to obtain health care is economic. Even though the Peruvian government has mandated free family planning services in public health centers, numerous facilities are underfunded and charge patients fees for other components of their visit, such as the doctor's consultation, thus putting the cost out of reach for the majority of the population.[8] In the case of childbirth, public health facilities are not allowed to charge patients for the actual delivery, but, in reality, patients are responsible for purchasing supplies like gloves and drugs, driving up the cost of the birth to at least US$25.[9] Additional expenses for transportation, loss of work time, and sometimes translation services, add up to make the cost of a visit to the health center out of reach for poor women. Yet health officials often ignore these hidden costs. Peru's overly centralized health care system translates to a disproportionate number of health facilities in urban areas, particularly in Lima, leaving rural women with even less access to services.[10] Yet, as Rossina Guerrero, a psychologist working at the feminist organization Flora Tristán, observes, severely impoverished areas exist even in Lima. "We say that in the rural areas like in the Andes, in the jungle, women have terrible access to services, but this is the case in many cities as well. Because of the poverty, women can't access these services."[11]

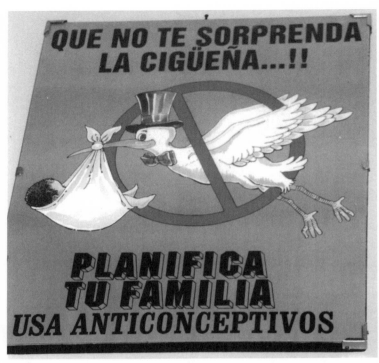

"Don't let the stork surprise you! Plan your family – use contraception."
Similar posters advertising contraception are abundant throughout Peruvian health centers, reflecting both the government's and donors' focus on family planning in recent years.

Compounding the barriers women face in physically reaching a clinic and financing their visit is the dwindling supply of contraceptives available in the health centers. Guerrero reports that the government has not considered family planning to be a priority in the past two or three years, leaving hundreds of health centers without a regular supply of contraceptives. Even just a few years ago, women could get eight or ten months' worth of contraceptive pills in one visit; now, with the shortage of contraception in the clinics, women can only obtain one or two cycles per visit.[12] The shortage forces women to return to the clinic every month or two—an unreasonable demand that undoubtedly contributes to the high discontinuation rate among women using modern contraceptives.

Partly as a result of the shortage of contraceptive supplies, health providers offer only a limited range of methods from which women can choose.

Dr. Miguel Gutiérrez, president of the Peruvian Society of Obstetrics and Gynecology and medical director for Pathfinder International, comments, "You can't impose on someone what method they are going to use. If you only have one method, you cannot say, 'Well, if you want to protect yourself, this is the only one we have.' "[13] Women who are unable or unwilling to take the one method offered are left with no viable family planning options.

For a woman to enjoy true access to health care, a range of variables must be in place beyond the availability of contraceptives in health clinics. Guerrero points out other barriers women face, such as discriminatory practices and physical or emotional abuse.[14] Even in the proximity of state-of-the-art medical facilities, a woman who is mired in an abusive relationship, with no economic independence and limited information about her body, will not likely be able to access health services.

Overall knowledge of contraception is high in Peru, with 98 percent of the population capable of naming at least one method, but myths about side effects and complications continue to surround modern family planning methods.[15] Inadequate counseling and follow-up care at health centers exacerbate the situation. Health providers frequently neglect to inform women of the common side effects of contraceptives and do not tell them that the side effects of hormonal contraception, like headaches and weight gain, may subside after a few weeks of use. Not surprisingly, many women stop taking the contraceptives once side effects occur, and they proceed to tell other women about their negative experience with the drugs.[16] Even though many women who use hormonal contraception do not experience any adverse effects, women's fear of side effects may be one of the most substantial obstacles to their use of modern contraception; traditional family planning methods are far more popular and trusted in Peru.

Indigenous women face the greatest challenges in accessing reproductive health care. Susana Chávez, a feminist activist and midwife at Flora Tristán, refers to the "double whammy" indigenous women experience—discrimination based on both race and language.[17] Though racism in Peru is diffused and underdetected, its effects are powerful. Yet few institutions exist to advocate for indigenous people's rights, unlike the proliferation of women's rights organizations and the official Ministry for the Promotion of Women (PROMUDEH). Tammy Quintanilla, a lawyer working with Movimiento El Pozo, points out, "Much of the racism is tied to language—you can hear it in the racial slurs and insults against indigenous people, people from the Amazon [. . .]. There are adolescents who tease their friends when they make mistakes, and instead of saying 'You are stupid, foolish, an idiot,' they say, 'You are indigenous.' "[18]

Chávez voices the sentiment that women who do not speak Spanish have "no power and no voice."[19]

Peru's maternal mortality rate of 185 deaths per 100,000 live births is one of the highest in the region, and in certain Andean and Amazonian areas, mortality rates are far higher.[20] Native people in the Amazon, comprising 40 percent of the Peruvian population, experience the highest mortality rates in the country. More than one respondent referred to their living conditions as "truly alarming," describing a situation in which women have almost no access to health care of any sort.[21] When indigenous women have demanded more support services for traditional family planning methods in public health centers, providers have frequently met their requests with scorn.[22] Indeed, more than one respondent felt that a fundamental reason that women in rural areas, particularly indigenous women, do not access health centers is because they feel mistreated and disrespected. "The theme of discrimination in health centers manifests itself in different ways—the announcements that are all in Spanish, the medical procedures, the consents, which are not designed for these women. They don't incorporate the cultural views of women who are not Spanish speakers," explains Rocío Gutiérrez of the feminist organization Movimiento Manuela Ramos.[23] Most health centers, even those located in remote areas in the Andes, do not have Quechua-speaking or Aymara-speaking staff, despite the dominance of those two indigenous languages in the area.

The biases of providers are another influence on women's use of family planning; health professionals may decide which method of contraception is best for a particular woman, rather than giving her all the information and letting her choose. One respondent, a well-respected doctor who has been practicing medicine for forty years, explains that he advises women who do not yet have children to only use barrier methods, like condoms, or traditional methods, such as withdrawal or the rhythm method. I observed him telling many young women that using hormonal contraceptives like the Pill or injectables may cause infertility. For older women who have had children, he recommends the IUD, informing women that they can have the same IUD for fifteen to twenty years (most IUDs should be used no longer than five to ten years). Likewise, this particular doctor advised one thirty-five-year-old woman that she need not worry about contraception because it took her two years to get pregnant with her first child, who is now one year old. The doctor reasoned that it would take her another two years to get pregnant, and by that time she will be thirty-seven and "out of danger." She seemed somewhat unconvinced by his explanation but nevertheless left the hospital without any contraception. Many doctors believe that poor, rural women are incapable of remembering to take the Pill every day, and so they only offer the longer term, provider-controlled methods to them. Providers' biases often interfere with women's ability to make intelligent and informed decisions for themselves.

Women attempting to use "natural," or traditional, family planning methods feel the added encumbrance of getting their partners' active cooperation, necessary for the two most popular traditional methods: withdrawal and periodic abstinence (the rhythm method). In a country where domestic violence and rape are staggeringly common, such cooperation may not be easily acquired. It was only in 1991 that lawmakers revised the penal code to recognize rape within marriage as a crime.[24] Although a recent law removed the requirement for women to obtain spousal or parental consent for family planning services, women trapped in abusive relationships still have little power to take care of their reproductive health needs.

Prostitutes are most vulnerable to sexual violence and among the least able to access health services. As Tammy Quintanilla, who works with an advocacy organization for sex workers, points out, "The majority of programs targeting prostitutes do so out of a desire to control the spread of STIs and HIV/AIDS, not out of a desire to make these women more autonomous and in control of their lives."[25] One study, by Movimiento El Pozo, found that nearly all prostitutes have children, and most cite meeting their children's material needs as the principal reason for their work.[26] These women are not in a position to bear more children, yet they often face unwanted pregnancies as a result of their work and the commonplace sexual violence directed against them.

Of the myriad obstacles Peruvian women face in accessing family planning services, perhaps the largest of all is cultural. Though most people accept family planning out of necessity, a number of societal barriers exist to its use. As sociologist Miguel Ramos explains, the Peruvian concept of masculinity is rife with contradiction; on the one hand, a "real" man is supposed to be a good provider, and this role is threatened when he has many children and the task of caring for all of them is too expensive. However, another aspect of masculine identity is the power to control women's sexuality, and a woman's use of family planning can jeopardize his ability to do so. Traditional *machismo* stirs up fear of women's disloyalty; a woman on birth control may have sex with as many partners as she chooses without risking an unwanted pregnancy.[27] Another *macho* stereotype is that men should constantly crave sex and their sexual desires should be met whenever demanded.[28] This sort of belief lends itself to men disrespecting their wives' fertile periods, which is problematic if the woman is using the rhythm method. A sense of ownership over women also impedes their husbands' willingness to let them access health services. The majority of Peruvian doctors are men, and most husbands do not want their wives' bodies to be touched by another man. Ramos notes that such an encounter raises the possibility of infidelity and teasing from the community: "'Hey look! Juancito is sending his woman to the health center so she can be touched!' They become the butt of jokes."[29] The societal pressure men feel to prove their manhood often runs counter to the best interests of their wives.

Studies have shown that in urban areas, family planning is usually seen as the woman's sole responsibility, and her partner is disinterested until they have the number of children for which he can provide.[30] It is also easier for urban women to attend a health clinic without their husbands' knowledge, and indeed many do. In contrast, women in rural areas have less autonomy, and the men tend to be more involved in their wives' reproductive health. Susana Chávez points out, "Women rarely get services from a health clinic [. . .] without going with their partners."[31]

Adolescent women also frequently experience men's unwillingness to be involved in family planning; among urban adolescents in particular, negotiating condom use is difficult. Societal norms dictate that sex should be spontaneous; being prepared with a condom in hand suggests an element of planning that people frown upon. Either the man or the woman may be deemed promiscuous if he or she proposes using a condom. Miguel Ramos articulates, "It's a bit of a game—the girls always have to be on the defensive, they have to say 'no' the first few times. The girls can never agree to have sex the first time he asks. In this rather perverse game, the use of a condom would signify that it's planned."[32]

Such dating games may be less common in the countryside, but a lack of contraceptive use with premarital sex persists, frequently due to the prevalence of sexual violence. In fact, one study in a rural area found that, for the *majority* of women, their first sexual experience was rape. In some areas of the country, Miguel Ramos points out, "there are cultural aspects that make it socially acceptable for a woman to be raped and then marry that man."[33] Until 1997, a man could avoid criminal prosecution for rape if he agreed to marry the victim.[34]

Traditional Peruvian culture also favors large families, and a portion of the population refuses family planning services out of their desire for many children. Chávez criticizes the sexual and reproductive rights movement for exclusively emphasizing the right to limit how many children a family has, even though "we have a population where there are people who want to have children."[35] The movement could be more effective if the message focused on a woman's right to decide how many children she has, regardless of the number, as well as emphasizing the health benefits of well-spaced births to both mother and child. While current family planning messages may resonate with couples who only want two or three children, psychologist Trixsi Vargas insists that women who want eight children are equally valid in their decisions, yet they are ignored in health messages.

Indeed, many women have eight children because only a few may survive.[36] While efforts at improving the accessibility of family planning are commendable, broader changes in living conditions and mortality rates must occur before women will have the number of pregnancies, and children, they desire. Such work must target the most disadvantaged sectors of the Peruvian population. As Susana Chávez points out, the fertility rate is declining, "but what persist are the disparities. In the rural areas, women still have double the number of children they want. [. . .] So the gaps remain—this has not diminished."[37] As the prior discussion on the multiple barriers to family planning illustrates, increasing women's access to such services will hinge on improvements of a wide range of variables, including those tied to the economy, culture, and politics, in addition to the health care system itself.

Catholic Influence on Reproductive Rights

As is the case in most Latin American countries, the Catholic Church wields considerable cultural and judicial power in Peru. Since the first days of Spanish colonialism in the 1500s, the Catholic Church played a pivotal role in shaping modern-day Peruvian society. Consequently, "There is a very popular sense of Catholicism among the people."[38] The Catholics carry weight within government circles as well. José Ugaz, a prominent lawyer, explains, "From a judicial perspective, the Peruvian government signed an agreement with the Church many years ago that said the Catholic Church would have a privileged position in the State."[39] Although this agreement was nullified during Alan Garcia's administration (1985–1990), the church maintains a tight relationship with government officials; a recent minister of health, a Catholic, famously declared, "My Constitution is the Bible."[40] The former prime minister, now an influential congressman, is also a conservative Catholic. With strong support from the religious right in the United States and the current Bush administration, factions of President Alejandro Toledo's conservative government have actively opposed dispensing the IUD and the Morning-After Pill (both labeled "abortifacients").[41] Predictably, Toledo's administration is also against making condoms available in high schools. Although a 2001 directive requires public health centers to offer emergency contraception, conservatives in the Ministry of Health have blocked the directive's implementation. The Morning-After Pill is currently only available in private pharmacies, at an expense of roughly US$8, an unaffordable cost for most people.[42] Conservative Catholics in the current government, following Bush's lead, have declared May 25 to be "Day of the Unborn," and they have succeeded in passing legislation protecting the "conceived."[43] This Catholic influence on politics persists despite the fact that many Peruvians support a secular state. Rossina Guerrero insists, "We think that faith should be a personal decision—my religious beliefs can't translate into political policies."[44]

The church's public stance on issues like sex education, contraception, and abortion run contrary to women's reproductive rights and public health concerns. Dr. Americo Mayorga of Arequipa laments, "The Catholic Church has always played a role against these things, even though they know that women who don't take care of themselves get pregnant, subject themselves to abortion, and die. . . . Even though the church knows all this, they only accept natural methods."[45] Interviewees expressed their frustration at the church's objection to any substantive reproductive health programs. The CEO of Inppares (Peruvian Institute for Responsible Parenthood), Dr. Daniel Gho Aspilcueta, comments on the Catholic Church's regular attacks on Inppares's work in reproductive health: "I always call them promoters of abortion, because if you deny people education and access to contraception, you are going to have more unwanted pregnancies, and obviously this leads to more abortions. I don't understand this. Why aren't they fighting against unwanted pregnancies? Because without unwanted pregnancies, there would be no abortions."[46] The Catholic influence in Peru is perhaps most visible when discussing this most volatile of issues: abortion. Though the church's power is not sufficient to mandate individuals' decisions in their personal lives (Peru has a high abortion rate, despite 80% of the population being Catholic), one activist makes clear, "There is a strong censorship from the church for any person to speak about abortion."[47]

Abortion

One of the greatest challenges to women's reproductive rights in this Latino country is the criminalization of abortion. Abortion is only legal in cases of saving the mother's life, and even then, a panel of three doctors must agree upon the medical diagnosis and the necessity for abortion and the husband must consent to the procedure.[48] Yet Peru's abortion rate is astronomical, and increasing. Official statistics on abortion are not kept, but the most reliable estimate of illegal abortions puts the current number at just over 350,000 per year, in a country with only twenty-five million people, up from 271,000 illegal abortions in 1994.[49] The consequences of illegal abortion in Peru are deleterious from both a women's rights and a public health perspective.

While women with resources have never had difficulty finding a doctor willing to provide a safe, illegal abortion, the majority of Peru's population, living in poverty, does not share this luxury. For those who cannot afford a safe abortion (starting around US$300), illegal abortion involves placing their health and lives at risk. Tammy Quintanilla explains that women use a variety of methods to abort by themselves, often inserting foreign objects into the vagina, such as chemicals, herbal infusions, branches, or tar. Some attempt to hit themselves or throw themselves down a staircase in order to abort.[50] Dr. Miguel Gutiérrez adds, "there are people who use ridiculous things to try to abort—like inserting soap in the vagina, using scissors, and who knows what else—things from the Amazon—and this puts the woman's life at risk."[51] Others go to backstreet abortion providers who conduct the procedures under unhygienic conditions. Only four blocks away from Lima's Plaza de Armas lies Avenida Tacna, where one block is lined with signs for treatment of *atraso menstrual* ("menstrual delay"). I entered one of the little shops and a man led me to a poorly lit back office. "What do you want?" he asked me. I told him I was looking for information about *atraso menstrual* and asked what his sign out front means. "It's for pregnancies. How many weeks do you have?" He proceeded to inform me that he could help women with abortions up to twelve weeks into the pregnancy, using a combination of tablets and an herbal concoction. The cost for the earliest possible termination was US$75.[52] Though I was surprised by the openness with which people advertise this illegal procedure (on the streets and in newspapers), one respondent assured me that the backstreet providers are not prosecuted—they make regular payments to local authorities and corruption keeps them out of jail.[53]

Nationally, 30 percent of all women undergoing an illegal abortion end up with complications, and many are too scared to seek help; only a fifth of women suffering complications go to a health center.[54] Those who go to the health clinics for treatment of postabortion complications rarely have a positive experience. Dr. Miguel Gutiérrez explains,

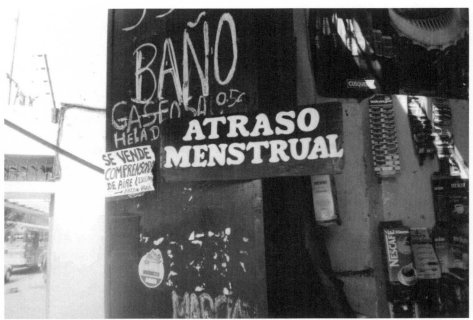

This sign openly advertising illegal abortions ("menstrual delay") is one of many along Avenida Tacna in downtown Lima, just blocks from the country's main police station and Parliament.

> We are working in the entire country with postabortion care, because women arrive at the hospitals with complications and they are treated badly sometimes, they don't get the best treatment [. . .]. They are not treated the same as women coming in with deliveries. And people tend to say, "Well, everything that is happening is your fault." So we try to get people to look at the whole picture, to see if these women are in abusive relationships, if they need a pap smear, if they have STIs, etc. We want staff to consider a woman who comes with complications from abortion as a human being.[55]

Several respondents noted that illegal abortions in Peru are safer now than they were a decade ago; in 1992, the complication rate was estimated to be significantly higher, at 47 percent.[56] The volume of abortion complications has diminished, even though the number of abortions is increasing. Of the four main causes of maternal mortality—abortion, hemorrhaging, infection, and preclampsia—abortion and hemorrhaging have historically vied for first place, but today, abortion comes in fourth place.[57] Perhaps the chief reason for this turnabout is the availability of prostaglandins in many pharmacies; fewer women abort using instruments—instead they use medications to induce bleeding. Furthermore, if a woman starts hemorrhaging from the abortion, she has a better chance of finding a health clinic that offers postabortion care now than in past years. Superior antibiotics have also saved the lives of many women suffering from postabortion infections.[58] Regardless, abortions for poor women remain unsafe; women living in extreme poverty have high abortion complication rates, around 44 percent.[59] Miguel Ramos observes, "The upper class or middle class has access to safe services, but for the poor, they have to put themselves in terrible situations. . . . It's a double violation against their sexual rights and their right to life."[60]

Although abortion is both illegal and commonplace in Peru, there are essentially no women or providers in jail because of it. José Ugaz notes, "The law is not applied in reality, and even when it is applied, it's usually poor women with few resources."[61] The vast majority of abortions go unreported because most are not complicated cases, and, even when complications do occur, health professionals have difficulty distinguishing between an induced abortion and a spontaneous abortion. By law, doctors are required to report any woman suspected of inducing an abortion, but most doctors have an aversion to the judicial process, and they do not want to be inconvenienced by it.[62] Beyond the time commitment inherent in filing a police report and testifying before a judge, doctors fear the corruption of the system; one doctor reports that a judge, in order to get a bribe, may accuse the health provider of provoking the abortion.[63] Even if both a patient and a provider are brought to court, the penalization of abortion disproportionately affects the patient. Dr. Gutiérrez observes, "There are more women prosecuted for illegal abortions than providers prosecuted, because the providers have the money to buy their way out of it."[64]

Although people generally accept that, as a private matter, cases of justified abortion exist, most still consider it a sin and a crime.[65] Surveys asking if people agree with abortion always reveal an overwhelmingly negative view of the topic. People state that they are against abortion, and then they translate their morals into law. Rossina Guerrero, psychologist at the feminist organization Flora Tristán, protests, "The problem of abortion has always been discussed from a moral perspective; it has rarely been discussed from a perspective based in public health, in human rights, in gender studies. It has always been debated in religious terms."[66] Feminist organizations like Flora Tristán are attempting to elevate the abortion debate and link it to other democracy-related topics. Guerrero continues,

In a country that doesn't allow women to really control their fertility, and that penalizes abortion, the result is negative, logically. While they are arguing about who's going to hell, who's going to heaven, women are dying. They always focus the debate on the life of the *niño*—and it's always the *niño* [male child], they never say *niña* [female child], do they?—and the debate doesn't center on the life of the woman. They don't talk about the conflict in human rights. We want the people making decisions to realize that these women have lives, they have histories and relationships and they have life goals. Abortion constitutes an example of an exercise of her rights.[67]

Cecilia Olea Mauleon of Flora Tristán is the coordinator of the September 28th Campaign, a movement begun in 1990 across Latin America to depenalize abortion. Though Flora Tristán is in favor of a liberal abortion law, some of their coalition partners only want the law loosened enough to allow victims of rape or incest to have legal abortions.[68] Working with several other nongovernmental organizations in Peru, Flora Tristán is attempting to raise public consciousness about illegal abortions. Though met with much resistance (abortion rights activists are often labeled *abortistas* [abortionists] and "enemies of the family"), the individuals engaged in the struggle for a more just law see cause for hope.

Compared to ten or twenty years ago, there is far more public awareness of the problem of abortion, as well as more sympathy in cases of rape, incest, or when abortion is medically necessary. A few high-profile cases have thrust abortion into the spotlight. Rossina Guerrero recalls, "Recently a seventeen-year-old girl had a life-threatening condition and the doctors refused her abortion, and she died a few hours after childbirth."[69] Publicity of such tragedies has garnered support from people for a more open abortion law. Given the currently deteriorated state of Peru's reproductive health services, Susana Chávez wonders if the public will realize the nonsensical nature of the abortion law: "If a woman goes to a health center now, she is not going to find a means by which she can control her fertility, and then if she becomes pregnant and has an abortion, the state will punish her for something for which they are largely responsible."[70]

Dr. Miguel Gutiérrez believes people need to understand that legalizing abortion is not equivalent to promoting abortion. The struggle must be centered on preventing unwanted pregnancies, while appropriately caring for women who are already in the position of facing an unwanted pregnancy.[71] Several respondents suggested that more awareness of the social injustice inherent to the abortion law will lead to increased protest. Dr. Daniel Aspilcueta of Inppares argues, "Decriminalizing abortion would mean that poor women who put their lives at risk to get illegal abortions could get the same care that women with resources get. It would mean that they are not any more severely punished than anyone else, and that they would not be afraid to get care for complications."[72] Peru's current abortion law clearly does not prevent abortions; it only serves to punish those women with the least resources.

Still, most politicians underestimate or deny the magnitude of the abortion problem, and the government is staunchly antichoice, partly because it is largely composed of conservative Catholic officials. Despite a clearly delineated separation of church and state in the nation's constitution, a visit to the Ministry of Health in Lima reveals a life-size statue of the Virgin Mary in the main lobby.[73] Abortion is still a taboo topic that most are reluctant to discuss. When I visited the Ministry of Health in 2003, an official helped me access statistics on family planning from the ministry's website. When I inquired about statistics concerning abortion, he fumed, "That is not open to the public!" and stormed off.[74]

In 1991, when revising the penal code, lawmakers engaged in a debate over whether to make abortion legal in cases of rape or fetal abnormality. The revisions did not pass, largely because the Catholic Church effectively blocked them.[75] The church wields considerable power in the upper echelons of government, and, as José Ugaz predicts, "No president is going to want to go against the Church—they would crucify him. So I don't think [the abortion law] is going to change in the foreseeable future."[76] Nevertheless, feminist activists continue to have hope, pointing to the small, yet concrete, advances made so far toward greater awareness of abortion.

Sterilization Abuses

While some Peruvian women are fighting for the right to control their fertility through access to contraception and abortion, others are defending their right to *have* children. Peru provides one of the clearest and most recent examples of abuse stemming from a population control agenda. Under President Fujimori in the late 1990s, hundreds of women were sterilized without their consent, sometimes even without their knowledge. The majority of these women were poor, rural-dwelling, indigenous, and often illiterate—the very same women who are least able to defend their rights. Many did not understand Spanish but were not offered adequate translation services.

The state policy was partly written by President Fujimori himself, according to José Ugaz, chief prosecutor during the Fujimori corruption scandal that led to the end of his presidency.[77] The new policy represented a dramatic departure from the country's previous sterilization law, under which a woman could only obtain a tubal ligation if she had four or more children, if she was above a certain age, or for medical reasons. In all cases, spousal consent was required.[78] The new sterilization policy lifted these restrictions. Fujimori's ardent promotion of the policy included intimidating doctors into meeting monthly tubal ligation quotas and offering financial incentives for exceeding the quota. Health officials in some instances offered poor women food in return for their agreeing to be sterilized; others pressured women daily in their homes to consent to the procedure. In many cases, health professionals did not inform women of other contraceptive options, nor did they tell them that sterilization is a permanent method. In some health clinics, temporary contraceptive methods such as injectables and the Pill were deliberately withheld from women in order to promote sterilization.[79] Although the government performed the sterilizations at no cost, health providers charged patients for follow-up care and treatment of complications, thus preventing untold numbers of women from returning to the hospital for assistance when they developed postsurgery complications.[80]

A few prominent feminist organizations were the first to bring the abuses to the attention of the public, revealing a coercive policy of the state and forcing a formal investigation by the Defensoría del Pueblo (a federal body responsible for protecting the rights of citizens).[81] In 1998, the government dropped all numeric goals for contraceptive use.[82] In a series of three publications written during and after the formal investigation, the Defensoría del Pueblo chronicles the stories of dozens of women who suffered under the stringent sterilization policy. One woman, in Piura, went to the local health center to receive her usual family planning method—injectables (Depo Provera). Health workers there told her they no longer offered injectables and that the only family planning method available was sterilization. They offered to give her food if she agreed to the procedure, and they advised her husband that he should force her to accept the surgery. The woman verbally agreed to be sterilized, though she never signed a consent form. She went home a few hours after the procedure, feeling "horrible," and died the next day from complications.[83] Another woman arrived at the hospital to deliver her baby and the doctor told her she had to pay ten Peruvian soles (US$3) for each of six prenatal visits she missed, as well as five soles for the birth certificate. The couple could not afford to pay sixty-five soles, and the doctor told them he would forego the charges if the woman agreed to be sterilized after her delivery.[84]

The Defensoría del Pueblo uncovered numerous cases of women's deaths from complications after their tubal ligation, when health providers denied them treatment because they could not afford to pay for it. In dozens of other cases, the woman was actually pregnant when doctors performed her sterilization; their inadequate presurgery assessment and failure to do a pregnancy test allowed such a mistake. Health officials frequently did not respond to investigators' demands to see the medical records of women who filed complaints, and, in many cases, they claimed that the medical records for a particular patient were lost.[85]

Though the Ministry of Health maintains that the family planning program during this time did not have any specific demographic goals, investigators from the Defensoría del Pueblo discovered evidence suggesting otherwise, namely in the paperwork that each health center was required to complete and return to the central government. On these forms, health centers had to provide a number for the "program goal for sterilization at this establishment," as well as the "number of patients *captured* for sterilization," or the "number of patients *submitted* to sterilization."[86] The investigators point out that if no demographic targets existed, there would be no need for these questions.

Rossina Guerrero elucidates the logic behind the abusive policy: "The abuses had a very strong component that linked poverty with contraception [. . .]. The fight against poverty—as all the politicians were saying—was linked to the decrease of the fertility rate. If you decrease the fertility rate, you decrease the poverty rate—that was the rhetoric they used, even though it's not necessarily that way."[87] Such rhetoric stems directly from the international discourse on population control.

The conservative sector of the newly elected Peruvian government seized the opportunity that the sterilization abuses of Fujimori's administration offered, using the scandal to support their own agenda by calling for an immediate end to all government-sponsored family planning.[88] Conservative politicians publicized inflated statistics of the women actually affected by the abuses and claimed that all women who were sterilized during this time period were victims. Some public figures used the scandal to undermine President Fujimori and to discredit surgical sterilization as a viable contraceptive option for women.[89] International media reported the inflated figures offered by the conservatives; one BBC article claimed that over 320,000 women were forced to be sterilized, when, in fact, only 773 people filed complaints with the Defensoría del Pueblo and the official investigation confirmed 300 cases of abuse.[90] The conservatives' use of a scandal that was originally highlighted by the women's movement threw feminist activists on the defensive; rather than focusing the controversy on women's right to resist sterilization, many groups have emphasized the legitimacy of voluntary sterilization as one of many contraceptive options. Dr. Daniel Aspilcueta, of Inppares, elaborates,

> It's true that there were abuses, but according to the most serious investigations, conducted by the Defensoría del Pueblo, they say there were not more than 300 cases [out of 300,000 sterilizations]. . . . It's certain that there were abuses, but they comprised less than 1 percent of the total program. So I ask people, "If I have a program, and 99 percent of the programs works, and 1 percent of the program doesn't work, is it a bad program?" With this, I would say that it is not an excellent program, it is not without flaws, but that does not mean we should get rid of it. The conservative sectors are taking advantage of this situation to oppose all methods of family planning.[91]

Feminist activists insist that, while surgical sterilization is a method with high potential for abuse, the solution is not to outlaw sterilization but to work toward informed consent. Susana Chávez relates, "Right now, there are sixty women in Piura who are demanding sterilization, and they have been refused this service for over a year—that is equally abusive."[92]

The sterilization abuse scandal in Peru, which garnered international press coverage, revealed the extent to which blatantly coercive population control policies still exist in parts of the world, regardless of the politically correct rhetoric about women's empowerment and reproductive health that has become popular since the ICPD in Cairo.

HIV/AIDS in Peru

HIV/AIDS, in the words of one women's health activist, is an epidemic "waiting to explode" in Peru.[93] Despite relatively high awareness of the disease, many respondents felt that Peruvians do not yet take the epidemic seriously and do not adequately protect themselves. Adolescents are particularly resistant to using condoms, as mentioned above, and condom use among married couples strongly implies infidelity and lack of trust or love in the minds of most Peruvians.[94] Although the size of Peru's HIV/AIDS epidemic is minuscule in comparison to the two African countries highlighted in this book, the number of people infected is nonetheless growing, and researchers have noticed "feminization" of the epidemic. Ten years ago, only one out of every fifteen HIV-positive people was a woman, but today women account for one out of three people living with HIV/AIDS.[95] Many HIV-positive women are married and believed they were safe from the disease because they are monogamous, not having known about their husbands' infidelity.

As the epidemic spreads and more Peruvians live with the disease, the Ministry of Health will be forced to revise its HIV services. Currently, treatment for any STI is provided free of cost, but HIV/AIDS treatment is deemed too expensive to offer for free.[96] Given the high poverty rate in the country, few HIV-positive patients can afford to pay for such crucial medication as antiretrovirals. Peru's fight against HIV/AIDS has far to go in terms of public education, accessibility of condoms and HIV tests, and life-skills training for men and women alike.

The Peruvian Feminist Movement

Though Peru's feminist movement gained strength since the 1970s, it remains overly centralized in Lima and is chiefly comprised of middle- and upper-class women. Tammy Quintanilla explains the challenges of feminist organizing in rural areas, "We do have feminist organizations in the districts—many of which don't recognize themselves as feminists—so yes, they exist, but they are few because there are such financial difficulties. They don't have the resources to live, to eat."[97] Women who must spend all their energy trying to survive have little time for formal feminist activism—a fact that contributes to the rather fragmented nature of the movement.

Most respondents were quick to agree that Peru has made many advances "thanks to the force of the feminist movement," though some believe women's rights activists alienated many people with their confrontational tactics in the beginning of the movement.[98] Dr. Miguel Gutiérrez criticizes the movement for using placards that read "Abortion is a right!" He explains: "The message that comes across is one of proabortion."[99] Instead, women's rights activists could emphasize "Yes to sex education! Yes to access to contraceptives! Yes to preventing women's deaths!" Considering the level of conservatism in Peru, the latter message may be better received. The backlash to Peru's feminist movement has been strong, and feminist organizations have had to respond to accusations of being radical and alienating. Miguel Ramos and Susana Chávez both praise the movement's increasing willingness and ability to form alliances with nonfeminist organizations working in a broad range of fields, such as public health, democracy, and human rights. Such coalitions bring greater visibility and legitimacy to the feminist movement.

Men's Involvement in Reproductive Rights

A quick survey of the reproductive rights movement in Peru reveals a predictable fact: Most of the actors are women. With men often making the decisions that affect women's reproductive health, the movement must find a way to better incorporate men in their efforts. First of all, as sociologist Miguel Ramos points out, there must be an effort not to discuss men in a purely negative light. "We need to view men not as obstacles to our objectives, but as partners in this work, as coparticipants, but not only as a means, not as objects. We need to recognize that men suffer, too, that they have fear and they need support."[100] Men, too, receive very little sex education, and at the same time deal with tremendous pressure from other men and their communities to adhere to societal norms of masculinity. Ramos continues, "The power of men is a contradictory power—there is authority, there are privileges, but we also see that this power comes with pains of very strong pressure to perform. We [as a society] should be saying, 'Look at what we are missing out by forcing men to act this way.' "[101]

Some organizations have chosen to work only with women, or only with children, in their reproductive health projects, yet, at the end of the day, most women and children go home to men who have disproportionate decision-making power and have not benefited from the education and sensitization of the development projects. Movimiento Manuela Ramos is one of the few organizations that have begun working with men, particularly in their adolescent program and through a women's health project called ReproSalud. In the latter program, the women participants themselves requested that their husbands be included. "They felt that [incorporation of men] was crucial for changes to be implemented in their own homes."[102] Prior to that, women were learning about domestic violence, but their husbands, including the abusive ones, were not.

How to get more men involved is a challenging question. Tammy Quintanilla of Movimiento El Pozo insists that the concept of what it means to be a man needs to change in Peruvian society. Today, there are a few men who understand this, and, Quintanilla believes, the feminist movement needs to identify these men and hold them up as leaders. "If there are no men in this movement, we cannot get far," she insists.[103]

Influence of the ICPD on Peru

In the words of one Peruvian women's health activist, the International Conference on Population and Development (ICPD) in Cairo was "one of the most important events of the last century."[104] The Peruvian government signed onto the Program of Action, and "it became a platform, a norm, which we could refer to when we were working for reproductive rights. Cairo clearly spelled out demands for the government, and this helped."[105] Before the conference in Cairo, topics like adolescent health and men's involvement in reproductive health received very little attention, and the government continued its focus on demographic targets. The conference in Cairo has changed that to some degree. An early draft of the 1998–2002 national population plan detailed the goal of reducing Peru's fertility rate to 2.5 children per woman, but, in the final version, the goal was to reach a "total fertility rate compatible with individual reproductive intentions."[106] The 1998 policy also explicitly states, "[R]eproductive health programmes should provide the widest array of services possible, without any type of coercion."[107]

Throughout the 1990s, President Fujimori's administration placed great emphasis on fertility reduction as a means of dealing with the problem of poverty.[108] While this population control focus led to abusive policies, as outlined above, it also served to create a favorable environment for realizing the goals set in Cairo and paved the way for feminists advocating better access to contraception.[109] With Fujimori's agenda, activists note that there was great change, with more family planning services and information available, "but the focus was always on converting people to a program in which the system imposed contraception on women."[110] Still, reproductive rights activists witnessed a mix of gains and setbacks under Fujimori; with Toledo's current government, gains are hardly visible.

Influence of International Politics

One of the contributing reasons for Peru's feminist movement remaining diffused and fragmented is the political situation thousands of miles away, in the United States. As in other developing countries, reproductive rights activists contend with the Mexico City policy, or Global Gag Rule, which prohibits organizations that receive U.S. funding from working on the issue of abortion. The policy effectively divides any feminist movement into two camps: those who continue accepting U.S. funds and those who do not. Miguel Ramos wonders

> how these organizations are working, like Manuela Ramos, since they receive a ton of money from USAID. How are they continuing their work? If they are working for women's rights, working to decrease

maternal mortality, and abortion is a crucial issue, how can they be silent about it? I don't know. This is a tremendous problem, that [the United States is] attaching such conditions to their aid.[111]

In the case of the feminist organization Movimiento Manuela Ramos, Bush's reinstatement of the Global Gag Rule sparked a fierce internal debate about whether or not the organization should continue accepting USAID funds. They were in the midst of various nonabortion related projects and did not want to abandon those communities before fulfilling their service commitments. Rocío Gutiérrez of Manuela Ramos explains, "This would compromise the health of many people. We already had contracts in many communities and we couldn't just break off." Yet deciding to continue as a USAID-funded organization has meant completely deserting their work on abortion. "Before the rule [. . .] we were one of the most active organizations working to decriminalize abortion in Peru."[112] The political beliefs of conservatives in the United States have effectively damaged the reproductive rights movement in Peru (and other developing countries that so heavily depend on U.S. funding).

Beyond the impact that the Global Gag Rule has on individual organizations, the policy splits the women's movement between those organizations that accept USAID funding and those that do not. Groups on both sides cannot form coalitions because of the gag rule. Tammy Quintanilla relates the struggle that CLADEM, a feminist organization, has experienced because they have refused USAID funds since the rule's inception in 1984. CLADEM's work has been far more difficult, given the scarcity of funding and their inability to collaborate with USAID-funded organizations.[113] Another major NGO working in the field of reproductive rights is Pathfinder International, which is based in the United States and carries out extensive postabortion care in Peru. As Dr. Miguel Gutiérrez reports, Pathfinder is unable to collaborate with local organizations that receive USAID funding and thus misses out on opportunities for the cooperation and mutual learning that come with working in coalitions.[114]

Aside from the specific consequences of the Global Gag Rule, the politics and desires of donor countries affect Peru's reproductive rights movement in a more general way. Despite the abandonment of population control terminology in the international discourse on reproductive health, many aid recipients still believe that donors are motivated by fears of overpopulation. Miguel Ramos, one of the few people researching men and reproductive rights, is concerned that funding for such research will disappear once Peru's fertility rate levels off and donors lose interest in the country. He cites Mexico as an example;

once the country successfully lowered its fertility rates and improved socio-economic indicators, the availability of donor funds shrunk rapidly.[115]

Other aid workers are afraid that, with fertility levels plummeting among certain sectors of the population (specifically, the urban, educated, privileged populations), national figures will mask the disparities within the country. Dr. Daniel Aspilcueta spells out,

> There is definitely still the need for [reproductive health work]. They look at the indicators and don't realize that those are just averages. The example I always use is that if you have one person who eats nothing, and another who eats half a chicken, their average is one-quarter of a chicken. One eats nothing, the other eats a lot, but their average isn't too bad. This is what's happening here—the fertility has decreased, contraceptive prevalence has increased, but there are sectors where fertility is still very high and contraception use is very low. They don't have access to their rights, to control their bodies and their lives.[116]

Although Peru's current fertility rate stands at only 2.9—a number that donors do not consider to be disastrous—a substantial portion of the population still lacks access to reproductive health services or the means by which they can control their fertility.[117]

Setbacks and Gains: A Look to the Future

Despite gains made after the ICPD in Cairo and the Fourth World Conference on Women in Beijing, Peruvian activists see a general slowing of their progress as the country experiences a conservative shift. As in the United States, reproductive health policies in Peru are intrinsically linked to presidential politics. Peru's 1993 constitution requires the state to be the primary health care provider in the country, and, as Rossina Guerrero points out, "In countries like ours where the state institutions assume management of health care, it's dangerous because the politics change and don't necessarily hold these areas as priority areas."[118] Meaningful advances on any reproductive rights front, like changing the abortion law, seem unlikely in the near future in Peru. Rocío Gutiérrez of Movimiento Manuela Ramos laments, "I don't think that in any other epoch we have had such a well-organized and powerful conservative sector."[119] Rather than pouring limited resources into the fight for decriminalizing abortion, many feminist groups are strategically focusing their attention on other equally crucial and more feasible goals. "We can fight more strongly for access to family planning services, the guarantee of the government to provide it, contraception for teenagers, emergency contraception," Gutiérrez observes.[120] Such work lays a solid foundation upon which other, more controversial gains may be made in the future.

Despite the sizable setbacks to their work and the glacial pace of advancement, reproductive rights activists seem to be optimistic overall. Traditionally, sexual rights, reproductive health, and women's rights in general were ignored; today, far more people are aware of grave problems like domestic violence, rape, sex trafficking, and clandestine abortion.[121] Rossina Guerrero adds, "We think that we have succeeded in getting abortion in the public consciousness in the past few years [. . .] and other groups that have never been talking about abortion are now denouncing the criminalization of abortion."[122] Public debate about the topic is the first step toward decriminalization.

Many respondents mentioned the need to sensitize the Peruvian population about their own rights, which politicians have historically neglected. "We have a history in which authoritarianism, circumstances of colonialism, discrimination, the politics of the governments that we have had—all this has generated a population that does not want to demand their rights."[123] Many Peruvians are accustomed to the presence of dictators, the use of a strong hand, and this is reflected in their interpersonal relationships as well, believes sociologist Miguel Ramos.[124] As Dr. Daniel Aspilcueta articulates,

> I think the topic of rights is incredibly important, and I think that the topic of rights starts with awareness of those rights, and demanding the exercise of those rights. This is a slow struggle, but it has to do with the perspective of liberty, of freedom, of making free, informed choices. When we accept these responsibilities that come with rights, when the government assumes responsibility for upholding these rights, then we will come to a better way of living. And what looks like a long path will not be so difficult.

Peruvian press coverage of international conferences highlighting human rights as well as local Peruvian stories of abuses have elevated the general awareness of human rights among the population, though much work in this regard remains to be done.

Conclusion

As in many Latin American countries, the challenges women in Peru face in exercising their reproductive rights are numerous and complex. Denied adequate sex education and access to a range of contraceptives, refused the right to legal and safe abortions, forced to undergo sterilization, Peruvian women have experienced a wide range of abuses of their reproductive rights. Larger economic, political, and social structures reinforce their subordinate position and weak decision-making power. Peruvians are currently coping with one of the most conservative governments in their recent history, but still society continues to slowly evolve in a positive direction. Public consciousness of women's rights seems to be improving, however slowly, and the feminist movement is slowly gaining ground.

4

Denmark

Background

Crouched on the peninsula of Jutland and seventy-eight islands in Northern Europe, the 5.4 million inhabitants of Denmark take great pride in their culture. This pride comes out strongly when discussing reproductive health and rights. Considered by many to be one of the most socially progressive countries in the world, Denmark does indeed boast a long history of advances in women's reproductive freedom. The government's interest in ensuring adequate reproductive health for women extends beyond its national borders; Denmark is one of the major donors to reproductive health programs worldwide as well.

In spite of well-deserved recognition for progress made, Danish activists point out areas in which society falls short of supporting full reproductive rights for its population. With an increasing (though still small) immigrant population, the need for wide-scale reproductive health programs has become even more pressing. The National Board of Health has stepped up sexual and reproductive health programs for immigrants, but the xenophobic tendencies of the current government hinder efforts to more fully support immigrants. Sexual education and resources for young people are still not wholly adequate, particularly in rural areas of the country. Women in Denmark may find their ability to make independent fertility-related decisions limited in an opposite way from what is seen in most other countries; women in certain circumstances may face societal expectations to have an abortion. As in other countries examined in this book, one finds activists in Denmark striving for a more just society, in which realization of one's reproductive rights is the norm for all women.

Fertility in Denmark

With an average of 1.7 children per woman, Denmark has one of the lowest fertility rates in the world.[1] Denmark's low fertility goes back decades; by 1933, the country was already at replacement level—2.1 children per woman.[2] Over the years, the government gradually adopted policies that prioritized the well-being of children, such as extended maternal and paternal leave, "which indirectly may have an effect on fertility if parents-to-be find life with children an attractive alternative."[3] Fertility began noticeably dropping in the 1960s as more educational and professional opportunities opened up for women. After an increase in the 1980s, fertility stabilized in the 1990s at its present rate.[4] Lisbeth B. Knudsen, a sociologist and demographer, is quick to point out that the declining fertility rates were coupled with declining abortion rates; in other words, the number of pregnancies dropped, not just the number of births.[5] Unlike in most countries, the Danish government has not heavily influenced fertility rates in one direction or the other. A group of scholars comparing family planning in the United States and Denmark concluded in 1990 that "Danish policy on reproduction and family planning has evolved on the basis of adapting legislation to the perceived needs of the population without promoting either growth or reduction. If there is a central focus, it is on the prevention of unwanted pregnancies and on the provision of accessible contraceptive services to all residents regardless of age or income."[6] Denmark does have one of the highest fertility rates of the Nordic countries, however—a point which people in the field attribute to Denmark's profamily policies, such as providing ample parental leave and affordable childcare.

Women in Denmark are generally expected to have professional careers and to be "active" outside the home.[7] Contrary to the reality in most countries of the world, a woman's decision to not have children is more or less socially acceptable, though Knudsen observes, "there are some female politicians with no children, and when they came out ten years ago and said why they have chosen not to have children, they had to also say how much they love children."[8] Family and friends may still pressure some women into having children, though this is slowly changing.

Danish reproductive health workers are proud of what they call "the Scandinavian way," referring to "a high degree of openness concerning sexual matters," manifested in compulsory sex education at an early age and easily accessible contraception.[9] As a report released by the Danish Family Planning Association (DFPA) details, "being a secular country, religious and conservative norms and values have no vital importance and influence on people's sexual behavior [. . .]. People's right to sexual self-determination is widely recognized, [and] imposition of shame or guilt in relation to sexual behavior [. . .] is rare."[10] The Danish approach to sex is generally pragmatic rather than moralistic. Sexuality is seen as a natural component of a healthy life and can be openly discussed in the media.[11] An example of Danes' view of a healthy sex life as a right may be found in their attention to assisting mentally and physically disabled people to this end. In some institutions for the disabled, staff members teach residents how to masturbate and provide them with sex aids. A few places even provide "surrogate sex partners," who are trained nurses.[12]

Asked if her culture has a liberal view towards sex, Lisbeth B. Knudsen answers, "Yes, yes, it's *Denmark*! And that's also why we say it's easy to talk about these things."[13] She points to the sex education children receive early in school as an example of this willingness to discuss sexual matters. Helle Samuelsen, an anthropologist at the Institute of Public Health, is more hesitant in her response: "I think that Denmark is often described as a country where sexuality is an open, almost a public issue, and to some extent it's correct but to [another] extent [. . .] it is an issue which is as private to us as to anyone else. So some issues can be discussed publicly, but when you talk about individual sexuality and so forth I think we are as restricted as anybody else."[14] Although Danes may be reserved in discussing their private lives, aspects of sexuality are present in public discourse to a much greater degree than in most countries.

Samuelsen believes that Denmark's secular nature may account for some of the culture's openness towards sexuality. "The majority of the Danish population [is] Protestant, but we are not practicing religion as you see in many Southern European countries or in the States. There are few people who go to church regularly." Another contributing factor may be the strong social support system in Denmark, in which public discussion about issues pertaining to social welfare, such as abortion, is common. For whatever combination of reasons, Danes do not shy away from discussions about sexual health, and this is perhaps most evident in their impressive sex education curricula.

Sex Education

Denmark has one of the lowest teen pregnancy rates in the world, undoubtedly attributable in part to the fact that sex education has been compulsory since 1970. A second law, the Public Health Act of 1975, requires age-appropriate sex education to be integrated in the schools by the third grade (age nine).[15]

There has never been a government-funded "abstinence-only" program targeting teenagers, as is found in the United States, and religious beliefs play a minor role in the formation of sex education policy.[16] Several factors contribute to Denmark's ability to foster a well-educated populace. Both the compactness of the country and its relatively small population facilitate dissemination of reproductive health information. The fact that Denmark is quite ethnically homogenous, with only a very small minority of non-Nordic immigrants, also makes information dissemination easier, because of both the ease of working in one language and the cultural acceptance in Nordic societies of discussing reproductive health matters. Again, the culture's open attitude toward sexuality creates an environment in which sex education is a normal component of the curriculum. It is generally expected that young people will be sexually active, and the legal age for sex is only fifteen.

However, despite the country's overall progressive attitude toward sexuality, the education that students receive does not always live up to the expressed values of society. Current legislation about sex education does not spell out how many hours of sex education are required or how extensive it should be. The education that students receive varies drastically from school to school, open to the interpretation of the individual teacher, who may not consider it a high priority.[17] Even though most students learn factual information about pregnancy, contraception, abortion, and sexually transmitted infections (STIs), they infrequently learn about the psychological aspects of relationships or discuss body image and other sexual health issues pertinent to teenagers.[18] The Danish Family Planning Association (DFPA) has recently started a program to "teach the teachers" about sex education in an effort to broaden and nationally systematize the sex education curriculum.[19]

In the meantime, the DFPA has implemented a program to help fill the gap; seventh through tenth graders come to their contraceptive clinic and listen to hour-long talks on sexuality and contraception. The clinic staff decided to specifically train young adults to be teachers, after finding that the age gap between doctors or nurses and students was too great for the teenagers to feel comfortable asking questions. The students' regular teachers are asked to leave for the duration of the lesson, "so our teachers are alone with the schoolchildren and it creates a totally different atmosphere," says Dr. Charlotte Wilken-Jensen, an obstetrician and head of DFPA's contraceptive clinic. Providing the sex education talks in a neutral environment by a third party seems to make the experience less awkward for everyone involved.

Few parents are resistant to their children visiting the clinic; most who do protest are among the immigrant population. Many immigrant children who come to the sex education talks do not participate as much as their Danish counterparts. These are the children that the teachers especially try to reach, particularly knowing that women of non-Danish ethnicity have higher abortion rates than Danish women.[20] Dr. Wilken-Jensen points out, "One piece of information that they always get is that the clinic is here, and that they are very welcome to come here."[21] By introducing teenagers not only to concepts in sex education but to the contraceptive clinic itself, the hope is that they will be more likely to visit the clinic when they become sexually active. This approach likely contributes to Denmark's high contraceptive prevalence among teenagers.

Access to Contraception

Along with the other Nordic countries, Denmark is famous for its excellent national health care system, which provides most health services free of charge to any resident. Eighty-five percent of the health care system is financed by taxes, making health care quite affordable for nearly the entire population.[22] Access to reproductive health services is impressive in scope and available through the primary health care system. A 1984 law mandates the availability of free contraceptive counseling to all citizens and residents, including minors, unmarried women, and women declared incapable of managing their own affairs without the consent of a guardian.[23] When speaking about public health issues in Denmark, the concept of "underserved" groups does not carry much weight, since everyone is covered under the national insurance plan and services are very accessible. Instead, attention is paid to "high-risk" groups, who are more likely to experience an unwanted pregnancy or a sexually transmitted infection (STI).[24] The DFPA has a clinic in Copenhagen targeting "high-risk" groups, such as prostitutes, the homeless, ethnic minorities, and teenagers. Services at the clinic are free, though there is a small charge for contraception. Efforts are underway to translate health materials into different languages for minorities, though funding for this is difficult to procure.[25]

Overall, contraceptive use in Denmark is very high; 78 percent of sexually active women currently use contraception.[26] Even among teenagers, contraceptive prevalence is impressive. A study of six hundred young men and women in rural Jutland (one of the most conservative parts of Denmark) found that 80 percent used contraception the first time they had sex. Another study of fifteen-year-olds elsewhere in the country came up with the same number.[27] Under Danish law, parents do not have to be notified when minors (under eighteen) obtain contraception, unlike other prescriptions or medical treatments.[28] Lisbeth B. Knudsen notes that the ease with which young people can get contraceptives "makes it easier to avoid an unwanted pregnancy—you can buy the condoms in the shops or go into the supermarkets and find them by where you pay—it's quite easy."

The Pill remains the most common contraceptive method used by women of all ages, with 26 percent of women using it, and some activists criticize general practitioners for not discussing the full range of contraceptive options with their patients.[29] Sterilization is not uncommon, at a prevalence of 5 percent, and, since 1974, more men have sought sterilization than women—the reverse of what is most often found in other countries.[30] Both the IUD and the diaphragm have fallen out of popular use in recent years, though the use of condoms has increased, largely due to the HIV/AIDS epidemic. During the 1980s, aggressive public education campaigns about HIV/AIDS were successful in raising awareness about the importance of faithful relationships and safe sex, yet the urgency of HIV/AIDS has since dissipated and condom use seems to have stabilized around 22 percent.[31] Lisbeth B. Knudsen explains that marketing campaigns have advocated condom use especially for relations with unknown partners; some Danes associate condoms with one-night stands rather than stable relationships. "Some people called it 'double Danish'—that you have the Pill against pregnancy and then the condom for STDs, because the condom has never been fully accepted as protecting against pregnancy."

The cost of contraception in general may present an obstacle to a portion of the Danish population, though it is affordable for the majority. At the DFPA clinic, a patient can receive three months' worth of pills for free, and after that a prescription costs about US$7.50 per month.[32] An IUD costs US$25 and may be used continuously for up to ten years. Though seemingly inexpensive for an industrialized country, these costs may discourage the poor, many of whom are recent immigrants, from seeking contraceptive services. Emergency contraception (EC), or the Morning-After Pill, has been available over the counter from pharmacists since 2001, though knowledge of the drug among the general population remains low.[33] EC is easily accessible through a general practitioner, and it is provided at a relatively low cost. Women have to pay out of pocket for both contraception and the Morning-After Pill in Denmark, but abortions are provided free of cost.[34]

Though young women's use of contraception without their parents' knowledge is not uncommon, decisions about contraceptive use seem to be made jointly by couples; women rarely use contraception without their partners' knowledge, as is seen in many other countries.[35] Helle Samuelsen ventures, "compared to many other countries, women in Denmark have a strong say in what to use and what not to use." Especially in stable, long-term relationships, people usually have an open discussion about which contraceptive to use and for how long.

Several factors in Denmark's society—from compulsory sex education at a young age, to easy access to contraception, to an expectation that sexual matters be discussed openly—contribute to the country's low rate of unwanted pregnancies and abortion. Since Denmark is doing fairly well in its coverage of sex education and contraception, reproductive rights activists pour much of their efforts into the issue of abortion. To fully understand the current situation in regard to abortion, a look to the country's history is helpful.

Abortion in Denmark in the Twentieth Century

Denmark has a long history of liberal abortion laws; as early as the 1920s, a handful of Danish activists were discussing the possibility of legalizing abortion.[36] In 1930, a change to the penal code made the prison sentence for an illegal abortion only two years, down from the eight-year penalty outlined in an 1866 law. During the 1920s and 1930s throughout Europe and North America, reproductive health and population issues were gaining attention in the political sphere, and a trend toward governmental involvement emerged. Issues like abortion and contraception came to be viewed as political issues that required a political response. Historian Sniff Nexoe wonders if the eventual loosening of Denmark's abortion law was less about sexual liberation and more about government control.

Despite the illegality of abortion, the practice was very common in the early 1900s. "If you wanted an abortion, you could get one. They were available—people ask[ed] around, girlfriends, family, if they had an interest in getting an abortion. But it took money and it took [. . .] determination."[37] Illegal abortion carried with it a heavy social stigma and the connotation of sexual recklessness or promiscuity, even though it was common among married women.[38] The illegal abortion industry thrived, with the majority of abortions being performed in the first trimester by qualified physicians. A study of abortions from 1952, in fact, found that the complication rate from illegal abortions was even lower than that for legal abortions.[39]

In the face of a well-established illegal abortion industry, police seldom prosecuted women for the crime. "In the beginning it was very difficult to prosecute women because it was a kind of crime which would be heard in front of a jury, and the jury had a tendency to acquit these women, even though they had actually admitted their guilt."[40] Lawyers viewed these acquittals as a threat to the penal system as a whole, since women were proven guilty of a crime and still escaped punishment. Considering that there were an estimated one thousand to twenty thousand illegal abortions a year during this time period, very few women actually went to prison.[41]

In 1932, the government created a nineteen-member commission of physicians, lawyers, politicians, and a nurse to look into the issue of abortion.[42] Lau Esbensen explains, "The formal argument to make the commission [. . .] was that the law that was already there didn't seem to work. For some reason, there seems to have been an enormous awareness that there were a lot of illegal abortions, and the number was rising."[43] The resulting commission recommended that abortion be made legal in four cases: medical indication (to protect the woman's health or life), ethical indication (in cases of rape or incest), eugenic indication (fearing fetal abnormalities), and social indication (when having a baby would be a social or economic burden on the mother). When the final law came into effect in 1939, it only included the first three scenarios, though the medical indication could loosely apply to conditions like depression and stress, thereby partly introducing a social indication. This was the first piece of abortion legislation in Denmark that was separate from the penal code.[44]

The 1939 law acknowledged abortion's legitimacy in some situations and shifted the dialogue about abortion from a judicial framework to a medical one, now associated with hospitals and doctors.[45] This rethinking, along with pressure to introduce a social indication, led the way to a series of new abortion laws, each more liberal than the last, in 1956, 1970, and 1973. The 1970 law opened legal abortion up to women who were over thirty-eight years old or who already had four children.[46] As political pressure to drop the abortion ban mounted, the most logical argument made was that 90 percent of women who applied for an abortion received one. "So it was a practical argument—if they are going to get it anyway, why don't we [legalize it]?"[47] In 1973, the same year that the U.S. Supreme Court decided *Roe v. Wade,* the Danish government passed its most liberal abortion law to date. This law allows for abortion on demand up to the twelfth week of the pregnancy. Women who are later than twelve weeks must submit an application to a panel (comprised of a gynecologist, a psychologist, and a social worker) to obtain permission on medical, ethical, eugenic, or social grounds.[48] The law does not specify an upper gestational limit to abortions, though in practice it ranges from eighteen to twenty-four weeks.[49] Thirty-some years later, this law remains in effect with only minor changes.

Present-Day Access to Abortion in Denmark

Denmark's present-day abortion rate is one of the lowest in the world, at around 13 per 1,000 women per year (compared to 84 per 1,000 women in Vietnam).[50] Abortion is easily accessible via a general practitioner and is usually carried out in a hospital under general anesthesia as an outpatient procedure and free of charge.[51] Compared to most countries in the world, Danish women seeking an abortion face very few logistical obstacles, which is partly evidenced by the fact that 97 percent of abortions in Denmark take place during the first trimester.[52]

Access to abortion is most difficult for minors and for women in their second trimester. Although it is legal to have sex at the age of fifteen in Denmark, the 1973 law specifies that women under eighteen require parental consent to obtain an abortion. A minor who does not wish to inform her parents may appeal to the same council that reviews cases from women in their second trimester, but rarely will her request for a waiver be granted. Dr. Charlotte Wilken-Jensen points out that young patients are better off when their parents know about the abortion and are able to support them. Most pregnant minors willingly tell their parents, and parental consent exemptions are only made in extreme circumstances. Dr. Wilken-Jensen relates the story of a young immigrant woman in Sweden who was recently killed for becoming pregnant outside of wedlock. "There's sometimes some risk that we don't—you know, [with] our tradition, we have a hard time understanding—that makes it necessary to give the permission without the parents. The council does that."[53] Most minors of Danish descent, however, would be denied the parental consent exemption, according to Dr. Wilken-Jensen, who sits on one of the councils.

Women further than twelve weeks into their pregnancy must go through a similar process to obtain permission for their abortions. The majority of women who obtain abortions in the second trimester have received a positive fetal diagnosis (of Down's syndrome or spina bifida, for example)—a circumstance in which the council always grants permission.[54] Dr. Wilken-Jensen elaborates, "Then there could be social reasons, and they should be real heavy social reasons. The further you are in the pregnancy, the [heavier] the indications should be. For the social reasons, we never go beyond eighteen weeks—it's not stated anywhere, but that's the practice." The restrictions on second-trimester abortions do not affect many people, however; fewer than five hundred abortions over twelve weeks are done each year in Denmark.[55]

For the past few years, women who have abortions early in their pregnancy have another option available to them; about one-third of abortions done today in Denmark are medical, rather than surgical, and that percentage is grow-ing.[56]* Medical abortions quickly became available after the procedure's introduction to the country, with nearly every hospital offering them today.[57] The majority of women who arrive at a clinic for an abortion are early enough in their pregnancy to do a medical abortion, despite the scheduling delays sometimes encountered.[58] Presently, most women undergoing medical abortions are required to remain in the hospital for the few hours it takes to miscarry, though some hospitals allow women to miscarry at home. Women who undergo a medical abortion at home rarely have complications. Dr. Wilken-Jensen predicts that someday, when the medical community is more comfortable with the procedure, all women will be offered the chance to go home. Such an option would drastically reduce the cost of the procedure to the state as well.[59] The number of complications and the chance of requiring a surgical evacuation of the uterus after a medical abortion is actually less than with surgical abortions, according to a recent study done in Copenhagen.[60]

One factor that often limits women's access to abortion in other countries—the shortage of doctors trained or willing to do the procedure—is not an obstacle in Denmark. Though doctors and nurses are not required by law to participate in abortions, they are required to at least refer patients to another provider, and each hospital is required to provide abortions.[61] When asked if abortion training is part of medical school, Lisbeth B. Knudsen answers, "Yes, of course"—a response that few Americans in the field would offer. Dr. Wilken-Jensen reports that, during her career, she has come across only two or three doctors unwilling to provide abortions, and none of them has been a gynecologist. Danish women seeking abortions are fortunate in that they do not have to contend with an antichoice medical community.

Opposition to Abortion

Abortion, a controversial issue in any part of the world, remains sensitive in Denmark, but not very politicized. Opposition to abortion in Denmark is weak and disjointed. It was a right-wing government that passed the 1973 law to legalize abortion, though some religious groups did protest, including the newly formed Christian People's Party (Kristeligt Folkeparti, KRF). While the Christian People's Party is still active today (it is the only political party

---

* Surgical abortion refers to the procedure done by a physician using instruments and vacuum aspiration to empty a woman's uterus. Medical abortion, available very early in a pregnancy, refers to a combination of medications that a woman takes orally and/or vaginally to induce an abortion.

formally opposed to abortion), its members seem to have abandoned the idea of overturning the 1973 law. Instead, KRF members concentrate their efforts on decreasing the number of abortions that occur by improving access to contraception and sex education. KRF politicians have also submitted proposals to increase funding for governmental programs designed to decrease the number of abortions.[62] The KRF's political platform states, "Legislation should be based on life beginning at conception," but this is immediately followed by "The efforts to reduce the number of abortions should be strengthened."[63] Johan Seidenfaden of the Danish Family Planning Association reports that the Christian People's Party often collaborates with the DFPA on their sex education and contraception programs. The two groups may have different platforms, but their goals are the same. While antiabortion groups in many other countries, including the United States, work to limit sex education and access to contraception, the KRF has no moral objection to educating the population about sexual matters or preventing unwanted pregnancies. They believe that abortion is morally wrong, but, perhaps recognizing that abortion has always taken place in society and most likely always will, they direct their energy into programs that will decrease the number of abortions.

Denmark's Right to Life is probably the most well-organized of the antiabortion groups. They have threatened to sue the government for making emergency contraception available without a prescription, though the lawsuit has not been filed to date.[64] As Sniff Nexoe explains, "[in Denmark] we do have this small antiabortionist movement as well, but it's very, very small and hasn't really got a loud voice in the debate—or there hasn't been any debate, that's actually the point!" The majority of Danes accept abortion as inevitable in society.

A few small antiabortion splinter groups have recently taken a turn toward the radical, by Danish standards, by calling abortion providers "baby-killers" and harassing the staff at the Danish Family Planning Association.[65] Dr. Wilken-Jensen, at Frederiksberg Hospital, has been targeted because her hospital is by far the largest abortion facility in Denmark, performing over eighteen hundred abortions per year (compared to five hundred by the second-largest abortion facility). "We receive ugly emails from the people who are against abortion, telling us all the terrible things that we should be subject[ed] to, threatening us: 'We know where you live, we know where you work.' And you get tough, but still, every time one comes in. . . . It's just recently—within the last year." To date, none of the antiabortion aggression has taken the form of physical violence like that witnessed in the United States.

The government has consistently supported the 1973 legislation in the decades since it was passed, and abortion is considered a public health or social issue instead of a political one. Sniff Nexoe mentions, "It's interesting because in Denmark it's really not a very controversial issue. Every now and then, you would meet a group of priests or something, making a small demonstration or speaking against abortion, but it's actually very rare." When asked whether abortion is ever a political issue during elections, Dr. Wilken-Jensen replies without hesitation, "No, never. It's part of life." Dr. Wilken-Jensen reports that surveys show 90 percent of the Danish population considers themselves prochoice.[66]

These strong prochoice beliefs do not always translate into complete acceptance of abortion, however. Danes highly support the legality of abortion, but do not always agree with abortion from an ethical point of view. Particularly with the advent of fetal diagnostics leading to selective abortions, as well as other new reproductive technologies, the debate over when life begins and other ethical issues persists.[67]

Social Stigma of Abortion

There is little social stigma surrounding abortion in Denmark compared to most countries. Facing an unwanted pregnancy, nevertheless, is always difficult; Helle Samuelsen remarks,

> Even though the access to abortion in Denmark is fairly easy compared to many other countries, the decision-making is still a hard choice for everyone. [. . .] I think that lots of people in Denmark are worried about the high level of abortion in Denmark, but it's not so much a political issue, it's more a social issue. People are worried about the social consequences and the consequences for the women themselves.[68]

Women undergoing abortions tend to blame themselves and feel poor self-esteem about the experience; abortion is a topic kept to oneself, a sort of private tragedy.[69] For this reason many activists would like the dialogue about abortion to include more discussion of the psychological or emotional side of the issue, rather than the purely legal.[70] Indeed, in recent years there does seem to be more frank talk of the emotions surrounding abortion, taking place, for example, in magazine articles that feature women's negative experiences with abortion. Lisbeth B. Knudsen speculates that even though most women feel they made the right decision, they feel free to discuss the aspects of abortion that were troubling to them because "it's the general opinion that the right to abortion will not be removed."[71] Some women feel able to express how difficult their abortions were, knowing that a strong opposition movement will not use their words against them to make abortion illegal.

Denmark's abortion rate is low compared to other countries, but it is regarded as high by many Danes considering the great degree of access to reproductive health information and contraception. Roughly one in five Danish women has had an abortion at some point in her life, though the abortion rate has recently been declining.[72] Religious arguments against abortion do not hold much weight in Denmark, but there is still some degree of social stigma surrounding abortion. "I think the kind of disapproval they would maybe meet would be, 'Why didn't you take more care?' But it's not the kind of disapproval saying, 'You're killing a life.' "[73] The stigma of abortion and unwanted pregnancy may be comparable to that of excessively drinking alcohol or using drugs, or other activities deemed irresponsible.

Societal Pressure to Have an Abortion

As some women getting abortions face a degree of social stigma, so too do women who decide *not* to have an abortion in certain circumstances. Danish women may find themselves pressured to have an abortion, particularly if they are young or receive a problematic fetal diagnosis. If a teenage girl gets pregnant, a standard reaction of her health provider may be to present abortion as the best choice for her. Sniff Nexoe points out, "This freedom to choose maybe is also a kind of an obligation to choose the right thing, which would be an abortion if you are a very young mother-to-be."[74] The source of pressure to have an abortion may be hard to pinpoint, as Nexoe notes, "Maybe it's not about one [single] person that is putting pressure [on her], but more the sense of what the right thing to do in society would be—if you are sixteen and pregnant, it's probably the best thing to choose an abortion." Dr. Wilken-Jensen describes teenage girls being thrown out of their homes for deciding to carry an unwanted pregnancy to term.[75] Women in this situation may also experience pressure from beyond their families and personal doctors. Lau Esbensen, a Ph.D. student at the University of Copenhagen's Center for Women and Gender Studies, explains, "There are many examples of women getting a very harsh response from the local authorities—they know that if these young women get their child, it will probably be quite expensive."[76]

Although the state will ensure that teenage mothers have a place to live and a way to continue their education—far more than what many governments do—there is little assistance for them beyond that.[77] Many teenage mothers heavily depend on the support of their families to cope. In some parts of the country, like Copenhagen, nonprofit organizations are starting to assist young mothers, but these centers are limited in their outreach and funding.[78] Only one-third of pregnant teenagers continue the pregnancy. [79]

Another scenario in which a woman may be expected to have an abortion is in the case of a positive fetal diagnosis, such as Down's syndrome. As fetal diagnostics become more readily available, the phenomenon of selective abortion increases. Women who receive a diagnosis for Down's syndrome during their pregnancy almost always choose to have an abortion; a 1986 study in southern Jutland found that nearly 90 percent of women in this situation terminated their pregnancies.[80] The local government in southern Jutland conducted a cost-analysis study, from which they concluded that encouraging amniocenteses for all pregnant women would be financially advantageous to the government, since the vast majority of women will choose abortion in the case of a fetal anomaly.[81] In 2002, an amendment to the 1973 abortion law added the requirement that women receive "supportive counseling" about their choice between abortion and delivery.[82] Dr. Wilken-Jensen is confident that pressure to have an abortion would not come from within the health care system. She believes the majority of doctors would give neutral advice, though they are guided by their knowledge of the implications of bringing up a disabled child. Pressure to have an abortion would come strongest from family and friends, and as Dr. Wilken-Jensen points outs, "You know, we don't have ten or eight children and say it's okay to have one or two that are not perfect— you get one or two children and you want them to be perfect."[83]

Lau Esbensen explains that there is very little debate about the ethical implications of selective abortions. Though some people would agree with Esbensen in calling the concept "ethically repulsive," a discussion about whether or not selective abortion is acceptable would undoubtedly turn to a discussion about abortion itself. Despite the prevalence of more frank discussions of abortion in recent years, some people still do not feel that the legal right to abortion is secure enough to open the debate up to potentially divisive topics. Esbensen argues that Danish society needs to open up to such a debate. He sees selective abortions as representative of a societal shift "from looking at the individual as irreplaceable, with some sort of eternal value [. . .] to seeing [people's] value as determined by their circumstances of life."[84] By assuming that a positive fetal diagnosis calls for an abortion, Danish society is essentially making a statement that disabled people are undesirable, that their existence should be prevented if possible. Esbensen, who is writing his thesis on this topic, believes that in this mindset, "You are not looking at a human being anymore; you are looking at a biological machine that is determined by [its] surroundings."[85] Though Esbensen raises valid ethical points, questioning abortion within an ethical framework inevitably spills over into a legal framework, which can be threatening to prochoice Danes.

The Reproductive Health of Immigrants and Ethnic Minorities in Denmark

Looking at reproductive rights in Denmark, one notices several areas that require ongoing attention, from designing a more uniform sex education curriculum nationwide to maintaining the low abortion rate. Meeting the reproductive health needs of a growing population of ethnic minority immigrants is perhaps the most pressing issue. In 1979, only 2 percent of the Danish population came from another country, compared to nearly 10 percent today (though some of those immigrants are from other Nordic countries).[86] Although abortion rates are declining faster among some ethnic minorities than among Danish women overall, non-Western women still generally have higher abortion rates than Danes.[87] Immigrant women from Iran, Vietnam, and Poland in particular experience more abortions than their Danish counterparts; Iranian teenagers, for example, have abortions at double the rate Danish teens do.[88] A study in Norway found that in a patient survey in which15 percent of the respondents were "non-Western," these women accounted for 25 percent of requests for induced abortion.[89] Minority women's access to health services in general is poorer, largely because of language barriers and their general marginalization in society. The Danish Family Planning Association is attempting to translate health materials into several foreign languages, including Turkish, Arabic, French, Spanish, and English, though funding for such projects is hard to secure, given the inability or unwillingness of the government to provide adequate resources for immigrant services. The DFPA also conducts trainings with doctors and health workers to offer counseling specifically for ethnic minorities.[90] The Danish government requires immigrants to take classes on Danish language and culture as part of their "integration," and the DFPA has been successful in visiting these classes and distributing information.[91]

Despite efforts of reproductive rights activists, however, immigrants remain a "high-risk" population and face a somewhat xenophobic environment in Denmark. The country's history is one of a largely homogenous population, with little racial or ethnic diversity. Adjusting to the influx of immigrants has not been a seamless process, as evidenced by the anti-immigration laws passed by the current right-wing government.

Setbacks and Gains: A Look to the Future

Partly in response to high abortion rates among ethnic minorities, the government passed an action plan in 1999 that included forty separate initiatives, all working to lower the abortion rate via increased access to information, counseling, and health services.[92] One way in which the DFPA is trying to coordinate sexual health information is through their new website, www.abortnet.dk, which is designed for both medical professionals and the public, though all the site's content is in Danish. Posted on the site is a combination of basic background information about abortion and contraception, as well as a database of new research and projects conducted throughout the country.[93] Efforts are also underway to provide abortion counselors with training in cultural competency so they may be better equipped to serve Denmark's ethnic minority population.[94]

One of the barriers to improving reproductive rights, even in a wealthy country like Denmark, is funding. The contraceptive clinic run by Dr. Wilken-Jensen through the DFPA nearly closed in 2001 due to a lack of funding from the municipality, but, as Johan Seidenfaden explains, "We managed to persuade them to continue and now we are obliged to focus mainly on what we call 'high-risk' groups."[95] Approximately 40 percent of DFPA's funding comes from the central government.[96] The financial barriers extend to individual people as well, who have a difficult time paying for their basic expenses in a country where the cost of living is so high.[97]

Finally, although many Danes are proud of their culture's openness to sexual matters, others are concerned that, in supporting the Danish liberal view of sex, people resist messages that focus on responsibility rather than freedom. As Lau Esbensen puts it, "We live in a society where people should express themselves freely, including their sexuality, and I'm all for that, but still you have to remind people that they should take their sexual lives seriously." In contrast to the United States, where it is often taboo to discuss sexuality and contraception openly, "in Denmark, we have reversed it, you could say, where it is considered moralizing to tell people they should take care of themselves. And that is another kind of taboo, which is just as destructive." Danish reproductive rights groups may best serve the population by continuing to emphasize a message of personal responsibility and safety, particularly considering the dangers attendant to sex, such as STIs and unwanted pregnancy.

Conclusion

With a relatively high level of sex education and contraceptive coverage, as well as widespread access to safe and legal abortion, Denmark deserves recognition for its respect for women's reproductive rights. Still, much work remains to be done to improve services for immigrant communities and to tackle complicated ethical questions that have come with new reproductive technologies. Lisbeth B. Knudsen points out that even if Denmark's sexual health indicators are impressive, commitment to these areas should not decline since there is always a new generation coming of age that needs the same degree of services and awareness. Denmark is in a unique position to provide an example for other countries by creating a society where women and men exercise their reproductive freedom openly. The extent to which this vision becomes reality will largely depend on the efforts of the reproductive rights movement.

5

United States of America

Background

In the country many consider to be the most powerful in the world, American citizens experience the highest poverty levels and largest gaps between rich and poor of any industrial country.[1] The educational and job opportunities, living standards, and health status of Americans are all heavily influenced by race, class, gender, and geographic location. Of the nearly three hundred million inhabitants of the United States, almost 20 percent live in poverty, according to a 1997 United Nations Development Program report, and that figure has been steadily increasing since the 1960s.[2] Poverty levels vary drastically by race; only 11.6 percent of whites live in poverty, while poverty rates for blacks and Latinos are 33.3 percent and 29.3 percent, respectively.[3] Though life expectancy in the country as a whole is 76.9 years, that figure plummets to 68.0 years for residents of the nation's capital, Washington, D.C., while black males in the District have a life expectancy of just 57.5 years.[4] Health indicators in the United States are far better than those in developing countries (the maternal mortality rate is just 9.9 deaths per 100,000 live births), but the United States ranks poorly in comparison to other developed countries.[5]

Throughout the 1990s, the fertility rate in the United States remained steady between 2.0 and 2.1 children per woman, just below replacement level.[6] Although the United States is a highly urbanized country, with just under 80 percent of the population living in urban areas, access to reproductive health care varies considerably depending on geographic location and socioeconomic level; sizable disparities persist.[7] Heavily shaped by the government's promotion of abstinence-only programs, the majority of sex education curricula throughout the country lack comprehensive information about contraception, abortion, and sexually transmitted infections (STIs). In general, contraception is widely available, though its high cost may deter some women from using it. Access to abortion is problematic for many women due to inadequate funding from the government and insurance companies, as well as a shortage of abortion providers. The United States' tumultuous history of racist reproductive health policies adds to the tension and sensitivity of the subject.

Troubling Roots: A Brief Look at the Politics of Race and Reproductive Health in the Twentieth Century

Given the United States' history of perpetrating genocide against American Indians, building the agricultural foundation of the country on the backs of African slaves, and numerous other abuses based on race, it is no surprise that, as Dorothy Roberts puts it, *"Reproductive politics in America inevitably involves racial politics."*[8] Medical professionals are not exempt from the country's history of racism; as early as the mid-1800s, Dr. J. Marion Sims, the "father of American gynecology," grew famous for his surgical discoveries that resulted from experiments on black female slaves using no anesthesia.[9] Roberts, a professor of law at Northwestern University, points out that black women's reproduction has continually been regulated to achieve social objectives in the United States. Examples are found as early as the antebellum period, with forced childbearing among slaves so their masters could make a larger profit. More recent welfare policies frame black women's reproduction as a cause of poverty and crime and therefore systematically attempt to reduce their fertility.[10]

The early movement for greater reproductive autonomy was also influenced by the racial politics of the time. Margaret Sanger, pioneer of reproductive rights, opened the first American contraceptive clinic in New York City in 1916.[11] Sanger spoke eloquently in terms of a woman's right to control how many children she has, but given the unpopularity of that message, many proponents of contraception instead framed their arguments in terms of controlling the fertility of minorities. In recent years, several racist quotes have been misattributed to Sanger, including that her aim was to "exterminate the Negro population."[12] Though Sanger did focus on low-income, minority, and immigrant populations, her motivation to help those women improve their lives through greater control over their fertility appears genuine. Sanger, in fact, was commended by W. E. B. DuBois, founder of the National Association for the Advancement of Colored People (NAACP), and by Martin Luther King Jr. as a passionate opponent of racism.[13] Sanger did support certain initiatives that most find objectionable today, such as incentives for the voluntary sterilization of people with disabling hereditary diseases and the tightening of immigration controls to limit the number of "diseased" and "feeble-minded" people entering the United States.[14] Sanger did not, however, subscribe to the racist views that the popular eugenics movement promoted at the time. In her work with the American Birth Control League (later renamed Planned Parenthood), Sanger attempted to establish the principle that a woman's right to control her fertility is a fundamental human right.[15]

Nevertheless, many vocal proponents of contraception in the early 1900s based their arguments on classist and racist principles of the eugenics movement, preying on whites' fears of "racial suicide" in order to enhance public acceptance of contraception. Angela Davis comments on contraception in the 1910s and 1920s: "What was demanded as a 'right' for the privileged came to be interpreted as a 'duty' for the poor."[16]

High-ranking politicians, including President Theodore Roosevelt, embraced the idea of eugenics and sought to implement their views through large-scale sterilization campaigns targeting "undesirables."[17] Forte and Judd note, "The USA became the first nation in the world to permit mass sterilization as part of an effort to 'purify the race.' By the mid-1930s, about 20,000 people had been sterilized against their will and twenty-one states had passed eugenic laws."[18] Between 1929 and 1941, the U.S. government carried out over seventy thousand involuntary sterilizations for eugenic purposes, mostly on epileptics, alcoholics, criminals, and the "feeble-minded."[19] The latter label was used not only to describe the mentally disabled but also to punish women for sexual "immorality." Some women who were deemed "promiscuous" and particularly those who became pregnant out of wedlock were institutionalized and sterilized during this time period.[20] The Nazis modeled their compulsory sterilization law on one enacted in California.[21] Since most of the sterilization policies only applied to state institutions, they disproportionately affected the poor.[22]

In addition to the poor, minority women were particularly vulnerable to compulsory sterilization programs. Even as late as the 1970s and early 1980s, minority women were victims of sterilization without informed consent. Teaching hospitals performed unnecessary hysterectomies, dubbed "Mississippi appendectomies," on poor black women[23] In 1972, a group of medical students at Boston City Hospital filed a complaint that doctors were performing unnecessary hysterectomies on black patients, and the director of obstetrics and gynecology at a New York municipal hospital stated, "In most major teaching hospitals in New York City, it is the unwritten policy to do elective hysterectomies on poor black and Puerto Rican women, with minimal indications, to train residents."[24] From 1970 to 1976, the Indian Health Service (IHS) sterilized one-quarter to one-half of all American Indian women aged fifteen to forty-four.[25] A study of American Indian sterilization discovered that some women struggling with alcoholism had complete hysterectomies, which doctors told them was "reversible."[26] In Montana, physicians performed tubal ligations on two fifteen-year-old girls during appendectomies, without the knowledge or consent of the girls or their parents.[27] The study also documents cases of doctors obtaining signed consent forms from women while they were under the influence of a sedative, on the same day as their delivery, or even the day *after* the tubal ligation.[28] One physician notes, "All the pureblood women of the Kaw tribe of Oklahoma have now been sterilized."[29] In 1976, Congress passed the Indian Health Care Improvement Act, which allows tribes to manage and control their own health care systems through the Indian Health Service (IHS); sterilization abuses apparently declined after many tribes took advantage of the act.[30]

The issue of sterilization divided the American reproductive rights movement along racial lines; while blacks wanted protection against abuses, whites were advocating for easier access to sterilization since in their experience it was difficult to find doctors willing to do the procedure.[31] In the 1970s, the American College of Obstetricians and Gynecologists (ACOG) recommended the "120-formula," meaning that if the woman's age multiplied by the number of children she already had equaled at least 120, she should be eligible for a tubal ligation. The woman still needed the endorsement of three doctors, including a psychiatrist, to actually obtain the surgery.[32] While white women encountered numerous obstacles to obtaining a tubal ligation, black women and other minorities experienced a number of coercive sterilization abuses. An organization of women of color called the Committee to End Sterilization Abuses recommended a series of guidelines, including informed consent in the preferred language of the patient, a thirty-day waiting period between counseling and the surgery, and refusal to accept a consent form signed during a woman's labor, immediately after a birth or abortion, or under threat of losing her welfare benefits. Planned Parenthood and NARAL, two prominent feminist organizations that were mostly white at the time, testified against these guidelines, but in 1978 the Department of Health, Education, and Welfare adopted most of them as mandatory for programs that provided sterilizations with federal funding.[33]

Examples of governmental institutions trying to dictate the fertility of poor women and minority women continues today; guiding such policies is the widespread belief that social problems are caused by reproduction and can be cured by population control.[34] Recent reports from welfare recipients, who are disproportionately black women, reveal that some are threatened with losing their benefits if they do not agree to sterilization; in South Carolina, one woman on welfare reported that her doctor refused to deliver her third child unless she agreed to a tubal ligation.[35] In some cases drug-addicted women have also been ordered by judges to be sterilized or to accept long-term, provider-controlled contraceptive methods, like Norplant or Depo Provera. Such court decisions violate women's right to make their own contraceptive decisions.

Sex Education

The United States has the highest teenage pregnancy rate of any developed country, though the rate is decreasing.[36] One million teenagers get pregnant each year in the United States, and 85 percent of those pregnancies are unintended.[37] By the age of twenty, 40 percent of American women have been pregnant (which is nine times higher than in the Netherlands).[38] About 35 percent of teenage pregnancies end in abortion.[39] Although teens in the United States are no more sexually active than adolescents in many other industrialized countries, they are less likely to use effective birth control and, even of those teens that do use birth control, one-third use it incorrectly.[40] The United States also holds the highest rate of sexually transmitted infections (STIs) among industrialized nations; one out of three people will have contracted at least one STI by the time they are twenty-four years old.[41] Although American youth are barraged with sexual messages from the mass media, they have little information about how to be sexually responsible or how to cope with an unwanted pregnancy.

The United States has a long history of "puritanical resistance" to recognizing sex as natural and healthy; many young people are sexually active but do not obtain contraception because they feel guilty about having sex in the first place.[42] Jane White, co-owner of an abortion clinic in Portland, Oregon, describes the "virginal standard: nice girls don't have sex." "We need girls to be able to say yes to sex—a choice, empowered. If it's a choice, she can prepare for sex."[43] Though it is widely believed in American culture that parents should be the ones to discuss sex with their children, studies report widespread discomfort and unwillingness among parents to do just that.[44] In the absence of national guidelines on sex education, curricula vary widely.[45] Only twenty states require sex education in schools, and of those, only ten require any information on contraception.[46] Less than 10 percent of American students receive comprehensive sex education that covers abortion, homosexuality, relationships, and STI prevention.[47]

Despite the high teen pregnancy rate, the government avidly promotes abstinence-only sex education, devoting $250 million to abstinence-only programs in 1996 alone.[48] A World Health Organization review of thirty-five sex education programs in the United States concluded that abstinence-only programs are less effective than comprehensive sex education programs.[49] Organizations that have published analyses supporting the effectiveness of comprehensive sex education include the American Academy of Pediatrics, the American Medical Association, the Centers for Disease Control, the Institute of Medicine, the Office of National AIDS Policy, the National Institutes of Health, the Society for Adolescent Medicine, and the Surgeon General of the United States.[50] Twenty-five studies have reported strong evidence that comprehensive sex education programs do not hasten the initiation of sex nor increase a teenager's average number of sexual partners.[51] Furthermore, teens who have received comprehensive sex education are significantly less likely to experience an STI or unwanted pregnancy.[52]

Despite the strong evidence in support of comprehensive sex education, both the national government and many state governments continue to push abstinence-only programs. In Mississippi, a law establishing abstinence-only sex education as the state's standard claims, "a mutually faithful, monogamous relationship in the context of marriage is the only appropriate setting for sexual intercourse."[53] Likewise, the Virginia legislature passed a bill (that the governor vetoed) requiring sex education programs to "present sexual abstinence before marriage and fidelity within monogamous marriage as moral obligations and not matters of personal opinion or personal choice."[54] Teachers in a North Carolina program in 1997 were instructed to only talk about contraception if students ask, and even then to emphasize failure rates. If asked about AIDS, teachers were supposed to tell students that it is only transmitted by IV drug use and "illegal homosexual acts."[55] Some abstinence-only materials incorrectly claim that condoms do not protect against sexually transmitted infections (STIs) and HIV/AIDS.[56] In one video used by some abstinence-only programs, a student asks, "What if I want to have sex before I get married?" The teacher responds, "Well, I guess you'll have to be prepared to die."[57]

Terry Daley of the Downtown Women's Center argues that sex education needs to happen "way before high school, before kids are sexually active," though U.S. society is generally not open to that approach.[58] She stresses that children "need to understand the awesome responsibilities of parenting" long before they become sexually active. In addition to the high number of unintended pregnancies among teens, Daley points out the substantial number of *intended* teenage pregnancies, "which are just as sad because these are young people who don't think they have any future except as parents." A study of Dominican women in New York concludes, "Especially where other means [besides childbearing] of claiming maturity are absent (work, education, home ownership, marriage, financial independence), motherhood seemed to become a rite of passage, a way to establish adulthood, offering something over which the respondents felt they were in control."[59] Roberts points out that teens may have babies because they have little incentive to avoid it; in the absence of clear educational and job opportunities, parenting may seem like the best option.[60]

Access to Health Services and Family Planning

Lacking a national health insurance program, the U.S. population relies on private practice office-based physicians, most of whom are specialists (only 16% of doctors are family or general practitioners), for the majority of their health care.[61] Eighteen percent of American women, including twenty million women of childbearing age, have no health insurance, and millions more are underinsured.[62] Access to health services varies widely by geographic location and income, which is correlated with race. One-third of all blacks and one-half of all black children in the United States live in poverty.[63] In the nation's capital, where 60 percent of the population is black, the poverty rate ranges from 7 percent to over 36 percent of the population, depending on the ward.[64] Ann Osborne, director of Little Rock Family Planning Services (LRFPS), claims that women's largest barrier to obtaining health services is poverty.[65]

Family planning in the United States is often expensive and not reimbursable by insurance companies; women pay 68 percent more out-of-pocket health care costs than men of the same age because of the cost of their contraception.[66] Most insurance companies do not pay for contraception, even when they cover other "optional" drugs for men, like Viagra.[67] Only half of the fifty states require insurers to cover contraception to the same degree as other prescription medications, and half of those states have special provisions that allow providers, plans, or employers to opt out on religious or moral grounds.[68] Poor people may also have difficulty finding a provider willing to accept their insurance; the number of obstetrician/gynecologists who accept Medicaid, the state-federal health insurance program for low-income people, is declining.[69] Although most states have significantly expanded their Medicaid coverage in recent years, women without dependent children are still ineligible for coverage in most states, regardless of how poor they are.[70] Minorities and poor women are most likely to use public family planning clinics or Planned Parenthood clinics, given their lower costs and, in the case of Planned Parenthood, sliding scale.[71] Rachel Atkins of Planned Parenthood of Northern New England explains that as the costs of health care rise, clinics like Planned Parenthood struggle to survive while providing patients with high-quality, low-cost services.[72]

As the U.S. population becomes increasingly diverse, language barriers prevent more and more residents from seeking health care. According to the National Latina Institute for Reproductive Health, over one-quarter of adult Latinos need translation services to access health care, but finding Spanish-speaking providers is often difficult, particularly in rural areas.[73] Bringing a friend or relative to the appointment to translate may not be a desirable option for women seeking reproductive health care, given the sensitive nature of the topic.

Contraception

Not until 1965 did the U.S. Supreme Court rule in *Griswold v. Connecticut* that the constitutional right to privacy includes the right to use contraception, though this ruling was limited to married couples only.[74] Amazingly, contraception was not legalized for unmarried women until 1972.[75] Today the contraceptive prevalence rate in the United States is 76 percent among married women—a relatively low number that partly reflects the multitude of barriers that women confront when trying to access contraception.[76] David et al. note that the average wait for Americans between becoming sexually active and using contraception is 1.5 to 2 years.[77] The leading birth control method in the United States is the Pill, chosen by 30 percent of family planning users, closely followed by tubal ligation, used by 27 percent of women.[78] Eighteen percent of contraceptive users report using condoms as their main family planning method. Women's contraceptive choices have expanded in recent years with the invention of two new hormonal methods: Ortho Evra (a contraceptive patch) and Nuva Ring (a vaginal ring), both of which work in a way similar to oral contraceptives.

Another new contraceptive method, Norplant, has been the target of much criticism from women's rights groups for its great potential for abuse. Norplant consists of a series of small match-like capsules that are implanted subdermally in a woman's arm and slowly release hormones over a five-year period. The Food and Drug Administration (FDA) approved Norplant in late 1990, despite formal opposition from the National Women's Health Network and Health Action International, representing hundreds of organizations in thirty-six countries that had concerns about Norplant's long-term safety.[79] In 2000, the FDA stopped distribution of Norplant to new users, citing concerns that certain batches of the contraceptive did not have adequate levels of hormones to be effective.[80]

Some women's rights activists argue that Norplant has been coercively imposed on poor women and minorities, much the way that sterilization was in the 1970s and earlier. During the ten years that Norplant was on the market, Medicaid paid for its insertion, and, in fact, more than half of Norplant users nationwide are Medicaid recipients.[81] Having the implants removed, however, has proven to be less accessible; women in Soperton, Georgia, report that Medicaid only pays to remove Norplant for "medical reasons." If a woman wanted to remove her Norplant earlier than two years from the date of insertion, she would have to pay $300 to cover the cost of removal and to reimburse the state for the original insertion.[82] Even when women complained of headaches, continuous bleeding, massive hair loss, and heart palpitations, some doctors called these symptoms "inconveniences," rather than "medical problems."[83] One American Indian woman in South Dakota who had Medicaid pay for her Norplant insertion wanted to have the implants removed after she gained sixty-five pounds. She was told that she could only have them removed if she agreed to have a tubal ligation.[84] A bill proposed (but never passed) in North Carolina would have required all women who get a state-funded abortion to be implanted with Norplant unless it was medically unsafe.[85] These fertility control efforts that disproportionately affect poor minority women make many feminists leery of the further development of long-term, provider-controlled methods like Norplant. Women should ideally have a wide range of contraceptive options to choose from, and the easily accessible option of removing provider-controlled methods like Norplant and the IUD should be included in the design of their insurance coverage.

Beyond the lack of information about contraceptives in many sex education programs, the prohibitive expense in some cases, and the lack of accessible clinics, Jane White also emphasizes that the number of unwanted pregnancies and abortions will remain high unless women's empowerment is promoted.[86] Until women have more control over when they have sex and with whom, they are unlikely to be able to prevent unwanted pregnancies.

Health professionals estimate that as many as 1.7 million of the 3 million unintended pregnancies that occur each year in the United States could be prevented by the use of emergency contraception (EC).[87] Emergency contraception is still not accessible to many people due to a lack of awareness, few providers, and the expensive cost in many areas. A recent survey found that only 31 percent of obstetrician/gynecologists prescribe EC more than five times a year; physicians of other specialties likely prescribe the drug even less frequently.[88] Just over half of states cover emergency contraception under their state Medicaid plans, and four states (Alaska, California, New Mexico, and Washington) allow pharmacists to dispense the drug without a prescription.[89] Many states are adopting "conscience clauses" that allow health providers, including physicians and pharmacists, to opt out of providing emergency contraception on religious or moral grounds. The refusal of many providers to counsel their patients about emergency contraception and offer a prescription for it likely contributes to the relatively high abortion rate in the United States.

Abortion in the United States before *Roe v. Wade*

Criminalization of abortion is a relatively recent phenomenon in the scope of U.S. history; common law in the American colonies and United States from 1607 to 1828 allowed women to have abortions at will.[90] Through most of the nineteenth century, abortion was legal until "quickening" (about four months) with little regulation.[91] In the 1870s, the American Medical Association launched a widespread campaign to criminalize abortion, partly in order to win professional power and restrict competition from midwives and homeopaths.[92] By 1900, in all American jurisdictions abortion was illegal except to save the women's health or life.[93]

Illegal abortions in the twentieth century, until their legalization in 1973, were common; many hospitals' emergency wards were full of women suffering complications from illegal abortions. Nationally, one thousand to five thousand women died each year of complications from illegal abortions, and hundreds of thousands more were injured.[94] Abortion deaths accounted for half of the maternal deaths of women of color and one-quarter of white maternal deaths.[95] Women seeking abortions during this time had few viable options. Ann Osborne of Little Rock Family Planning Services tells her personal story:

> When I was eighteen, I had an illegal abortion on a metal desk, in Boston, performed by a man I had never seen before. [. . .] I almost died, and ended up in the ICU, almost dead. And when I woke up from that, the physician who was caring for me happened to be an Irish Catholic obstetrician gynecologist. He said to me, and this is absolutely true, "If you don't tell me who did this to you, I'm going to let you die

here." I swear to God. And I said, "I'm not going to tell you." . . . [Later,] I wrote a letter to the medical society about that physician. I had his privileges suspended for a period of time.[96]

Many women who survived illegal abortions report neglect and abuse, including molestation and rape, at the hands of their provider.

Other women who were in Osborne's position—pregnant and scared—ended up carrying their unintended pregnancy to term; Terry Daley's story is one that many women of her age experienced. Growing up in a poor family in the 1940s, Daley never expected she would be able to go to college, but she received a full scholarship to Willamette University in the late 1950s. In her third year of college, she became pregnant, had to drop out of school, and lost her scholarship. Daley explains that she had virtually no sex education and had never used contraception before. "I had the vague idea that a woman got pregnant when she wanted to have a child." Daley's doctor gave her a thumbnail sketch of death by illegal abortion—her first exposure to the concept—and she had her first child in 1961, at the age of twenty-one.[97]

Both Osborne and Daley lament the fact that most young women today do not understand what it was like before abortion was legalized. Ann Osborne remembers, "When *Roe v. Wade* passed, I felt very, very strongly that people who had gone through this really had to stand up and speak for what they believed in. But the young people today who, let's say, have had surgical abortion or medical abortion—they don't know what it's like to have to find a network to have an illegal abortion."[98] Since young American women have lived their entire lives in a country in which abortion is legal, many take the right for granted and do not prioritize reproductive rights when voting.

Many factors converged to lead to the legalization of abortion. As women delayed marriage and childbirth, increased their attendance in higher education, and joined the labor force in greater numbers, the pressure to be able to control the timing of childbearing grew.[99] Both feminist activism and political pressure from population control advocates contributed to the legalization of abortion. In 1969, the National Association for the Repeal of Abortion Laws (NARAL) was established as the first single-issue abortion rights organization.[100] On January 22, 1973, the U.S. Supreme Court legalized abortion in a historic 7–2 decision, emphasizing that the decision to terminate a pregnancy belonged in the private relationship between doctor and patient. As one doctor relates, "The deaths [from illegal abortions] stopped overnight in 1973 and I never saw another abortion death in all the eighteen years after that until I retired."[101]

However, a series of court decisions after *Roe v. Wade* restricted women's access to abortion. The Church Amendment, passed shortly after the *Roe v. Wade* decision, allows individual or institutional health providers that receive federal funding to refuse to perform abortions on religious or moral grounds. By the late 1970s, over half the states adopted similar provisions, and many included refusal clauses for contraception and sterilization as well.[102] The 1977 Hyde Amendment prohibits the use of federal funds to pay for abortions except in cases of rape or incest, or to save the woman's life. The number of federally funded abortions dropped from almost three hundred thousand in 1977 to fewer than three hundred in 1992.[103] In 1980, the U.S. Supreme Court ruled in *Harris v. McRae* that states are not obligated to fund abortion services.[104] Then, in 1989, in *Webster v. Reproductive Health Services,* the Supreme Court granted greater latitude to individual states to restrict abortion services, as long as those restrictions did not present an "undue burden" on the women seeking services.[105]

Abortion Today: Obstacles to Access

The United States has one of highest abortion rates in the industrialized world, though the rate has been declining and recently hit its lowest point in twenty years.[106] Partly as a result of inadequate sex education and poor access to contraception, more than half of all pregnancies in the United States are unintended, and half of those unintended pregnancies—1.5 million per year—end in abortion.[107] By age forty-five, nearly half of all American women will have had at least one abortion.[108] Given the polarized nature of the topic in the United States, it is no surprise that women face numerous obstacles in attempting to obtain an abortion. Access to abortion, in the words of one activist, is "currently in a state of crisis."[109]

The financial expense of an abortion is formidable to many women even though, correcting for inflation, the cost of an abortion in 1991 was half of its cost in 1973.[110] Though a woman's blood type, gestational age, and choice of anesthesia all influence the price, generally a first-trimester abortion costs at least $300 to $500.[111] Because the Hyde Amendment prohibits the use of federal Medicaid funds to pay for abortions, individual state legislatures decide whether or not they will fund the procedure for poor women. As of 2003, only nineteen states use their own funds to subsidize "medically necessary" abortions for Medicaid recipients. In the context of these states, "medically necessary" is broadly defined to include a woman's socioeconomic reasons for having an abortion, such as the negative mental and financial impact of carrying an unwanted pregnancy to term. Of these nineteen states, only four have such a policy on a voluntary basis; the other fifteen have been ordered by state courts to fund these abortions.[112] Taking a more conservative approach, four other states pay for abortion only in cases of fetal anomalies or to save the woman's life; the remaining twenty-seven states provide no abortion coverage.[113] People who depend on the federal government for health care, such as military personnel and their families, government employees, many American Indians, and Peace Corps volunteers, all lack any coverage for an abortion.[114]

Poor women are three times more likely to have an abortion than women who are better off financially, making the dearth of public funding for abortions particularly problematic.[115] Even today, some poor women who live in rural areas and lack Medicaid funding end up performing abortions at home by using quinine pills, taking brewer's yeast, or drinking turpentine.[116] Black women are disproportionately affected by the lack of public funding for abortions; not only do black women experience higher poverty rates than white women, but they also account for 24 percent of abortions done in the United States, even though they make up only 12 percent of the population.[117] Securing sufficient funds for an abortion in a timely manner is exceedingly difficult for many women with few resources.

Perhaps the most pervasive obstacle to obtaining an abortion is simply women's lack of awareness and information. Given the prevalence of anti-abortion campaigns that utilize scare tactics and myths to frighten people from having abortions, it is no surprise that many women, even those who show up in abortion clinics as patients, harbor devastating beliefs about abortion. Some women believe infertility, extreme illness, or even death are all common complications of abortion, and many women do not realize that a physician will be performing the surgery. Abbie Adams, a clinic worker in Albuquerque, observes, "Women come and [. . .] just have these horrid ideas about what an abortion is, and when I tell them, if they're in the first trimester, it's a five-minute procedure, we use strong medications, we dilate the cervix, which is a hole you already have . . . you can see the relief on their faces. They expected us to cut open their stomachs. 'Is this legal?' We have women asking that all the time."[118] Many women also do not realize that abortion services are confidential, and they do not know how to find an abortion clinic.

The combination of ignorance and denial delays many pregnant women in getting an abortion. Ann Osborne explains that, after moving to Arkansas from working many years in Boston, she notices more patients in Arkansas who are fourteen or fifteen years old and twenty weeks pregnant, yet they are "so imbued in denial" that "When you ask these patients how long they've known they are pregnant, they'll say two or three days."[119] Adams points out that some women know so little about their bodies, "it's very easy to pretend that you're not pregnant if you don't want to be."

Pregnancy resource centers, also called crisis pregnancy centers, are a particularly prevalent source of women's myths about abortion. These religiously based organizations advertise in newspapers and billboards, asking, "Pregnant? Need help?" Many attract young, pregnant women and girls by offering free pregnancy tests or even, in some cases, ultrasound examinations. Although a urine pregnancy test takes only five minutes to complete, women at pregnancy resource centers are commonly told that the results will take an hour or more to obtain, during which time they can have a free counseling session. "Counselors" at these centers emphasize fetal development, stressing how much the woman's "baby" can do at a given gestational age. They usually describe abortion procedures in grotesque language and exaggerate or outright lie about possible complications from abortion, including future miscarriages, infertility, hemorrhaging, uterine perforation, and infection. Staff at crisis pregnancy centers exaggerate the "inherent dangers of abortion," despite the fact that a first-trimester abortion is one of the safest surgeries performed in the United States—far safer than a tonsillectomy, appendectomy, or a full-term delivery.[120] One center even told their clients that the chance of contracting breast cancer increases by 80 percent after having an abortion. One counselor said, "You know when you occasionally see really young women with breast cancer? Well, usually those women have had an abortion." Pregnancy resource centers also describe sexual dysfunction, suicidal thoughts, and "anniversary syndrome" as comprising "postabortion syndrome," despite numerous studies, including one by the American Psychological Association, refuting the syndrome's existence.[121] At a center in Beaverton, Oregon, a counselor inquired about the opinion of a client's boyfriend, adding, "It's the father's decision, too!"[122] Under President Bush's Compassion Capital Fund, some of these pregnancy resource centers received federal funding.[123]

Although religious teachings against abortion make the decision to terminate a pregnancy more agonizing for many women, religion does not seem to stop women from having abortions overall; one out of six abortion patients in the United States is evangelical or born-again Christian, and nearly one-third are Catholic (Catholics comprise 25% of the general population).[124] Prochoice religious organizations like the Religious Coalition for Reproductive Choice (RCRC) and Catholics for a Free Choice (CFFC) attempt to help women struggling to reconcile their religion with their personal needs.

In addition to lacking factual information about abortion, many women are also at a disadvantage because of poor self-esteem and not being accustomed to prioritizing their own health. Ann Osborne remarks that self-esteem issues "loom very large" for her patients in Little Rock, Arkansas.[125] Brittney Camp, a counselor at Little Rock Family Planning Services, believes that some women's dependence on men is one of their greatest obstacles to reproductive freedom, moreso in some parts of the country than others.[126] She relates that even when she asks patients questions directly, they sometimes can hardly answer without looking to their boyfriend or husband for approval or confirmation. Growing up in Arkansas, Camp describes the environment: "Women are subservient to men, and men make the decisions. [. . .] I think a lot of that comes from the church because they preach to them, you know, women are supposed to be servants to the men. [. . .] That's how I was raised. It's not so much antichoice as it is antiwoman." Taught to be obedient and to look to men and religious leaders for direction, some women are not empowered to make their own reproductive decisions. Camp continues, "There's a church on every corner, and they're preaching about how bad abortion is." At the extreme end of this spectrum, women who are in abusive relationships face particularly difficult challenges when it comes to fulfilling their reproductive health needs.[127]

Since the Supreme Court left it up to individual states to decide what abortion restrictions to impose (as long as they do not present an "undue burden"), the most intense battle over access to abortion has been carried out in state legislatures. Though the majority of Americans are prochoice, many support restrictions on abortion that "sound good" but actually end up hurting women.[128] Parental consent laws, for example, seem logical to many people but frequently delay the process of obtaining an abortion; second-trimester abortions for minors in Minnesota increased by 18 percent after the state passed its parental notification law.[129] The majority of minors seeking abortions (61%, according to a 1991 study) willingly talk to their parents about it, and many of those who choose otherwise have valid reasons for their decision, such as fear of violence in the family.[130] Furthermore, the majority of minors who do not tell their parents do consult another adult other than clinic staff. Twenty-three states require parental consent for an abortion, and another twenty require parental notification.[131]

Mandatory waiting periods, which twenty-one states have in effect, generally require women to wait twenty-four hours after their initial visit to a clinic before they can have an abortion.[132] Such laws suggest that women make their decision lightly and they need a legal barrier to keep them from having abortions spontaneously. Terry Daley argues that mandatory waiting periods are "humiliating, patronizing, insufferable." As an abortion clinic worker, she testifies that women rarely call her clinic until they are completely sure of their decision.[133] Mandatory waiting period laws, like Alabama's Women's Right to Know Act, require women to make two separate visits to an abortion clinic in order to have mandatory fetal development counseling before the appointment for their actual abortion.[134] In most states with this kind of legislation, the mandatory counseling emphasizes fetal development and includes graphic photographs.

Another thirty-one states have banned so-called partial-birth abortions, and President Bush signed a federal ban in 2003.[135] The procedure that "partial-birth abortion" supposedly refers to is "dilation and extraction" (D&X), which comprises a very small percentage of second-trimester abortions each year. However, the nonmedical language of these bans could be interpreted to apply to all abortions, even those in the first trimester. In *Stenberg v. Carhart*, the Supreme Court found one such ban, from Nebraska, unconstitutional because the definition of the procedure was imprecise and because the ban did not include an exception to protect the woman's health.[136] A few other courts have struck down similar bans as unconstitutional, and in July 2005 the U.S. Court of Appeals for the Eighth Circuit ruled the federal ban unconstitutional; time will tell whether the ban is eventually overturned.[137]

Thirty-six states have laws establishing regulations that only apply to abortion providers and clinics; these regulations usually relate to zoning, building codes, record keeping, and administration, despite the lack of medical justification for this.[138] One such bill, proposed in Oregon in 1999, would have specified the exact measurements of the waiting room for each abortion clinic in the state, essentially requiring major renovations for no reasonable medical reason.[139]

State restrictions on abortion are discriminatory because they single out providers and patients seeking abortion in a way that does not apply to any other medical procedure. Such restrictions also affect women of varying socioeconomic levels differently. In New Mexico, Abbie Adams reports, only minors who are on Medicaid are required to obtain parental consent for an abortion.[140] Poor women living in rural areas, far from the nearest abortion clinic, are most affected by mandatory waiting periods because they must take additional time off work and find housing for a night in order to make two visits to the clinic.

For the millions of women who live anywhere but in a large metropolis, finding a doctor willing to provide abortions is a difficult feat; 90 percent of providers are located in urban areas.[141] Sadly, 87 percent of all U.S. counties have no abortion provider, and that number increases to 97 percent in rural areas.[142] The future picture of abortion providers looks bleak; half of all abortion providers today are over fifty years old, yet few younger doctors are being trained to provide abortions.[143] Only 12 percent of ob-gyn residency programs have routine abortion training, half offer abortion training as an elective, and over one-quarter (27%) have no opportunity for training at all.[144] Medical Students for Choice is a national organization attempting to increase the number of physicians trained in abortion services, and the great need for their work is evidenced by the rapidly declining number of providers. In 1983, 42 percent of obstetrician/gynecologists provided abortions, but that number dropped to 33 percent by 1995; likewise, the number of hospitals providing abortions halved between 1982 and 1996.[145] The result is that many women have to travel far distances to reach an abortion clinic. At Little Rock Family Planning Services, 35 percent of patients come from out of state, often traveling from as far as Mississippi and Tennessee, two of the most poverty-stricken states in the country.[146]

Abbie Adams of Abortion and Counseling Services notes that her clinic in Albuquerque is one of only three in the entire state of New Mexico. Living in a state that is very large geographically, with a small population, women in New Mexico often travel hundreds of miles to reach a provider. New Mexico is one of the few states that funds abortions through its Medicaid program, and at least half of the patients at Adams's clinic are Medicaid recipients. The combination of barriers to accessing abortion care often result in women arriving at the clinic beyond the clinic's twenty-one week cut-off date. Adams explains that in those cases, they can only refer patients to clinics in Boulder or Kansas City for an abortion, but Medicaid does not fund abortions across state lines. Those women are left with the near-impossible task of quickly coming up with a way to pay for an abortion out of pocket—an expense that is usually over $1,000.[147]

Although 89 percent of abortions in the United States are performed in the first trimester of the pregnancy, a number of women end up having second-trimester abortions. In addition to the numerous barriers to accessing abortion care in a timely manner listed above, Jane White notes, "In my experience, people in the second trimester are people who don't have control over their lives." She points out the need for more drug treatment centers and domestic violence shelters to help women regain control over their lives and pay more attention to their bodies and health.[148]

Antiabortion Violence

One of the factors that surely contributes to the declining number of doctors willing to provide abortions is the recent history of violence against providers and clinic workers. Throughout the 1980s, antichoice groups organized regular clinic blockades and picketing, and stepped up their actions with bomb threats and vandalism. More than 80 percent of abortion clinics experienced some form of harassment during this time.[149] The situation worsened in the 1990s, with seven murders of physicians and clinic workers and seventeen attempted murders.[150] Since 1977, there have been 15,087 *reported* instances of violence or harassment against abortion doctors and clinics, and the actual number is likely to be much higher.[151] As Rachel Atkins of Planned Parenthood notes, "We went from a time when women had to fear dying from an abortion to fear being shot and murdered in their attempt to seek legal health care."[152]

Jane White describes her experience at the Downtown Women's Center in Portland, Oregon. In the late 1990s, someone shot a bullet through the window of the operating room in the early morning hours; no one was present at the time. The clinic has also received bomb threats, as well as threatening phone calls and mail. In the past, the clinic had many protesters, but after staff obtained a court injunction against specific individuals, the protesters stopped coming. The Downtown Women's Center is fortunate in that the clinic is located on the ninth floor of a large medical building in downtown Portland; the majority of passers-by do not even realize they are there. Still, the clinic currently has video camera surveillance of the hallway outside their clinic, and a patient must have her name on the appointment list to be buzzed into the waiting room. A heavy steel door separates the waiting room from the interior of the clinic, and staff installed bulletproof glass at the receptionist's desk and in the operating room.[153]

The security measures taken by staff at Little Rock Family Planning Services in Arkansas are even stricter; a rather intimidating security guard stands watch at the door to check the photo ID of every person entering the clinic and to search everyone's personal belongings. Patients walk through a metal detector and may also be whisked by the security guard with a handheld metal-detector wand. Once in the waiting room, patients must be buzzed in a second time to reach the rest of the clinic, where they may not bring their purses or bags. Patients and their partners are personally escorted to the restroom, between exam rooms, or out of the clinic; no one is allowed to walk around the clinic unaccompanied. LRFPS occasionally has protesters, and they have experienced a few "minor bomb threats," which never materialized. Like the Downtown Women's Center, LRFPS had a shooting, but at a time that no one was present in the clinic.[154]

The threats and violence extend beyond the confines of abortion clinics; many abortion providers find themselves targets even in their own homes, threatened by the small minority of the antichoice movement that believes violence is a justifiable tactic. Ann Osborne, a provider in Boston and then in Arkansas, had U.S. Marshals living with her and her husband for six months in 1994 after John Salvi shot and killed Osborne's administrative assistant, Leanne Nichols. (Salvi also killed Shannon Lowney in a shooting at a different clinic on the same day.) Even Osborne's daughter, who was a college student at the time, was threatened.[155] Antichoice groups also targeted Dr. Curtis Boyd, a provider in Albuquerque and northern Texas, as well as his children.[156] In January 1998, Eric Rudolph bombed an abortion clinic in Birmingham, Alabama, killing security guard Robert Sanderson and nearly killing nurse Emily Lyons. Larry Rodick, president of Planned Parenthood of Alabama, remembers the tense atmosphere that followed, particularly since Rudolph was a fugitive for more than five years.[157]

On January 22, 1995, the American Coalition of Life Activists (ACLA) unveiled a poster at their annual protest in Washington, D.C., which read, "Guilty of Crimes against Humanity—The Deadly Dozen." Below, the names and home addresses of thirteen prominent abortion providers across the United States appeared in bold type, just above the phrase "$5,000 Reward—Abortionist." To the targeted doctors, the message of this hit list was clear: Stop performing abortions or your life will be in danger. Dr. Elizabeth Newhall, medical director of the Downtown Women's Center and the only female physician on the "Deadly Dozen List," soon received a phone call from an FBI agent of the Domestic Terrorist Task Force. Following the FBI's recommendations, Dr. Newhall began to wear a bulletproof vest and disguises to work, varying the route she took each day. She also invested in additional locks and window coverings for her home. The other doctors on the list took similar precautions, and several accepted protection offered to them by U.S. Marshals. Planned Parenthood of the Columbia/Willamette spent an estimated $500,000 on security measures taken as a result of the "Deadly Dozen List."[158]

In 1997, ACLA members contributed to the formation of a website called the "Nuremberg Files," which listed over two hundred abortion providers nationwide. Information listed about providers included home addresses, phone numbers, and often descriptions of their cars, license plate numbers, the names of their children, wedding anniversary dates, and other personal details. Many of the files also contained photographs of the doctors and their homes. The site's creators claim the files were produced to collect information about abortion providers for use in future "war crime trials," such as those held in Germany following World War II. The website lists the "abortionists" under titles such as "baby butchers" and "murderers," with pictures of bloody aborted fetuses dripping down the side. The website drew attention in October 1998 when the name of Dr. Barnett Slepian was dramatically crossed out after he was killed by a sniper in his home in Buffalo, New York. The names of other murdered abortion providers were crossed out on the list, while those wounded were shaded in gray. Dr. Warren Hern testified, "I felt like a hunted animal . . . like I could be shot at any time." Dr. Elizabeth Newhall adds, "Suddenly, I felt real visible to individuals who might not be quite balanced."

Two abortion clinics and four physicians filed a lawsuit against ACLA and fourteen individuals, seeking financial damages and an injunction against ACLA's actions. The case was the first civil suit to go to trial under the federal Freedom of Access to Clinic Entrances Act of 1994—a law that prohibits physical or psychological intimidation of anyone seeking or providing abortion services. A federal court in Portland found the defendants guilty and awarded the plaintiffs $109 million. After a series of appeals, the original verdict stands, and the Supreme Court has refused to hear the defendants' appeal.[159] Though not ordered by the court, the Internet Service Provider (ISP) of the Nuremberg Files website refused to host the site shortly after the first verdict in 1999; unfortunately, mirror sites of the original remain online.

Providing abortion services has become a job that necessitates security measures few professions require. More than one interviewee for this chapter declined a photograph for security reasons. Of the abortion providers who have been so heavily targeted, few probably ever thought their job would require such bravery. Jane White recalls, "When protesters were outside Dr. Belknap's house, he said, 'That's my badge of courage. That tells me I'm doing the right thing.'"[160]

A solution offered by many to better protect providers is integrating abortion care into hospitals to avoid the currently segregated state of abortion care in stand-alone clinics. Eighty-seven percent of abortions in the United States are currently provided in a clinic; less than 7 percent are provided in hospitals.[161] Moving abortion services into hospitals would not only provide a stronger shield for providers and patients against bombings and shootings, but it would also shift the procedure into the realm of comprehensive care.[162] Integrating abortion care into hospitals seems unlikely to happen anytime soon, however, given the increasing number of secular hospitals merging with

Catholic hospitals. Providing services to eighty-eight million Americans per year, Catholic hospitals represent the single largest group of not-for-profit hospitals in the country.[163] While 81 percent of abortion providers were located in hospitals in 1973, that number dropped to just 36 percent in 1996.[164]

Additionally, Jane White believes that the American Medical Association and other professional societies should encourage more doctors to take a little heat. "If everybody says they're a Jew, you can't kill the Jews."[165] Today the overwhelming majority of abortions are performed by a handful of doctors; only 2 percent of all obstetrician/gynecologists perform twenty-five or more abortions per month.[166] It is specifically because there are so few doctors willing to provide abortions that those doctors have been relatively easy targets for the violent faction of the antichoice movement. Another way to increase access for women and to lessen the pressure on already-practicing providers is to expand the pool of health professionals eligible to perform first-trimester abortions. Given adequate training, this could include physician assistants (who can currently provide abortions in some parts of the country), nurse practitioners, and nurse-midwives. The majority of relevant professional medical societies have endorsed such an expansion, including the American College of Obstetricians and Gynecologists, the American Academy of Physician Assistants, the American College of Nurse-Midwives, and the National Association of Nurse Practitioners in Women's Health, among others.[167] A 2004 study that compared complication rates of abortions performed by physician assistants and physicians found no statistically significant difference.[168]

Given the numerous obstacles impeding women's access to abortions, including insufficient financial resources, misinformation, legislative barriers, and the declining number of providers, it is clear that access to abortion is truly in a state of crisis. Terry Daley finds it amazing that, despite the abundant and frightening myths circulating about abortion and despite being required to navigate an intimidating security system at many clinics, women still show up at her clinic's door.[169]

Sexually Transmitted Infections (STIs) and HIV/AIDS

Detailed discussion of STIs and HIV/AIDS is beyond the scope of this chapter; however, with the highest rate of sexually transmitted infections (STIs) in the industrial world, the United States still has much work to do in STI education and prevention.[170] Beginning with inadequate sex education, American youth, particularly those who live in impoverished areas, are vulnerable to contracting a sexually transmitted infection. Women suffer more frequent and more serious complications from STIs than men do.[171] Rates of STIs and HIV/AIDS reflect national health disparities among different racial groups. Though blacks comprise only 13 percent of the U.S. population, they account for 77 percent of all gonorrhea cases and 50 percent of new HIV cases.[172] Prevalence of HIV/AIDS is twenty-one times higher among blacks than among whites.[173] Likewise, though the national HIV/AIDS rate in 2000 was 14.6 cases per 100,000 people, in the District of Columbia (with a 70% minority population), the rate was more than ten times the national rate, at 152.9 per 100,000 people.[174] In fact, AIDS is the fifth leading cause of death in the nation's capital. Both in D.C. and nationally, the number of deaths from AIDS has been declining, partly because of increased awareness of the disease and improved antiretroviral therapies, yet much work remains to be done.[175] Despite two decades of experience with HIV/AIDS, the U.S. government still lacks a comprehensive national AIDS policy.[176]

Minority Women's Health

Sometimes referred to as the "South within the North," pockets of industrialized countries like the United States resemble conditions found in developing countries; minority women living in impoverished areas of the United States experience a much lower health status than their wealthier, white counterparts. American Indians are perhaps the most disadvantaged minority in the United States. A violent history of genocide, broken treaties, coerced sterilization, and forced schooling to "Americanize" Indians has left the Native population of the United States suffering. Pushed onto reservations and given what have often been inadequate health services, members of the three hundred American Indian tribes tend to suffer from many illnesses and health conditions, like cardiovascular disease and some types of cancer, at greater rates than the general population.[177] The disadvantages that American Indian communities experience extend to reproductive health and rights as well. The scope of this disadvantage is difficult to gauge, largely because of the dearth of research on American Indian women's sexual and reproductive health. When studies do take race into account, they usually look at differences between blacks, whites, and Latinos, seldom looking at American Indians.[178]

In one study of 130 American Indian young women aged fifteen to twenty, 81 percent reported not using contraception the first time they had sex.[179] A 1982 study demonstrated that American Indian adolescents have less knowledge about sex than whites or Latinos.[180] Abbie Adams of Abortion and Counseling Services in Albuquerque, New Mexico, notes significant differences between the races in terms of access to reproductive health services and abortion in particular. Adams's impression is that few of the Native women in that area know abortion is an option for them, and even fewer know that Medicaid provides transportation if needed.[181] Many American Indian women are in a difficult position to exercise their reproductive rights, given the numerous economic, educational, and geographic barriers they face.

Latinos represent a sizable minority in the U.S. population; there are currently 35 million Latinos in the United States, and by 2050, an estimated one-quarter of the American female population will be Latina.[182] Like American Indians, Latinas face many obstacles to accessing reproductive health care, including language barriers, poverty, limited access to services, discriminatory treatment, lack of awareness of health risks, and lack of health insurance. Latinas have the highest uninsured rate of any ethnic group in the United States, at 42 percent and rising.[183] Latinas' unintended pregnancy rate is twice that of whites, as is their teen pregnancy rate.[184] Though an increasing number of reproductive health organizations now translate their publications and services into Spanish, finding bilingual health providers is still a challenge in most parts of the country.

African American women also experience worse reproductive health indicators than the national averages. The infant mortality rate, for example, is 6.9 deaths per 1,000 live births nationally, but the rate for blacks is more than double that, at 14 deaths per 1,000 births.[185] Black women are more likely to live in poverty, have an abortion, and contract an STI than their white counterparts.[186] The recent trend of meting out criminal sentences to drug-addicted pregnant women also disproportionately hurts black women, who are more likely than whites to be reported for drug abuse because of their more frequent contact with institutions like public hospitals, Medicaid officials, and probation officers.[187] Between 1985 and 1995, two hundred women in thirty states were charged with maternal drug use. The charges ranged from "distributing drugs to a minor" and "child abuse and neglect," to "reckless endangerment," "manslaughter," and "assault with a deadly weapon." Since drug distribution laws in many states do not apply to fetuses, women in more than one case were convicted on the argument that they delivered crack cocaine to their babies through the umbilical cord during the sixty seconds after birth before the cord is cut.[188] Nationally, 11 to 25 percent of newborns are affected by their mothers' illegal drug use.[189] A 1991 study found nearly equal rates of illegal drug use during pregnancy among blacks and whites, yet black women are ten times more likely than white women to be reported.[190]

Recent cases convicting women of child abuse for using crack cocaine during pregnancy unjustly single out these women for punishment even though some women use other harmful substances, like alcohol and cigarettes, during pregnancy.[191] Such legislation pits the rights of the fetus against the rights of the mother. Ironically, very few drug rehabilitation centers accept pregnant women, even though it is during a woman's pregnancy that she may be most receptive to changing her life.[192] A number of professional societies have come out publicly against criminal prosecutions of drug-addicted pregnant women; these groups include the American Medical Association, the American College of Obstetricians and Gynecologists, and March of Dimes. They all believe that such prosecutions will drive pregnant drug users away from much-needed treatment and prenatal care.[193]

One organization that exemplifies the approach of targeting minority drug-addicted women is CRACK (Children Requiring a Caring Community), now known as "Project Prevention." Established in 1997 by Barbara Harris, a middle-aged homemaker in California, CRACK offers to pay drug-addicted women $200 if they agree to be sterilized or use long-term contraceptive methods like Norplant, the IUD, or Depo Provera. In the case of Depo Provera use, the $200 is paid over the course of one year to provide an incentive for women to continue getting shots every three months.[194] The woman must show proof of narcotics abuse and proof of the procedure done by a physician in order to receive her money. In the first five years of the program, 1,050 women participated, of whom only half were white.[195] Quoted in an early interview, Harris states, "We don't allow dogs to breed. We spay them. We neuter them. We try to keep them from having unwanted puppies, and yet these women are literally having litters of children."[196] CRACK has received tremendous media coverage, most of which has been positive.[197] The well-known conservative radio talk-show host Dr. Laura Schlessinger has been one of CRACK's staunchest supporters since the program's inception.[198]

CRACK intentionally places billboards in predominantly black and Latina neighborhoods. One such advertisement reads, "Don't let a pregnancy ruin your drug habit."[199] Scully points out that none of the birth control methods that CRACK finances protect women against STIs or HIV/AIDS. Furthermore, hormonal contraceptive methods require screening for contraindications, regular pap smears, and monitoring for side effects—all services that poor, drug-addicted women are unlikely to get. The CRACK program assumes that drug-addicted women will always be drug addicts and that treatment options are not worthy of being pursued.[200] Such a program is a continuation of "the idea that procreation is the cause of social problems, and therefore social problems can be solved by controlling the fertility of the victims of those social inequities."[201] That philosophy, still seemingly well accepted in the United States, affects a wide range of policies both in the United States and abroad.

Influence of the ICPD

The United States is the largest contributor to population programs worldwide and therefore has great influence on the reproductive health of millions of women around the world.[202] Historically, an important part of the United States' strategy for addressing poverty and underdevelopment was mass distribution of contraception, assuming that "the population problem would yield to a technical fix—birth control—rather than requiring attention to the social, economic, and cultural circumstances that influence fertility decisions and behavior."[203] In the past ten to fifteen years, however, the United States has, to some extent, incorporated the broader definition of reproductive health and rights presented at the 1994 International Conference on Population and Development (ICPD). In the first two years after the ICPD, the United States led the donor community in financial support of the Cairo agenda; the United States' contribution of over $600 million per year in 1995 and 1996 represented 49 percent and 47 percent of the total global population assistance.[204] In the few years immediately following the ICPD, the United States devoted a large portion of the budget for USAID's Center for Population, Health, and Nutrition to carrying out the Cairo agenda.[205] USAID's spending on maternal health jumped from between $10 million and 15 million annually before the ICPD to $50 million per year after the conference.[206] Likewise, funding for USAID's Women in Development office more than doubled from 1992 to 1996, and grew in "size, validity, and vitality."[207]

Despite initial signs for optimism, however, a conservative political environment in the United States soon led to dramatic cuts in funding for women's reproductive health abroad. In 1996, a Republican-controlled Congress slashed family planning assistance by 35 percent, and in 1999 Congress eliminated all funds for the United Nations Population Fund (UNFPA).[208] Funding for population activities in 1998 was just 70 percent of 1995 levels.[209] For the United States to fulfill its share of the ICPD's plan, funding for reproductive health would need to triple.[210] An important step toward reducing poverty in developing countries would require not only an increase in U.S. funding for foreign aid, but the appropriate use of that foreign aid in programs that have a tangible impact on the poorest segments of the population. The United States currently ranks last out of twenty-two major donor countries in terms of its percentage of GNP devoted to foreign aid, funneling just 0.1 percent of the gross national product to development overseas.[211]

The influence of the ICPD today can be seen in the expanded scope of the Demographic and Health Surveys (DHS) that USAID funds in developing countries. In the past, the DHS focused exclusively on family planning, but USAID has broadened more recent surveys to include other reproductive health and women's empowerment issues. Jacobsen argues that the United States still focuses excessively on quantitative markers such as a country's total fertility rate, instead of adequately paying attention to qualitative indicators, like quality of care, accessibility of services, and the participation of nongovernmental organizations.[212] Between the conservative climate in Congress and the continued efforts of population control advocates, advancing the Cairo agenda has proven to be a slow and challenging task.

The Mainstream Reproductive Rights Movement

Since the 1970s, the mainstream reproductive rights movement in the United States has for the most part narrowly focused on the legal defense of abortion, neglecting issues of equal importance that disproportionately affect poor women and women of color. The term "reproductive rights," coined at the end of the 1970s, has become synonymous in many people's minds with "abortion rights."[213] Even the framing of the abortion issue as a matter of "choice" is seen as problematic by many: "The language of choice spoke to those in the society who thought of themselves as having choices, not to those who did not."[214] Dorothy Roberts believes that the mainstream reproductive rights movement is not well equipped to handle issues that do not fit into the mold of defending the right to legal abortion.[215]

In 1977, when Rosie Jimenez became the first woman known to die from an illegal abortion after the Hyde Amendment cut off federal funding for abortions, not a single one of the national organizations took up the issue.[216] Fried and Clarke point out that the mainstream reproductive rights movement may not have considered Jimenez to be a very sympathetic character; as a single, Mexican American mother on welfare who had been pregnant several times before and lived in a border town known for illegal drug trafficking, Jimenez was not someone with whom the majority of women's groups wanted to align themselves. Jimenez's illegal abortionist received just three days in jail and a $100 fine.[217]

Roberts emphasizes that there has always been a strong reproductive rights movement among women of color; in 1941, the National Council of Negro Women was the first national organization to officially endorse birth control, for example.[218] In the 1950s, Dr. Dorothy Brown, the first black female surgeon general in the United States and a Tennessee state representative, became the first state legislator to introduce a bill legalizing abortion.[219] The mainstream movement is gradually recognizing that the work of women of color has not been a marginal part of the movement, yet Roberts points out that "until very recently, [some groups] not only focused exclusively on abortion rights, but sometimes worked in opposition to women of color and their efforts to address a broader range of issues, especially coerced or abusive birth control practices based on the population control ideology."[220]

Women of color organizations have been more adept at looking at broader reproductive health and rights issues, placing these issues in their social context of poverty and racial discrimination.[221] "There's a concern about being impelled to have an abortion because you can't afford another child as much as the concern about not being able to get an abortion if you want," Roberts notes.[222] As women of color gained greater leadership roles in the reproductive rights movement, more organizations began to emphasize the right to safe childbearing, the right to affordable health care, and the right to refuse sterilization, for example.[223] The reproductive rights agenda has slowly broadened, with more emphasis now on access to education, job opportunities, childcare, housing, and health care.[224]

As the women's rights movement has continued to evolve in the United States, various organizations are becoming more practiced at collaborating and forming alliances, which, Roberts believes, are crucial to the future of the movement. Although women of color have organized for better reproductive health for just as long as white women, Roberts notes that it is only recently that different women of color organizations have formed visible and influential coalitions, such as the SisterSong Women of Color Reproductive Health Collective.[225] As an example of the power of coalitions, Roberts points to lessons learned during the organization of the 2004 March for Women's Lives in Washington, D.C.:

> When it was first being organized by Planned Parenthood and NOW [the National Organization for Women], there wasn't much excitement about it. I understand at one point it wasn't even clear if it was going to happen. And then there was a lot of discontent—it was first going to be called the March for Choice, which connotes abortion rights, and a lot of groups said, "We're not going to support this, if it's another example of this exclusive focus." So they opened it up and included the National Black Women's Imperative and the National Latina Institute for

Reproductive Health as key organizers, and that changed it to the March for Women's Lives, and that was critical in building broad-based support, including support from organizations like the NAACP [the National Association for the Advancement of Colored People], which had never supported the march before.

Organizations like Third Wave and Choice USA have been pivotal in their focus on multiracial organizing that includes attention to a broad range of issues.[226] As reproductive rights activists see links between various issues like abortion, welfare reform, antipoverty, and antiracism, more people will be brought into the movement, which is imperative in this time of increasingly strong attacks on reproductive freedom.

Opposition to Reproductive Rights

A variety of antichoice pieces of legislation have gradually chipped away at the legal right to abortion. During the 1999 legislative session, over four hundred antichoice bills were introduced across the country, forty of which were enacted by Congress and various state legislatures.[227] Although the majority of Americans support the legal right to abortion, backing for legal restrictions is increasing, particularly among young people.[228] Legal restrictions like parental consent, mandatory waiting periods, and "partial-birth abortion" bans disproportionately burden poor, rural, minority, and teenage women. As Fried and Clarke point out, the slow erosion of access does not immediately have an impact on white, middle-class women, making it difficult to mobilize those prochoice supporters.[229]

In addition to blatant restrictions on the provision of abortion services, antichoice organizations have been successful in attacking reproductive rights in less direct ways as well. The antichoice movement is trying to establish a legal foundation for fetal rights through a variety of tactics. Politicians who are against abortion have recently supported bills limiting stem cell research and punishing crimes against the fetus or "unborn child." President Bush's Children Health Insurance Program (CHIP) includes language that guarantees a fetus's right to health insurance.[230] A recent case of a woman prosecuted for refusing a cesarean section is yet another example. These are all ways to promote the idea that the fetus has the same legal rights as a child, apart from the pregnant woman. "One of the ultimate goals of this promotion of fetal rights is to destroy the right to abortion, because at some point, the more the fetus looks like a person, with rights equal to the woman's, the more abortion looks like murder."[231] Roberts points out that if the reproductive rights movement myopically focuses on legal restrictions to abortion, it will fail to see that these other moves also counter the right to abortion, perhaps even more powerfully.[232]

The recently conservative political climate has slowed the progress of the reproductive rights movement. During his two terms, President Bush has tried to restrict reproductive rights in a number of ways, from reinstating the Global Gag Rule, to banning "partial-birth abortions," to trying to take possession of the medical records of women who have had abortions using the drug mifepristone.[233] The Bush administration quietly removed information about condoms from the National Institutes for Health website and, through financing abstinence-only sex education programs, promotes misinformation about condoms not being safe or effective.[234] Many of these attacks are subtle enough that "without a lot of public knowledge, they are just moving things backward."[235] Beyond having an antichoice president and Congress, antichoice politicians have been successful on a state level as well. Rachel Atkins of Planned Parenthood points out, "A lot of the backslide on abortion has been at the state level. So if you still have antichoice legislators controlling the state legislations, it won't improve much."[236] Prochoice activists must garner support at every level of government to stem the tide of new legal restrictions on abortion.

Opportunities for Future Gains

One way in which the reproductive rights movement will, hopefully, continue to gain strength is by its greater inclusion of men. Jane White points to the need for men to be leaders in bringing other men to the movement. Remembering a civil rights protest at which a white man asked what he could do to help, White relates that the organizer told him to go to his own people and educate them. Women in the movement can support, financially and through volunteering, the few men's groups already existing, but men will be the most effective ones drawing other men into the movement.[237] Terry Daley emphasizes the need to get men more involved from an early age, when they are still children, by providing a solid education in sexual and reproductive health and rights, as well as a model of gender equality in the home.[238]

Few reproductive health programs currently exist that specifically target men, with a couple notable exceptions. The Young Men's Clinic in New York City has provided medical, social work, mental health, and health education services to adolescent and young adult men since 1987.[239] The clinic attempts to create a male-friendly atmosphere in which men can feel comfortable discussing family planning and STIs. Similarly, the Man2Man program in North

Central Philadelphia targets men for reproductive health education and services.[240] Recognizing the dearth of reproductive health and pregnancy prevention services available to young men, public health experts designed fifteen weekly, two-hour-long sessions delivered to groups of adolescent boys by an adult male facilitator. The program includes attention to personal development, life skills, fatherhood, relationships, and health and sexuality. Dorothy Roberts insists that as the movement makes connections between reproductive rights and broader social issues, more men will get involved. She points to the March for Women's Lives' outreach with the NAACP as evidence of this.[241] Drawing more men into the discussion on reproductive rights could considerably boost the strength of the movement.

Conclusion

Given the considerable wealth of the United States, it is inexcusable that such wide health disparities persist within the population. One's access to health care is largely dependent on socioeconomic level and geographic location rather than need, and the religious beliefs of those in control dictate to a large extent what reproductive health services and information are made available to women. The United States has the potential to provide comprehensive sex education, a wide range of contraceptives, and accessible abortion services to its population, but a myriad of political barriers stand in the way. During this time when conservatives dominate both national and state political bodies, it is incumbent on the reproductive rights movement to be more inclusive, drawing in people working on a broad range of social justice issues. Without more collaboration between activist organizations, the current political forces will continue to erode women's ability to exercise their reproductive freedom.

6

Vietnam

Background

With seventy-eight million people, Vietnam is the second most populous nation in Southeast Asia, and it is a country that has witnessed great changes in recent history.[1] In the past fifty years, Vietnam has moved from colonial rule to division into separate republics with differing political systems, and then to reunification under a socialist government. In the 1980s, the country implemented sweeping free-market reforms (*doi moi*).[2] Vietnam is an anomaly in the world of population and reproductive health; despite being an impoverished country with a mostly rural population and low education levels, Vietnam's reproductive health indicators are far better than those in countries of a comparable socioeconomic level. The gross national product per capita is just US$375, yet the country's maternal mortality rate is relatively low, at 100 deaths per 100,000 live births, and its infant mortality rate is only 18 deaths per 1,000 live births.[3] In the past thirty years, Vietnam has also experienced one of the fastest demographic transitions in the world, resulting in very low fertility rates.[4]

Yet despite its relatively favorable health indicators, the health status of Vietnamese people is far from ideal. Access to basic health services remains limited for segments of the population, particularly for the ethnic minorities living in mountainous areas. Sex education is only recently being integrated into the curriculum, though it still lacks comprehensive information about contraception and abortion. Women's contraceptive options have been limited since the onset of major family planning programs in the 1950s and 1960s; the IUD was practically the only modern contraceptive method available to women in some parts of the country until recently. Vietnam also has one of the highest abortion rates in the world; in a woman's lifetime, she will have an average of 2.5 abortions.[5] The government has historically been heavily involved in formulating and implementing strict population policies to guide the demographic changes of the country.

Vietnam's History of Population Policies

Vietnam ranks 151 out of 174 countries for gross national product per capita, and only 13 percent of the population is urban-dwelling.[6] Yet, unlike many other developing countries with largely rural populations, Vietnam's fertility rate is among the lowest in the world, at 1.9 children per woman—below replacement level.[7] This represents a rapid decline from a fertility rate of four children per woman as recently as 1987.[8] Demographers cite several factors involved in Vietnam's dramatic fertility decline, ranging from a relatively long history of family planning programs to the country's more recent, well-publicized population policy. Vietnam started its first family planning program in the early 1960s, well before most developing countries, and the government has consistently devoted substantial resources to its implementation. Many governmental and nongovernmental bodies, such as the Vietnam Family Planning Association (VINAFPA); the Committee on Population, Family, and Children (CPFC); and the Women's Union, have all tackled the issue of family planning together, working toward similar goals.[9] An intense information, education, and communication (IEC) campaign using mass media has always been a central component of the family planning program, particularly in regard to the use of the IUD and, to a lesser extent, the Pill and condoms.[10] Vietnam has also traditionally had a solid primary health care system, even during difficult economic times.

Perhaps the principal reason for the drop in fertility is Vietnam's adoption of a restrictive population policy in 1988, modeled on China's one-child policy but more lenient, allowing each family to have one or two children.[11] An amended version of the population policy is still in place today, and the policy has been very effective at lowering fertility rates nationwide. At the national level, the old population policy required each family to have no more than two children, but did not include specific fines or incentives. The government left such details to the district and commune levels to decide individually.[12] Local authorities enforced the population policy in various ways, often through fines ranging from 60 to 800 kilos of paddy rice per child born in excess of the policy's dictates (equivalent to one month to one year's worth of earnings), depending on the locality.[13] Likewise, women were offered bonuses ranging from 120 to 400 kilos of rice if they agreed to be permanently sterilized.[14]

During IUD insertion campaigns, village health workers received monetary bonuses for every IUD they inserted, and in some areas the local authorities read the names of married women with children who did not use IUDs over the loudspeaker system in the village, in an attempt to persuade them to join the campaign.[15] According to Dr. Vu Quy Nhan, director of research at the Population Council, the government delayed the salaries of its employees, including teachers and health providers, who did not follow the population policy and, in some cases, denied them promotions or even fired them.[16] Several large companies also adopted this practice. In an annual competition, the government awarded select companies the Labor Medal for their work promoting the population policy, and employers rewarded select female employees for "good realization of the population-family planning programme."[17]

Since this population policy was the subject of widespread criticism by international rights groups, the government has downplayed the system of fines and incentives that possibly propelled the policy forward. Dr. Nguyen Kim Cuc, formerly employed by the Ministry of Health and now vice president of VINAFPA, insists, "We only go to motivate them—not any punishment!"[18] When asked about the incentive system, she denies its recent use and vaguely refers to the use of incentives "maybe," in the 1960s and 1970s. Other professionals associated with the government express a similarly uncritical allegiance to the population policy. Do Thi Thanh Nhan of the Vietnam Women's Union (a governmental body) expresses, "We are very happy to see the major changes in our country, economically, socially, politically. It's thanks to the Party and state policies."[19]

Dr. Nguyen Kim Cuc claims that the population policy has generally been well accepted in urban areas but less popular in rural and mountainous areas, where people need a larger labor force for their agricultural lifestyles. Yet even in rural areas the demand for children is changing; since the economic reforms (*doi moi*) of the 1980s, the majority of Vietnamese have far less land than before. A major incentive for having many children in the past was the need for help on the family farm, but with less land allotted to each family, having fewer children is now more economically sound. Tine Gammeltoft, a medical anthropologist, argues that the drive to reduce fertility rates also came from below, from the communities, and not merely from the government in Hanoi:

> There [are] all these messages about having only one or two children but take really good care of them and invest really well in them—send them to school, give them good clothes. It just makes sense to people, that it's a way out of poverty. [. . .] The aspiration was already there, maybe, for

the small family, and then the government put it into policy and made it look like it was the government, but it wasn't only from the government. It came from below, too.[20]

Still, the need for fines and incentives to enforce the population policy demonstrates that it was not universally accepted.

Only in 2003 did the government abandon the one-or-two-child policy, though it continues to urge families to have a "responsible" number of children, promoting the message *mot hoac hai con* ("one or two children") and equating small families with happy families in their mass-media campaigns.[21]

Much ambiguity about the new policy remains at all levels of government.[22] Part of the confusion about the new policy stems from the government's own indecisiveness. After publishing an ordinance in May 2003 stating that people

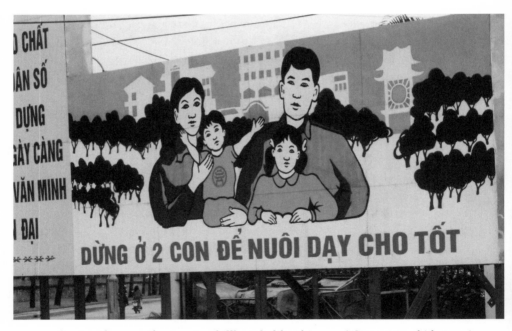

Scattered across the country, billboards like this one ("Stop at two kids to raise your children better") portray not only the government's efforts to encourage small families, but also its attempt to address son preference. Government-funded public health campaigns frequently display a happy family with one boy and one girl.

were free to have as many children as they desire, the government withdrew that statement and claimed that people are still required to limit the number of children they have, though a specific number is not given.[23] *Vietnam Population News*, a government publication, reported a Population Ordinance dated May 1, 2003, which declared that the old population policy was in effect and the new ordinance prohibits "communication and information dissemination that are against the population policy."[24] Another new policy excluded any fines or penalties for having more than two children.[25]

The impetus to change the population policy undoubtedly stemmed at least in part from the move toward a broader reproductive health perspective after the International Conference on Population and Development (ICPD), in which the emphasis of the population field shifted from demographics to human rights.[26] As Sita Michael Bormann of the United Nations Population Fund (UNFPA) in Vietnam explains, "The government realized that it's not possible to have a two-child policy while talking about reproductive rights."[27] This internal conflict of interests for the government, between its desire to stem population growth and its recent participation in dialogue about reproductive rights, contributes to the mixed messages sent to people about the current population policy.

Family planning "motivators" at the grassroots level have had difficulty explaining the new policy to the rural populations they serve.[28] Dr. Vu Quy Nhan of the Population Council explains, "At first, when the population policy changed, some people in rural areas began to say, 'We have no limitation!' They were used to getting clear messages about how many children to have, but now the government is trying to incorporate the ICPD idea that families can decide for themselves."[29] Many policy makers were initially apprehensive that, in the absence of a strict guideline from the government, families would choose to have many children. Sita Michael Bormann maintains,

> It takes awhile for people's mentality to change, though, and for people to not be afraid anymore of the consequences of having more than two children. We are a long way off from implementation of these ideas. But when people do understand the new policy, that they have more freedom to decide on these matters, we do not expect a sudden population explosion—we think people will still choose to have small families.

How, exactly, people are able to fulfill their wishes of having small families depends largely on their access to sex education, contraception, and abortion. Reproductive decisions are also heavily influenced by the country's cultural background and history with both Confucianism and communism.

Cultural Influences in Vietnam:
Confucianism and Communism

Vietnam's spiritual influences are often referred to as the "triple religion"—Confucianism, Taoism, and Buddhism.[30] Though perhaps not as ingrained in the culture as is the case in China, Confucian ideology has permeated Vietnamese culture for over one thousand years.[31] Central to Confucianism is the virtue of *li*, or hierarchical order. Five hierarchical relationships are particularly important in Confucianism: between ruler and minister, father and son, husband and wife, older and younger brother, and friend and friend. Swidler clarifies, "The essence of the relationship was that of superior-inferior."[32] Likewise, communism's emphasis on service to the state complements the Confucian principle of *li*.

The "success" of Vietnam's strict population policy is likely related in part to Vietnam's Confucian and communist influences. The communist structure of the government creates a powerful network of social control, particularly through the Women's Union, Farmer's Union, Youth Union, and mass media. The Women's Union receives all of its funding from the government and is charged with advocating for the general welfare of women. According to Sita Bormann Michael, the government is very efficient in delivering messages to the population, and the population is accustomed to taking those messages seriously.[33] Daniel Levitt of USAID echoes a similar sentiment, describing the effectiveness of the government's information system down to the commune level. "The chain of command is relatively clear and apparently respected. In disseminating guidance and protocol, Confucian influence comes out strongly. People generally follow directions and deviation is not encouraged."[34]

Vietnam's experience with Confucianism and communism has undoubtedly shaped the women's rights movement as well. Although Vietnam's early communist government discussed women's rights, Quach Thu Trang of Population Development International notes that the promotion of these rights was generally to serve the country rather than the individual. "For example, during the war time, gender issues were promoted to have more resources for fighting against enemies. Then during the time of country reconstruction, gender issues were mentioned aiming to have more resources for economic development."[35] Introducing the topic of women's rights for the sake of women themselves has not been easy in Vietnam. As Quach Thu Trang points out, "Human rights in general is a very new concept. It still seems foreign and strange." Introducing the concept of sexual and reproductive rights to Vietnam has been particularly difficult because the country has historically not spoken in the language of "rights" as most Westerners understand the term. Quach Thu Trang continues, "We've had years of strict communist culture, in which there hasn't been much emphasis on individual rights" beyond discussion of those rights to further the state's goals. Some scholars argue "Confucianism will [. . .] have to move to replace its human subordinationism with egalitarianism (while still recognizing the real differences in persons), especially with regard to women."[36] This "New Confucianism" attempts to move the traditional virtue of *li* away from its emphasis on hierarchy and instead focus on equality. The extent to which this transformation takes place will affect women's ability to control their own reproductive health and fertility.

Sex Education

Very little sex education is offered to Vietnamese children in school, and most of the information given focuses on anatomy and conception, but lacks details about how to prevent conception or how to avoid HIV/AIDS and other sexually transmitted infections (STIs). Only through IEC (information, education, communication) campaigns on television and in pamphlets do people obtain more complete reproductive health information, but this type of dissemination does not reach many adolescents and people living in mountainous areas, where televisions are scarce.[37] A written policy mandating sex education exists at the national level, but in reality there are few schools that include any sex education at all, though this seems to be slowly changing.[38] Even in those that do provide sex education, as Nina McCoy of Family Health International explains, "The whole emphasis is on responsibility—the teachers are terrified to talk about biology."[39] The government introduced "population education" into the curriculum in 1984, but information about STIs, family planning, pregnancy, and abortion was not included.[40] The Women's Union has done extensive work in promoting sex education, but their focus tends to be on encouraging abstinence and faithfulness rather than disseminating concrete information for sexually active teenagers.[41]

Women born in the 1950s knew very little about sex until after they were married; to speak of sexuality was like "committing a crime."[42] In traditional Vietnamese culture, women rarely discuss sexual matters, but this tradition does not accommodate the needs of young women today, who are under pressure to have sex to an extent they never have been before.[43] Professor Le Thi Nham Tuyet, director of the Research Center for Gender, Family, and Environment in Development (CGFED), notes that Vietnamese people today see myriad sexualized images in the mass media, yet they lack solid information about sexual and reproductive health.[44]

Though sex education is very limited in Vietnam, the situation seems to be slowly improving. Le Thi Nham Tuyet explains, "Years ago, the teachers and parents did not want to show children books about sex education, claiming that the books teach children how to go out and have sex. But now, they think it's necessary to give the materials to their children."[45] Still, many parents in both rural and urban areas refuse to discuss sex with their children, preferring that the information be provided in school. Nina McCoy recalls the sex education program spearheaded by the Red Cross:

> When the Red Cross started doing an assessment, they thought it would take hours and hours to convince the parents that their kids should get sex education in the schools. And they found that parents want the schools to do this! Not like in the U.S.—it's the other way around! It's the teachers who are not ready to do this. In the South, in some of the more rural and Catholic provinces, we ran into more opposition, but elsewhere it wasn't a problem. We never once had a parent pull their child out of the program here in the North. We had 10,000 kids go through that program. I think part of the success was because it was the Red Cross behind it, and they're run by seventy-year-olds, right there, and they loved it! They had never had any of this education either, in their entire lives! The program was designed for youth, but it ended up pulling in people from all ages.[46]

The Red Cross cleverly circumvented the resistance of teachers to implementing a sex education curriculum by utilizing another of the community's teaching sources—its own volunteers, who are mostly elderly women—to run the program. The Population Council implemented another creative program, in which they organized soccer teams for adolescent boys and included a teaching component about HIV/AIDS, sexuality, and contraception. The program successfully increased awareness of sexual health among the boys and decreased their negative attitudes toward people living with HIV/AIDS.[47]

Until recently, the government paid little attention to sexual health and sexual rights, and did not consider the subject a priority in primary or secondary education.[48] The national guidelines on reproductive health have traditionally ignored adolescents, and there are few places youth can go to get information and counseling related to their reproductive health.[49] Dr. Vu Quy Nhan estimates that about 70 percent of policy makers favor sex education, and 30 percent are against it; what form that education takes is a more complicated question.[50] Just in the past few years have the Ministry of Health and Ministry of Education and Training been willing to discuss the subject of sex education; both ministries are working with UNFPA and VINAFPA to pilot a sex education curriculum in a few provinces. UNFPA hopes to replicate the program throughout the country.[51] Even the sex education curriculum developed by UNFPA is not wholly comprehensive, however, focusing on biology and omitting sensitive topics like abortion.[52] The authors open the curriculum with conservative, "safe" topics, gradually expanding to more sensitive subjects. The curriculum includes demographics and issues related to "family life, how to be a good wife, then biology, family planning, sexuality."[53] Though the content has expanded since the program's inception, it remains incomplete, yet is still controversial.

The task of persuading provincial authorities to support sex education was formidable in the beginning of UNFPA's program, but health professionals have made progress convincing the community that adolescents need this vital information, particularly in the face of widespread myths about sex and in the presence of a growing HIV/AIDS epidemic.[54] Even once the curriculum is approved by local authorities, however, convincing the teachers to adopt the curriculum is a tremendous challenge. Teachers are reluctant to teach what is perceived as an embarrassing and awkward subject.[55] Scheduling problems also arise; Nina McCoy points out that "even if you get the teachers trained and excited to teach it, there's no time in the day—they are already cramming so much into their classes." Realizing the goal of a solid sex education curriculum will require structural adjustments in the education system as a whole to give the subject the space and resources it deserves.

Some sex education proponents argue that schools are not the most appropriate place for sex education. Particularly since *doi moi*, which opened up greater job opportunities for youth, more and more adolescents are dropping out of school to work.[56] Others argue that the subject material could be effectively delivered in the schools, but in a less embarrassing manner, if an outside party—a teacher specialized in sex education—visited the schools for that purpose only.[57] Such is the model at the Danish Family Planning Association's clinic in Copenhagen, Denmark.

Professor Le Thi Nham Tuyet emphasizes the need to develop educational materials suitable to a particular community's local culture and lifestyle. Given the diversity of Vietnam's population, from the mountainous to coastal regions, and the differences in age of marriage and fertility rates, CGFED is conducting a study of the traditional customs of people in different parts of the country, hoping to integrate traditional values into the new sex education curricula. "Otherwise, it is a waste of money, to get materials to them that don't fit the people there. They live in different conditions and should have different materials."[58] A curriculum designed with an affluent, urban Kinh population in mind may be of little relevance to a poor, rural, Hmong community.

Access to Health Services and Contraception

Even if comprehensive sex education becomes available to the Vietnamese population, a substantial barrier to reproductive health exists: access to health services and contraception. Health conditions and access to health care in Vietnam vary tremendously between urban and rural areas. Nguyen Thi Bich Hang, country representative of Marie Stopes International (MSI), reports that in one province where MSI works, 70 to 80 percent of the women who receive MSI's services have symptoms of malnutrition and anemia. Many have five or six children, yet they have little access to even the most basic health services.[59] The estimated maternal mortality rate in the Central and Northern Highlands is three to four times the national average.[60] Though the government and international nongovernmental organizations (NGOs) have recently invested far more resources into the development of rural health centers than previously seen, much work remains to be done.[61] Awareness and knowledge of reproductive health issues remains low in remote areas, which is particularly dangerous since HIV infections have been reported in all sixty-one provinces of the country.[62] Reproductive tract infections (RTIs) are also extremely prevalent in mountainous areas, where the supply of water is limited and hygiene is inadequate; studies show that 20 to 70 percent of Vietnamese women have an RTI at any given time.[63] Dr. Nguyen Kim Cuc of the Vietnam Family Planning Association (VINAFPA) explains, "Women must work in the water [in rice paddies] all day long, even during menstruation, so the water is not clean and there are many gynecological problems." The situation has improved in recent years, partly due to the work of the Women's Union on improving access to gynecological exams and maternal care, but the wide disparities between rural and urban persist.[64] Of the twenty-five hundred women who die each year in Vietnam because of pregnancy and childbirth, 90 percent live in rural areas, and 90 percent die of preventable causes.[65]

Vietnam's health disparities are also strikingly split along ethnic lines. The country's majority ethnic group, the Kinh, enjoy higher health indicators than the fifty-three other ethnic groups—75 percent of whom live in the remote mountainous regions of the country.[66] Though some ethnic minority groups live in urban areas and enjoy the same access to health services as the

Kinh, others, like the Hmong, continue to live in remote areas and to deliver their babies at home, without medical assistance.[67] The infant mortality rates for the Gia-rai, Hmong, and other minorities are up to three times higher than the rates for the Kinh, and the Hmong's fertility rate is 7 children per woman, compared to the national average of 1.9.[68] Ethnic minorities make up just 14 percent of the population, yet they represent 30 percent of Vietnam's poor.[69] In the mountainous regions of Vietnam, only 9 percent of communes (counties) have a doctor, and not a single doctor lives in any of three mountainous provinces in the North (Lai Chau, Lao Cai, and Son La).[70] Given the size and rough terrain of the mountainous regions, even in those communes that have a health station, transportation to the center may require a full day of traveling. Upon reaching these remote health stations, people often find that none of the providers speak their language and all of the health materials are in Kinh. Few people in the ethnic minority population can speak Kinh, and even fewer are literate. The economic cost of traveling to the health center and obtaining services remains substantial.[71]

The government has recently approved several policies that recognize and support ethnic minorities. When the *doi moi* free-market reforms went into effect, health centers serving disadvantaged populations (mostly ethnic minorities) were exempted from the policy of charging user fees.[72] Ethnic minorities were allowed to have three children per couple under the old population policy, rather than two.[73] In 2002, 17 percent of representatives to the National Assembly were ethnic minorities, meaning that they have even greater representation in the government than in the general population.[74] Still, infrastructural and economic barriers have impeded the government's attempts to diminish health inequities in the country.

Nationwide, the quality of care in health centers is generally lacking. The majority of government hospitals in both rural and urban settings are overloaded with patients and understaffed, making adequate counseling difficult to provide. One development worker describes contraceptive counseling in Vietnam as "abysmal."[75] Inadequate counseling contributes to Vietnam's high rate of contraceptive discontinuation; if women are not counseled that they may temporarily have certain side effects while using the IUD or the Pill, they are more likely to discontinue use when they experience such side effects. Part of the problem stems from the population's reluctance to attend small health centers; people have more faith in the large hospitals and flock there for care, not realizing that basic family planning and reproductive health services are easily provided by well-trained nurses and midwives at the commune level.[76] Although national contraceptive prevalence is quite high, at 79 percent, this number ranges from 83 percent in the Red River Delta to just 66 precent in the Central Highlands.[77]

Public health centers supply roughly 90 percent of the modern contraceptives used in Vietnam.[78] As seen in other countries, the NGO sector in Vietnam has stepped in to try to compensate for the shortfalls of government health services. Marie Stopes International (MSI), with its eight clinics nationwide, is attempting to carve out a middle ground between the expensive private sector and the inadequate public sector, providing health services at prices comparable to those found in public health centers but with the perks that the private sector offers. MSI has created a sustainable model that is as cost efficient as the government health services, but with higher quality of care. Since 1989, MSI has been offering reproductive health services, including abortion, that emphasize comprehensive counseling, informed choices, and a high quality of care. The staff at MSI encourage an atmosphere in which clients are encouraged to ask their doctors questions—something that is not common in Vietnam.[79] A comparison between MSI's model and the government's health services—in terms of the level of counseling, the range of choices, and the amount of question-asking by patients—can provide a clue to the low quality of the government's health services.

Although there is no official policy that prohibits unmarried women from obtaining contraception, the reality is that adolescents have little access to contraception until they marry.[80] No official gynecological services exist for girls under eighteen years old, even though there are three hundred thousand deliveries and abortions each year to women of this age group.[81]

Contraception in Vietnam: Limited Choices

Beyond sex education and physical access to a health facility that provides contraception, people need a range of contraceptive options to attain optimal reproductive health and autonomy. For many years, the two main forms of birth control in Vietnam were the IUD and abortion.[82] Even today, the IUD is by far the most common modern method used, despite many women's physical intolerance for it. In 1994, Vietnam shared the highest IUD prevalence in the world with China and Cuba, with 33 percent of married women using one; by 2002, 38 percent of married women used the IUD.[83] When Vietnam started its family planning program in the 1960s, the IUD was the only contraceptive method offered, and this situation remained unchanged throughout the economically difficult, postwar years in the 1970s.[84] Only in recent years have other methods become readily available, but a 2000 study showed that just 39 percent of family planning clients were counseled about more than one contraceptive option during their visit to the health center.[85]

The reasons for Vietnam's continued high IUD use are numerous. The IUD has the advantage of anonymity: "A woman with an IUD can still appear 'normal' [having periods], as if she were not using contraception."[86] A forty-year history of heavy IUD use has also created a habit difficult to break, even if the IUD is not the most suitable method for many women. The biases of health providers themselves are most likely the greatest influence on high IUD usage. Numerous studies have found that provider bias is strong; providers prefer the IUD to the Pill, partly due to a lack of faith that women will remember to take the Pill every day. Nguyen Kim Cuc of VINAFPA, a provider herself, relates:

> The government only buys the IUD, and when the IUD is inserted in the uterus and [the woman] can't get pregnant, it's easier for the people because their education is limited and they don't understand anything. They want to have any contraception but they don't do anything every day—it is easier for them and they like to get the IUD.

The fact that informing and educating women is not always a priority for providers is itself a barrier to reproductive autonomy, since women are not given the tools to think of themselves as in control in the first place. Providers also favor the IUD because of a strong population control agenda. As a result of the country's population policy, providers had financial incentives to insert IUDs, but none to prescribe the Pill or condoms.[87] The government has favored this long-term, provider-controlled method for the realization of its demographic goals, often paying little attention to contraindications for IUD use, such as the presence of a reproductive tract infection.[88]

Negotiating condom use within a marriage is an improbable option for most women; the spread of HIV/AIDS among monogamous wives of migrant workers is testament to this sad fact. Since the government's promotion of condom use has only been in relation to HIV/AIDS prevention, most men associate condoms with one-night stands or casual relationships; condoms are seen as useful for disease prevention, but not for contraception (which makes it difficult for women to request their use).[89] Most men believe that condoms reduce sexual pleasure as well, and few men use them, even though condoms are rather inexpensive, at 200 dong apiece (roughly equivalent to US$0.12). Although the Women's Union has tried to socially market condoms to men, emphasizing men's responsibility in pregnancy and STI prevention, the method remains quite unpopular.[90]

The perception of condoms as a method only for casual partners, along with men's reluctance to use them, leaves women with few options. As Tine Gammeltoft asks, "What's left, if the provider advises you not to use the Pill, and if your husband refuses to use a condom?"[91] Yet another reason for the IUD's popularity above all other methods is the fear of hormones and the idea that Western medicine is dangerous, particularly when taken regularly. "The Pill and Depo Provera are considered medicine. So then you have no choice but the IUD and abortion as a back-up."[92]

Nevertheless, the Pill and condoms are slowly gaining popularity in rural areas, particularly with the spread of HIV/AIDS, though as of yet there is little information known about the methods and myths abound.[93] Many women prefer the Pill because of the ease with which they can start and stop taking it without the help of a health provider, in contrast to IUD insertion and removal.[94] The government exercises strict control over what contraceptives are available in Vietnam, often refusing to import contraceptive methods that are approved in other countries. For example, only three-month injectables are currently available in Vietnam, even though many women prefer one-month injectables because they are associated with fewer side effects.[95]

Unlike in many other countries, religious influences in Vietnam generally do not present an obstacle to women obtaining contraception. The majority of the Vietnamese population is Buddhist—a religion that does not forbid contraception. The Catholic population may feel pressure to abstain from abortion, but they usually do not object to use of the IUD.[96] Those women who choose to use traditional birth control methods for religious or personal reasons comprise 20 percent of family planning users, but they receive very little, if any, information about withdrawal and the rhythm method in public health sectors.[97] Counseling and support for women using traditional methods should be integrated into the family planning program to help these women control their fertility in the way they choose. Emergency contraception is technically legal in Vietnam, but it is not very accessible and few people are aware of it.[98]

Abortion

Vietnam has consistently had the highest abortion rate in the world, tied with Cuba and Romania, with a lifetime total abortion rate (TAR) of 2.5 abortions per woman, according to studies in 1992 and 1994.[99] Though abortion statistics vary, an estimated 800,000 to 1.4 million abortions occur each year in Vietnam.[100] A UNFPA report documents that 40 percent of all pregnancies in Vietnam end in abortion.[101] Abortion only became a crime in Vietnam during

French colonial times and was legalized again in the 1945 constitution, though the procedure did not become widely available until the 1960s.[102] Physicians, physician assistants, and trained midwives can all legally perform abortions.[103] While the government has not openly promoted the use of abortion as birth control, its policies have certainly encouraged the practice by limiting access to alternative contraceptive methods while simultaneously making legal abortion accessible and inexpensive. Le Thi Nham Tuyet argues that Vietnam's drastic drop in fertility is not good news, as it is treated, but is rather an indication of the rising rates of abortion among adolescents.[104] Ironically, abortion is more accessible to adolescents than contraception is, in terms of finances and physical access to providers, according to Drs. Nguyen Kim Cuc and Nguyen Thi Hoai Duc.[105]

Despite the large number of abortions in Vietnam, or perhaps because of it, Vietnam has been fortunate to avoid the massive mortality and morbidity (illness) often associated with abortion in developing countries. Since the inception of the family planning program in the early 1960s, there have been few contraceptive options available; indeed, in the early years, "there was basically the IUD, with abortion as a back-up."[106] Because abortion has been legal in Vietnam for decades, medical professionals in the public sector have performed the vast majority of abortions, and with few complications. Access to abortion has greatly improved since the 1960s; when abortion was first legalized, shortly after the country's independence, a woman needed a letter of demand signed by her husband, in addition to a letter of approval by the head of the village. Today, regardless of a woman's marital status, no additional consent beyond her own is needed for the procedure.[107]

Vietnam's high abortion rate partially stems from inadequate sex education but it also results from women being highly encouraged to use the IUD, even though it is not the most appropriate method for everyone. One study of IUD users found that nearly half of them report that the IUD decreases their ability to work, which is particularly notable considering the importance of farming and providing for one's family.[108] There is a widespread belief that the Western-made IUD is too "big" for Vietnamese women, and that it causes weakness and fatigue.[109] Women who cannot tolerate the IUD or choose not to use it are left with few viable options for contraception. The low use of other modern contraceptive methods, coupled with the prevalence of less effective, traditional methods like withdrawal, leads to a high number of unwanted pregnancies.[110]

The fact that the previous population policy offered health providers financial incentives to perform abortions (and to insert IUDs) also undoubtedly contributed to high abortion rates.[111] There has historically been very little postabortion contraception counseling, which leads to repeat abortions; one study found that of the women having abortions in the public health sector, nearly half had already had at least one prior abortion.[112] The quality of abortion services in general is quite low; a 2000 study found that in many health centers gloves and instruments were not properly disinfected, and a substantial portion of health providers did not wash their hands between patients. Almost one-third of providers performed abortions with contaminated gloves, and another 5 percent without any gloves. Only 10 percent of providers explained what they were doing before starting a pelvic exam. These findings are particularly troubling given the fact that these providers were aware of the study and knew they were being observed.[113] Another study found that one-third of abortion patients did not receive any contraception counseling whatsoever.[114]

In an attempt to address these problems, the Ford Foundation has funded the Comprehensive Abortion Care program (CAC), with technical assistance from Ipas, an international reproductive rights organization. The Ministry of Health and the Institute for the Protection of the Mother and Newborn (IPMN) have cooperated in implementing CAC, which includes training providers in improved techniques for first- and second-trimester abortion, counseling, infection prevention, and monitoring of services. According to Lisa Messersmith of the Ford Foundation, the CAC program is "revolutionizing the way abortions are performed in Vietnam," raising the standards of care in clinics throughout the country.[115] In the last five years, the Ministry of Health and other policy makers have recognized that abortion can be harmful to a woman's health; more resources are now being directed to prevent abortion via increased education and access to contraception.[116]

Abortion in Vietnam is not necessarily stigmatized, but it remains a sensitive topic. Tine Gammeltoft conducted a reproductive health survey of four hundred women, and only twenty-eight women responded to the sole question that was about abortion. "The rest just didn't answer—didn't answer anything. So that tells a little about how sensitive it is, and how uncomfortable many women feel having to undergo those abortions."[117] Abortion may be stigmatized among adolescent girls; if a teenage girl gets pregnant, her parents and members of the community would probably be angry because of taboos against premarital sex, according to Dr. Nguyen Kim Cuc. But if a married couple has an unwanted pregnancy, the woman would not be looked down upon for having an abortion. The stigma of abortion seems to be less of a societal issue and more one of personal guilt. An old saying that refers to the psychological stress of abortion states, "One abortion is like three deliveries."[118]

Women will almost certainly choose to have an abortion in the case of a fetal diagnosis that is anomalous. If the anomaly is related to the baby's extremities, a couple may choose to continue the pregnancy, but "if something is wrong with the head, it's very unacceptable."[119]

In the Vietnamese language, a clear distinction exists between "menstrual regulation" (an abortion performed in the first six weeks of pregnancy) and abortion (performed after six weeks). In the case of "menstrual regulation," one word used to describe the embryo is "bean seed," whereas the word for abortion literally means "sucking out the fetus."[120] Since many menstrual regulations are done within days of a woman missing her period, without confirmation of pregnancy, it is possible that many abortions done in Vietnam are for women who are not even pregnant. Approximately 45 to 60 percent of abortions in Vietnam are menstrual regulations.[121] Many women believe that using the rhythm or withdrawal method with menstrual regulation as a backup is better for their health than using the IUD or the Pill, given the perception in some areas of modern contraception being dangerous.[122] As the availability of medical abortion grows, a woman's ability to "regulate" her period will become even easier. Preliminary studies show that women prefer the method for its greater privacy, as well as the fact that they can avoid physical contact with a physician.[123] Currently, the Ministry of Health has only approved the use of medical abortion at a few selected hospitals, but in reality, the necessary drugs are available directly from pharmacists.[124]

Although the Vietnamese government has been chastised, with just cause, for its excessive focus on abortion as a population control method while neglecting women's total reproductive health needs, it is true that Vietnam has established a system whereby women have a right to choose whether or not to have a baby. Lisa Messersmith reminds us, "Vietnam needs to be praised for maintaining and securing that right for women. Asia in general is not very open to reproductive rights like abortion. [. . .] Vietnam has [been] and can play an incredible role in the region for advancing women's right to terminate a pregnancy she doesn't want."[125] Abortion is quite accessible and affordable, and Vietnam deserves recognition for this achievement, even if the government has had less than ideal motives in the past.

Son Preference

Preference for sons remains strong in Vietnam and is a major cause of continued high fertility in some areas; one study estimates that the total fertility rate would drop by 10 percent in the absence of son preference.[126] Most families with more than two children are families who had two daughters and continued bearing children until a boy was born. Women are generally under tremendous pressure from their in-laws and husband to produce a son.[127] If a woman does not give birth to a son, her husband may marry a second wife. In 1996, local courts saw 49,711 divorce cases, of which 17.5 percent were related to a couple's inability to bear a boy; having a son is therefore a kind of insurance against polygamy and divorce.[128] A woman who does not bear a son may be disgraced with the label *khong biet de*, or "unable to give birth."[129]

By tradition, girls leave the house when they get married and are not considered long-term members of the family.[130] A traditional Vietnamese saying is "A family with ten daughters has no children."[131] In the absence of sons, familial privileges and obligations fall to a paternal nephew rather than to a daughter.[132] Mothers often breastfeed sons longer than daughters, and girls do not have equal access to education or health care as they grow up.[133] Nationally, 29 percent of boys fifteen to nineteen years old are in school, compared to 20 percent of girls.[134] Son preference varies by location, however, with some urban-dwellers discarding the tradition.[135] In most rural areas, families want at least one son, and preferably two. Son preference also varies by occupation; as Dr. Vu Quy Nhan points out, fishermen rely on other men for labor, and thus have a difficult time accepting daughters.[136] An answer to son preference, Dr. Nhan suggests, includes introducing other kinds of work in which daughters can bring income to the family, like work in a factory that produces handicrafts.[137]

Abortion based on the sex of the fetus is illegal in Vietnam, though there is speculation that it does occur, however infrequently. The 1989 and 1999 censuses in Hanoi and Ho Chi Minh City show no altered sex ratio at birth, unlike reports from China and India, but Vietnam is the only Southeast Asian country with a higher five-year mortality rate for girls than for boys.[138] Though the government has actively tried to alter the preference for sons through mass-media campaigns that show happy families, each with one daughter and one son, cultural traditions are slow to change. Rumors about how to conceive a boy abound: "Take iodine to get a boy, have intercourse on this day to get a boy."[139] Women commonly obtain an ultrasound during their pregnancy for the specific purpose of knowing the sex of their baby, not in order to have an abortion if the child is male, but so they may mentally prepare themselves for the birth. Anthropologist Tine Gammeltoft notices that women are quick to deny wanting to know the sex of their baby, even when that is their sole motivation for obtaining the ultrasound.[140]

The HIV/AIDS Epidemic

Vietnam's HIV/AIDS epidemic is just now gaining momentum, and the government's overall response to the epidemic has been disappointing. The first case of HIV was detected in Vietnam in 1991, and its prevalence doubled every year between 1994 and 2000; today there are an estimated 160,000 people living with HIV/AIDS.[141] By the late 1990s, the government was under pressure from international organizations to be proactive about HIV.[142] The government established the National AIDS Bureau, separate from the Ministry of Health, with branches at every level of government, down to the provincial level. Such an approach has proven effective in numerous countries, but, shortly after establishment of the bureau, the government merged the National AIDS Bureau with the "social evils" campaign. The AIDS committee is now housed within the Ministry for Prevention of Prostitution, Drugs, and Social Evils. In the minds of many Vietnamese, HIV/AIDS is not *linked* to the "social evils"; it *is* a social evil. The government has played a large role in perpetuating this idea. Daniel Levitt notes, "Beginning in the mid-nineties, the government imposed a mass-media campaign that linked HIV/AIDS with sex work, drug use, and death, incorporating graphic images that tend to stick in people's minds with strong associations. It is only recently that the central government has taken initial steps to de-link HIV from so-called 'social evils,' but the imagery remains on many streets throughout the country."[143] The campaign has had terrible effects on people living with HIV, many of whom are isolated from their communities and even from their families.[144]

Interlacing HIV prevention with the "social evils" campaign has been disastrous; not only does it heighten the stigma against HIV-positive people, but the legal ramifications have impeded much needed prevention work. Family Health International has faced difficulty with their prevention programs in which community members distribute condoms. "The anti–social evils campaign interferes with the implementation of these projects because possession of many condoms can lead to the person's arrest. The social evils campaign can also force sex work into more hidden and unsafe environments."[145] In a country where possessing large numbers of condoms is a crime, efforts to control a growing HIV epidemic are constrained, to say the least.

Commenting on the lumping together of prostitution, drug use, and HIV/AIDS, Nina McCoy of Family Health International points out, "They're not wrong that these things are associated—of course they are!—but not solely, and it's not because it's evil, it's because it's a problem." McCoy notes that the epidemic is still concentrated enough among drug users and sex workers in the major cities that the greater population can continue to ignore it. Yet the epidemic is quickly becoming generalized, with rising infection rates among adolescents, and once the upper class is affected, McCoy believes, the population will wake up.[146] Most donors are only focusing on the concentrated epidemic, targeting the most vulnerable and marginalized populations, such as drug users, but in doing so, they ignore the general population, which is also at risk. McCoy criticizes many donors' vertical approach to HIV/AIDS work, separating it from their work on poverty alleviation, despite the interconnected nature of the issues.

At the time of the government's backslide in HIV/AIDS prevention and control, both UNAIDS and UNDP had weak leadership, according to McCoy, and the international NGOs were not strong enough in their protestations. Now, after much criticism, the government is slowly changing its tactic, pouring more resources into HIV prevention and reframing the issue. McCoy notes, "They essentially lost four years to work on the epidemic, and that means they lost their window. There were only 5,000 tested cases then, and now it's [sic] 80,000 tested cases, which realistically means 250,000 people infected." Today the government is backpedaling and attempting to minimize the stigma of HIV, though the AIDS committee remains linked to the social evils campaign. Daniel Levitt of USAID reports,

> There are studies that focus on HIV stigma and discrimination that have found that even when people's knowledge levels of HIV are high, and they have a solid understanding of its modes of transmission, they may still refuse to patronize a café that is attended by someone who is HIV-positive, for fear of transmission through a teacup. In some communities in Vietnam, they will not allow someone who has died of AIDS to be buried in a community cemetery. Some people in the Office of Government, National Assembly, and Ministry of Health are making the effort to change public perceptions of people living with HIV/AIDS, by shaking the hands of HIV-positive people, and by visiting hospitals and clinics, trying to lessen the stigma attached to HIV, but it's quite difficult to market [. . .] HIV/AIDS warning messages that simultaneously support people living with HIV/AIDS. It's no easy task, and the stigma still remains, often most manifest in the health sector.[147]

Tine Gammeltoft adds, "It is actually changing—you can see in the street, there are posters and it probably doesn't change much, but just the fact that they're there—'Don't avoid people with HIV' and things like that. Which of course doesn't work, but it's a sign at least that the government is going in other ways."[148] The government's shifting position appears inadequate to stem the rising tide of the epidemic, however.

Vietnam's near future with HIV/AIDS looks grim; prevention efforts have been too small and too late. Although USAID markets condoms in Vietnam and has donated over twenty million to date, condoms are still an unpopular method.[149] A widely accepted motto is that love and trust translate to unprotected sex.[150] The Vietnamese government and donors must be more proactive in educating the population about HIV/AIDS and fully supporting both prevention and treatment programs.

Men's Involvement in Reproductive Health Issues

Asked what the largest obstacle is to reproductive rights, many professionals in the field felt that Vietnam's male-dominated society was the answer. Levitt relates,

> As you leave urban centers in Vietnam, education levels drop dramatically and there's a marked gender differential between men's and women's education levels and literacy. [. . .] While one doesn't need an education to make healthy choices about contraception [. . .], it certainly helps, as most demographic transitions have shown. Additionally, if a family has two children, one boy and one girl, and can only send one to school, the boy will go and the girl will not.

Men's involvement in women's health in Vietnam is complex; on the one hand, men are often the decision-makers of the family, even when it comes to family planning and reproductive health. Yet, on the other hand, some men consider family planning to be "women's business" and completely withdraw from the decision-making process. Particularly in rural areas, there is the deep-rooted cultural belief that family planning is a women's responsibility, as evidenced by the high rates of tubal ligation compared to vasectomy (5.9% and 0.5% of the population, respectively).[151] Women state that they want to endure the "painful" experience of sterilization to save their husbands from it, even though vasectomy is a much simpler procedure. Myths about vasectomies abound, such as the idea that a man will lose his sexual libido or become dull or stupid after being sterilized.[152]

Quach Thu Trang of Population Development International (PDI) points out that many development organizations perpetuate the idea of reproduction as solely a woman's domain by not involving men in their reproductive health activities. The Women's Union is the only sponsor of most reproductive health-related events—not the Farmer's Union or the Youth Union, even though the involvement of the latter two groups would bring more men into the discussion. Quach Thu Trang explains, "We just focus on the women and bring them all the training and information, and the whole audience is women, so automatically the men think that this is not their task, their duty, and [our] way of approaching [it] also supports their thinking." Population Development International has tried to collaborate with the Farmer's Union and Health Department to counteract this phenomenon. They also encourage the women in their programs to share the information they learn with their husbands.

In the name of women's "empowerment," men tend to have no or very little involvement in reproductive health matters. If a woman gets pregnant and she already has two or three children, she may go get an abortion without even discussing it with her husband, informing him of her decision later. This means that she carries the full burden, and he is left out of the picture entirely. Men very rarely accompany their wives to the family planning clinics—they see family planning as the woman's domain, especially if they have not yet had the two or three children that they want.[153] Studies have revealed that some men think abortion is an excellent contraceptive, and they assure their partners, "I will help you if you get pregnant," meaning they will pay for the abortion.[154] Some men prefer to use abortion as contraception rather than using a condom.[155] Men are not always indifferent about abortion, however; some studies show that men are genuinely concerned about the toll an abortion takes on their partners.[156]

Tine Gammeltoft conducted a study of women who received an anomalous fetal diagnosis during their pregnancy. The study revealed that, in these situations, the decision about whether or not to terminate the pregnancy is often made by male elders in the family or community. "Hanoi is a bit different, but as soon as you get ten kilometers outside of Hanoi, the decision is made by male elders, not by the woman, not even by the husband. The father-in-law [makes the decision], or maybe the two fathers-in-law together, so the two families agree, but the woman herself is not the primary decision-maker."[157]

In the past several years, reproductive health organizations have become more adept at targeting men, realizing that they may be the ones making reproductive health-related decisions. How, exactly, to get men more involved is a complicated question. Many professionals in the field recommend getting men involved as early as possible, from the time they are students and first become sexually active.[158] Levitt suggests finding "agents of change"—people who can be leaders. "You have to locate inspirational men who have influence in their community or among their peers. What has worked with respect to the HIV epidemic? Many people point to the leadership in Uganda, noting that it was effective to see the president himself talking about HIV/AIDS, safe practices, and support for positive people on public television."

Sita Michael Bormann notes the rapidity with which public dialogue has moved from beginning to discuss women's rights to discussing men's involvement. "In most countries, that progression is spread out over decades—people begin talking about women's rights, then gender, and then men's involvement. Here, it has happened so quickly; talking about men doesn't make sense to a lot of people who are just starting to think about women—it's like it's contradictory." Research on men's involvement in reproductive health is just beginning. Likewise, though domestic violence and alcoholism are common in Vietnam, they have not been well researched and not much is known about their effects on women's reproductive health.

Influence of the ICPD on Vietnam

The 1994 International Conference on Population and Development in Cairo had a tangible impact on Vietnam; the country has since begun to slowly move away from coercive population control policies toward a more holistic reproductive health-based approach that includes attention to reproductive tract infections (RTIs), infertility, and maternal and child health. The government has started to loosen its strict prohibitions on new contraceptives coming into the country, and there is more focus now on adolescent sexual and reproductive health.[159] The sentiments of the ICPD's Program of Action are, for the most part, well reflected in Vietnamese national policies today. Sita Michael Bormann explains, "Now we are in a long period of pushing the government to follow through on what they've signed [ICPD, Beijing Declaration on Women]."

Many professionals in the field argue, however, that the changes since the ICPD have come late and remain superficial. The National Committee on Population and Family Planning (NCPFP) changed its name to the Committee on Population, Family, and Children (CPFC), but the committee's emphasis remains disproportionately centered on population control. Though there is now more focus on other reproductive health issues than before, the concept of reproductive rights is difficult to find in official documents.[160] The "mobile IUD insertion teams" have been renamed "mobile family planning teams," though, as discussed earlier, few contraceptive methods are available other than the IUD.[161] Even as late as 1998, the leading headline of *Population-Family Planning News* (published by the NCPFP) read "Population Control Results Promising."[162] Despite the fact that the ICPD particularly discouraged quotas or demographic targets, Vietnam's Population Strategy 2001–2010 reads, under Implementation, Stage 1 (2001–2005): "Every effort will be made to achieve firmly sustainable fertility reduction, especially in areas with high fertility, in order to reach replacement fertility [2.1 children per woman] for the country as a whole by 2005 at the latest."[163] If a national government publication includes a statement that runs so counter to the ICPD's declarations, then it is likely the sentiments of the conference are not deeply felt at local levels of government.

The effects of the ICPD have not filtered down to an implementation level in many parts of the country, though Gammeltoft insists that the commitment to the ICPD is in many ways sincere. "This emphasis on the family, and on children, is sincere enough. People understand that it's the future, and to invest in the future you have to invest in the children. [. . .] It's not just for the donors."[164] Still, the shift from a strict one-or-two-child population policy with clearly delineated fertility goals to a more comprehensive vision of reproductive health and rights will take years to materialize.

Other International Influences on Vietnam

Several major international organizations have a strong presence in Vietnam, where they are visible for their work on reproductive health. These organizations include UNICEF, UNFPA, WHO, AusAID, the World Bank, the Asian Development Bank (ADB), Japan International Cooperation Agency (JICA), Pathfinder International, and Save the Children, to name a few.[165] As is the case in most developing countries, the politics of donors inevitably influence the activities of local NGOs. The donors control the funding, "So people tend to say what the donors want them to say, and then they [the NGOs] still do what they want for the most part. They use the donor-speak and know what is the right way to talk about things."[166] A major obstacle to progress mentioned by several development workers is donors' refusal to replicate projects. Though there are dozens of successful pilot projects conducted by both local NGOs and the government, they are seldom replicated because the donors "want to be funding something new, something 'cutting edge.' "[167]

Relatively speaking, U.S. politics do not influence reproductive health in Vietnam as much as in other developing countries, largely because USAID does not fund any reproductive health activities in Vietnam, with the exception of Safe Motherhood projects and HIV/AIDS work.[168] Why exactly USAID has decided to bypass Vietnam in its reproductive health work is unclear, though a few hypotheses circulate. One interviewee thought USAID might not be involved in Vietnam because of their perception of abortion practices in the country.[169] Another speculated that it could be from a misreading of the statistics. "Nationally, Vietnam looks pretty good, but when you get down to the provincial level, you get some stats that look like sub-Saharan Africa numbers, especially in the Central Highlands and Northern mountainous regions."[170] Yet another hypothesis is that the U.S. government pulled out of reproductive health work in the early 1990s following ethically questionable studies conducted in Vietnam using the potentially carcinogenic chemical quinacrine to sterilize women. Fifty thousand women were sterilized by inserting quinacrine hydrochloride pellets into their uteruses, causing inflammation and scarring sufficient to permanently block the fallopian tubes.[171] Whether or not USAID was involved in these studies is uncertain, but regardless, the agency may have abandoned reproductive health in order to avoid being associated with any reproductive health-related abuses. Now there is a general feeling among donors that countries in Southeast Asia have family planning under control. Daniel Levitt points out, "While HIV funds are as much as quadrupling, MCH [maternal and child health] funding has remained stagnant, or even dropped in some places."[172]

U.S. politics do influence Vietnam in the form of the Global Gag Rule and President Bush's refusal to pay dues to the United Nations. The latter decision resulted in a substantial budget cut for the United Nations Population Fund (UNFPA), though the Dutch embassy in Vietnam stepped in and offered to partially compensate for the loss.[173] In the past few years, organizations receiving funding from the United States have also been under pressure neither to support certain interventions focused on commercial sex workers, nor even to implement harm reduction programs with drug users, like needle exchanges and promoting condom use. As Levitt points out, "There is a great deal of debate in America and among aid workers about whether or not these regulations are based on public health best practices or the politics of dogma. Unfortunately, current evidence is not always at the forefront [of policy-making]."

The "Nongovernmental" Sector

The lack of a true nongovernmental sector in Vietnam is troubling and inhibits the full progress of the reproductive rights movement. Nongovernmental organizations (NGOs) were banned until the early 1990s, and even then they were only allowed as research institutions. The Research Center for Gender, Family, and Environment in Development (CGFED) was one of the first such institutions, and it remains one of the few "independent" NGOs today; unlike the majority of NGOs, CGFED was not established by retired government officials. In contrast, the Reproductive and Family Health Center (RaFH) was founded by Dr. Nguyen Thi Hoai Duc, who worked at the governmental Institute for the Protection of the Mother and Newborn for thirty years, then worked directly for the Ministry of Health, and then retired to set up RaFH.[174] Likewise, the vice president of VINAFPA retired from the Women's Union and was invited to her current position by the chairwoman of the governmental Committee on Population and Family Planning.[175] Many development workers interviewed emphasize that they would not call the NGOs "nongovernmental" organizations as much as "local" organizations.[176]

Lisa Messersmith notes that one of the greatest challenges the reproductive rights movement faces is "the lack of a legal framework that allows for independent nongovernmental organizations to become advocates for change." Strict legal regulations on nongovernmental organizations impede the development of any social movements outside the rubric of governmental bodies, such as the Women's Union. The approval process for NGOs is a long and frustrating one, full of confusing rules based on a 1957 law. Several respondents noted the difficulty that NGOs face if they do not have the support of the government. With the highly organized and effective system of government, NGOs that are not approved will encounter obstacles at every level of government, down to the commune level.

Even though the government controls NGOs and must approve of all their programs, local organizations are still in a position to conduct projects that the government never would. Tine Gammeltoft points to Le Thi Nham Tuyet of CG-FED: "[S]he's saying things that the government could never, ever say [. . .]. She can say things that are not on the government line."[177] Though development workers in NGOs must be careful in their conduct, they do have more freedom than government officials to express opinions that do not perfectly match those of the government.

The Vietnamese government seems to be slowly loosening its regulations as it becomes more secure. Since Renovation (*doi moi*, in 1986), the government has made drastic changes. The law that outlines the process for NGO approval is slated to be rewritten by 2007, which will hopefully open up the process to larger numbers of ordinary citizens who are not affiliated with the government.[178] In the past five years, the government has allowed more open debates about issues surrounding gender equity, and the National Assembly debates are now televised to the public.[179] Even with these signs of openness, however, it will take a long time for this government, so accustomed to a high level of power, to relinquish any significant amount of control to a truly nongovernmental sector.

Feminism and the Reproductive Rights Movement in Vietnam

Vietnam has a notable history of strong, independent women in the public sphere, particularly in comparison to some neighboring Asian countries, like China. Throughout the Nguyen Dynasty and French colonial rule, women were able to inherit property, which led to their relatively higher social status compared to women in most other Confucian societies.[180] The 1945 constitution stipulates, "Women are equal to men in all respects," and calls for paid maternity leave and equal pay between the sexes for equal work.[181] "Vietnamese myth, legend, and history are full of stories of strong and brave women," for example, the famous Trung sisters, who led a revolt against Chinese invaders in 43 B.C..[182] Vietnam's history also includes indigenous matriarchal cultures that existed centuries ago.[183] In the past few decades, women have made their mark on the national level, now filling leadership and political roles; an impressive 27 percent of members of the National Assembly are women (compared to 15% women in the U.S. Congress), and, as of 2004, Vietnam had a female vice president and five female ministers.[184] The Women's Union has been at the forefront of the women's movement in Vietnam, conducting gender awareness workshops and trainings. Vietnamese women have also been involved in local organizations that advocate for women's rights.

However, as several women's rights activists point out, the representation of women in powerful positions rapidly declines as one moves down to the provincial and commune levels, let alone in the home.[185] On the surface, gender equality in Vietnam looks impressive, but upon closer scrutiny, one sees that men dominate in sensitive situations, as in relation to sexuality. Women are not often in a position to negotiate on equal terrain how many children they have or when and under what circumstances they have sex (which is particularly important in HIV, STI, and pregnancy prevention).[186] Women may be able to raise their voices politically through the Women's Union, but whether or not community leaders respect their voices is another issue.[187] Despite a constitutional guarantee of equal pay for equal work, jobs have become increasingly segregated in Vietnam since the economic reforms, and women employees do not earn as much as their male counterparts.[188] Women working in the health field, for example, make an average of 350,000 dong per month, compared to the salary of 500,000 dong per month that men in the health field make.[189] The preference for sons, as well as the preferential treatment that sons receive in terms of health care and education, is one "symptom of inequality."[190] Population Development International (PDI), an NGO working in Vietnam, has designed projects that combine work in family planning, income generation, agriculture, protection of the environment, and credit and savings projects. As Quach Thu Trang, reproductive health program officer at PDI, explains,

> We like to have an intervention on different factors, because if we just provide women with knowledge or information on reproductive health, but they have no power or no financial [means] to make decisions, [they cannot go far.] If women could contribute to the family income in a more substantial way, they could claim a louder voice in the family for the right to make health care decisions.

Most women currently rely on their husbands for their economic subsistence, which, along with social and cultural factors, contributes to their position of limited power to make decisions for the family.

The Women's Union, in its portrayal of women's role in society, outlines five "duties" of women: keeping the family happy and harmonious, keeping the children healthy and well-behaved, remaining active in study, participating in the economy, and participating in community activities. Quach Thu Trang criticizes this vision: "We expect too much of women—how can they do all that at once?" Though women have entered the workforce in the past few decades in numbers never seen before, they are expected to carry out their jobs in addition to the full-time work of maintaining their families and homes. One of the largest challenges that the women's movement in Vietnam faces is the fact that women are not aware of their own rights. When asked about women's rights, "They say things like they have the right to take care of their family—but that's not the right that's being threatened!"[191] Likewise, women in rural areas who have very little access to health care report high levels of contentment in health surveys, despite the low quality of care offered to them. Part of the reason for this may be the women's low standards and part may be "courtesy bias," when participants merely tell the researchers what they believe is the desired response.[192] Women's rights activists are attempting to sensitize the population so that women will raise their standards.

Another challenge for the women's rights movement is an internal one: the inadequate understanding of reproductive rights even within the movement. Most people, including the reproductive health workers in the nongovernmental sector, do not see the connection between reproductive health and reproductive rights. "They have more than ten years of experience, yet even they can't explain reproductive rights very well. So if you think about how difficult it is for them, imagine how it is for the rest of the people."[193] To the average Vietnamese, the concept of reproductive rights is a foggy one at best. As Tine

Gammeltoft illustrates, "Like the young woman who was pregnant [with a positive fetal diagnosis] when the two old fathers [in-law] were deciding what to do—if she was to stand up and say, 'You know, I have my reproductive rights, and I would like to have this child, even though you say I should have an abortion.' That's just unthinkable!"[194] Much work remains to be done to sensitize the population in regard to the concept of reproductive rights.

On an official level, perhaps the most useful exercise for the women's movement would be to consider gender when forming any policy, whether it is related to transportation or agriculture or manufacturing. Policy makers should ask, "How does this affect women? Are there going to be women peer educators? Does the local leadership include women?"[195]

Since Vietnam is so progressive on a legislative level, with gender equality spelled out in official documents, the next focus of attention involves changing cultural traditions and kinship systems, a process that takes far more time than signing a policy into law.[196] With their history of fending off foreign opponents (China, France, and the United States), Vietnamese people tend to be proud and nationalistic, and they will not necessarily adopt models from other countries just because they are the norm elsewhere.[197]

Conclusion

Vietnam has a history of dynamic changes in relation to its economy, political system, and culture—the field of sexual and reproductive health and rights presents no exception. The past fifty years have seen drastic changes in women's reproductive health, ranging from lower mortality and fertility rates to increased access to health information. Yet many challenges remain in this poor country, particularly for the ethnic minorities and other people living in the mountainous regions.[198] Vietnamese women are still far from living in a culture in which their reproductive autonomy is a priority, made possible by comprehensive sex education, access to a wide range of contraceptives, and the right to have as many children as they choose. As it moves into the twenty-first century, Vietnam is experiencing a shift of perspectives, from focusing entirely on the community and allegiance to the state to focusing on individual rights. The challenge for Vietnamese activists will be to carve out a Vietnamese definition of individuality and human rights, improving women's reproductive freedom while preserving the myriad benefits of their traditional culture.

7

Jordan

Background

Bordering Syria, Iraq, Saudi Arabia, and Israel, Jordan is a small country with 5.3 million inhabitants and a relatively stable political history.[1] Jordan gained independence in 1921 and became "Trans-Jordan" in 1923, but it was not until 1950 that Trans-Jordan and the West Bank merged to form what is now called the Hashemite Kingdom of Jordan. In 1967 Israel occupied the West Bank of Jordan, and, in 1988, the West Bank was "administratively disengaged" from the Kingdom to facilitate the establishment of a Palestinian state.[2] What remains of Jordan was divided into twelve governorates (districts).

Jordan is a lower-middle income country with a medium ranking on the human development index (HDI).[3] The gross domestic product per capita is US$3,347, and recent increases in unemployment and poverty have resulted in the diminishment of the middle class.[4] Since 1946, Jordan's population has been one of the fastest growing in the world; between 1994 and 2004, the population grew at an average rate of 4.3 percent annually. Most of Jordan's population growth is due to immigrants from the Arab-Israeli wars in 1948 and 1967, as well as the return of over two hundred thousand Jordanians during the 1990 Gulf War.[5] Jordan's population nearly doubled in fifteen years, from 1979 to 1994.[6] Approximately 98 percent of the population is Muslim, and scholars note, "Religion permeates every aspect of individual, family and social life in Jordan."[7] In contrast to Vietnam, Jordan is unique in that the country enjoys high education levels with a mostly urban population (80%), yet it has a relatively *high* fertility rate.[8]

Fertility

Jordan's fertility rate was the highest in the Middle East in the period from 1960 to 1965, at 8 children per woman. By the mid-1990s, it stood at 5.1, and the 2002 Population and Family Health Survey shows the fertility rate has dropped quite dramatically to 3.7 children per woman.[9] Until recently, there has been no sizable family planning program, and people tend to have large families, despite the country's relatively high HDI ranking and universal knowledge of contraception (100% of Jordanians know at least one contraceptive method).[10] The latest Population and Family Health Survey also reveals that though the total fertility rate is 3.7, the desired fertility rate is just 2.6, indicating that an unmet need for family planning exists.[11]

Jordan formed the National Population Commission/General Secretariat in 1988 (now called the Higher Population Council), but even they would not dare to use the term "family planning," which was taboo until the early 1990s. Only "birth spacing" was deemed acceptable.[12] Jordan does not have a history of population control programs, perhaps because of its small size and status as a relatively new country.[13] Prior to the International Conference on Population and Development (ICPD), the government avoided the issue of family planning because it was so sensitive. They relied on indirect policies and socioeconomic development to address the population issue. These policies were vague and implicit; only in recent years has the government established clear population policies. Family planning use was already on the increase, partly as a result of the economic crisis in the late 1980s and its attendant spike in the cost of living. Jordan's peace treaty with Israel in the early 1990s may have also boosted family planning use, since Jordanians did not feel as threatened as before, though the extent to which regional politics influences fertility is unknown.[14]

Sex Education

Adolescents in Jordan have a low level of knowledge about sexual matters; there is essentially no sex education in schools. What little information trickles through usually comes after puberty, which is too late in the opinion of Dr. Basma Khraisat, director of Family Health International's Impact Project in Jordan.[15] A 2000 study showed that 57 percent of young women experienced shock and fear at their first menstruation, having never been told what to expect.[16] Approximately 4.3 percent of women are pregnant or already have a child by the time they reach the age of twenty; though this number is small in comparison to other countries (like in the United States, where 40% of twenty-year-old women have been pregnant), it still represents a sizable portion of the young population that needs access to reproductive health services and information.[17] Dana Khan Malhas, national program officer for the United Nations Development Fund for Women (UNIFEM), explains,

> Sexuality and issues related to it are still considered a taboo subject in all of the countries of the region. Strict social norms hence result in reluctance to [provide] education about issues related to sexuality and health related topics to men and women alike, but mostly to women, which results in young women being either afraid or reluctant [to get] information about sexual matters due to the stigma and the direct link of such questions with sexual activity.[18]

Though discussing sexual health has historically been taboo in Jordan, Seifeldin Abbaro of the United Nations Population Fund (UNFPA) points out that, with the information revolution, most young people have access to a multitude of informal sources for information about sex.[19] Given that situation, many believe it would be better for young people to learn correct information about reproductive health from their teachers, rather than picking up misinformation from unreliable sources.

In 1997, UNFPA collaborated with the Ministry of Education to incorporate population education, including basic elements of sexual health, general hygiene, and demographics, into the curriculum.[20] Although textbooks include information about sexual maturation and anatomy, teachers often tell students, "Go read it at home."[21] When the curriculum is modified to include topics on sexual reproduction, many teachers are embarrassed and skip over it; both teachers and students are shy to discuss such subjects.[22] In the future, UNFPA plans to involve teachers to a larger extent in the development of the sex education curriculum, attempting to design the curriculum in a way that maximizes their comfort teaching the sensitive material. An evaluation of the current curriculum hopes to pinpoint why exactly, beyond embarrassment, teachers shy away from teaching the reproductive health components. Teachers may be reluctant to teach reproductive health matters because of a fear of backlash from parents, whom they believe are against sex education.[23] In fact, a study conducted by UNFPA found that most parents are receptive to some degree of sex education, though they are reluctant to directly discuss the topic with their children because of its sensitive nature and also because of their own lack of education about sexual health.[24] Still, youth prefer to get information about sex education through the media and health centers, studies report.[25]

Young people's main source of information related to sexual health is peer-to-peer communication, as well as the Internet and satellite television; UNFPA is working to develop peer education programs to improve the accuracy of the information passed from friend to friend.[26] UNFPA has also contributed to the expansion of reproductive health information taught in Jordan's medical schools.[27]

Seifeldin Abbaro argues against the model of the Danish Family Planning Association, in which a third party comes in to teach sex education to students. "I don't think we should encourage people to think of this element of education as an external element." He points out that Islam calls for the collection of knowledge, and there is much history in Arab cultures of addressing these issues of basic human nature. Religious leaders in many mosques, in fact, discuss sex quite openly, though adolescents, and girls in particular, are unlikely to be present.[28] Reproductive health workers like Abbaro wish to re-emphasize that aspect of their cultural heritage, teaching young people about the changes that happen during puberty and the naturalness of sexual feelings. Abbaro advocates a system that informs young people while highlighting the need to act responsibly, to understand and manage one's needs. Addressing these issues with a cultural lens becomes extremely important, Abbaro argues, because otherwise, sex education will continue to be viewed as an external, Western import. Abbaro feels that Jordanians need not look beyond their own culture and religion to find discussion of sexual health matters. Finding a way for regular teachers to incorporate sex education into their curriculum is also ideal in terms of continuity; if students have questions about sex education later, they will not be able to find the external teacher who came in for an afternoon to teach the subject.[29]

Access to Health Services and Family Planning

Numerous obstacles impede women's access to reproductive health services and particularly to family planning. A lack of awareness among women about their reproductive health and sexuality persists. Women generally cannot get such information from the mass media or from their families. More than one health development organization is conducting door-to-door counseling with local field workers, with the belief that this is the best way for women to get sensitive information in the privacy of their own homes.[30] Commercial Market Strategies, an international reproductive health organization, reaches two hundred thousand women of reproductive age per year with their outreach program.[31]

Health centers in both urban and rural areas are physically accessible—generally located within five to ten kilometers of each other—but they are often overcrowded, understaffed, and have limited hours of operation.[32] Contraception and childbirth services are free in public health centers, but there are other costs related to obtaining family planning, and women are usually dependent on their husbands for money.[33] Many women only go to the health centers for antenatal care or if one of their children falls ill; they do not regularly attend for their own health.[34] Asma Bishara, program director of Johns Hopkins University's Center for Communication Programs, emphasizes the need to "connect women with the health facilities and to make her sure that this facility is for her *own* health."[35] Bishara points out that even when a woman is persuaded of the need to pursue health care for herself, she may encounter resistance from her mother-in-law, sisters, and husband.[36]

Once women do reach a health center, they may not successfully obtain health services due to their strong preference for female physicians. A recent survey of three hundred women asked them what they would do if they went to a health center for an IUD insertion and only a male physician was present. Three-quarters reported they would leave the health center without the IUD, and 87 percent said they would prefer a female midwife to a male doctor.[37] Nouf Al-Omari, a nurse with Commercial Market Strategies (CMS), reports that CMS and others were successful in their advocacy to change the national policy so that trained midwives could do IUD insertions.[38] Dr. Ayman Abdel-Mohsen of Primary Health Care Initiatives (PHCI) emphasizes the usefulness of midwives:

> There is a treasure in this country that is called the midwife [. . .]—a hidden treasure. They are from the community; they represent the very social class that attends to the clinics; they have the ability to talk the very same language as the clients; and they are very well motivated and they are stable—they stay at their clinics, they don't jump from one clinic to another. So we are putting a very big investment in midwives.[39]

Efforts are currently underway to train more midwives to perform IUD insertions, but a shortage of female providers persists. Since only about 10 percent of public health providers are women, many patients choose the private sector to ensure that they are seen by a female provider.[40]

Beyond the dearth of female providers, another weakness of the public health sector is its inadequate counseling, including premarital, prenatal, and postnatal counseling. In most clinics today, a woman does not receive any postnatal contraceptive counseling until she returns with her newborn for vaccinations several weeks after the delivery.[41] As Seifeldin Abbaro points out, some women may already be fertile again before that time. The current state of reproductive health counseling in Jordan does not aid women in making informed decisions related to childbearing. Additionally, in the recent past, a lack of privacy and shortage of supplies in public clinics deterred women from attending; a 1994 study found that 13 percent of health centers lacked gloves at the time of the study, 65 percent did not have speculums, and 55 percent lacked an autoclave for sterilizing instruments.[42] Today, health centers appear to be much better stocked, partly due to funding from USAID through Primary Health Care Initiatives (PHCI).[43]

Despite Jordan's diverse population of Bedouins, Palestinians, Circassians, Chechens, and others, health inequities along ethnic lines are difficult to find. Perhaps more important in determining who has the best access to health care is level of education and job opportunities.[44] Unlike in many countries, where the rural population is poorest, in a highly urbanized country like Jordan, the urban poor are perhaps equally marginalized.[45] The United Nations Relief and Works Agency (UNRWA) is charged with providing free health care to the 1.7 million registered Palestinian refugees in Jordan. Twenty-three health centers are available for their use, though the additional 500,000 refugees who are not registered are ineligible to use the free services.[46]

One of the organizations that have attempted to assist the urban poor in Jordan, the Arab Women Organization (AWO), opened two clinics in the mid-1990s with funding from UNFPA in order to serve disadvantaged populations. One of the clinics is located in Wadi Abdoun, an impoverished part of Amman that officials discourage people from living in and have thus neglected from a health care perspective.[47] AWO has tried to increase accessibility of their clinics to women by housing in each clinic a public library where children can stay and read books while their mothers are seen by clinic staff. The organization also trains women from these neighborhoods to make home visits, talking to other women about their health and the benefits of child spacing through the use of family planning.[48] Though a small organization, AWO provides a good example of a nongovernmental organization trying to improve poor urban women's access to reproductive health services, including contraception.

Contraceptive Use in Jordan

The Jordanian government established the National Population Commission (NPC) in 1973, but officials at the NPC did not publicly state their support of family planning programs until 1987. Though the message then was couched in terms of the health benefits to mother and child, it still sparked controversy, even within the Ministry of Health.[49] To mention "family planning" (*tanzim al-osra*) was largely taboo in Jordan until the early 1990s, when growing dialogue about reproductive health gradually raised people's awareness of the issue and family planning became less controversial to mention. In 1993, the government adopted its first National Birth Spacing Program and described it as a program "that deals basically with the health of the mother and child"—again, trying to avoid controversy.[50] Today family planning is still mostly discussed from the perspective of maternal and child health, or from an economic point of view, rather than one of human rights.[51] Dr. Zuhair Al-Zu'bi of UNRWA believes the message that health professionals send to the population must stress that family planning is not necessarily for limiting the number of children a family has, but for spacing their children.[52] The World Health Organization and local NGOs have collaborated to push this message, since Islam prohibits birth limitation. Although birth spacing does of course indirectly limit the number of children a family has, the term "birth spacing" (*muba'ada*) is far more acceptable to the population than "birth control."[53] A 2000 study by CMS found that the term "family planning" is also now acceptable.[54] Dr. Abdel-Mohsen explains their approach at Primary Health Care Initiatives, "We are trying to have her understand and appreciate the value of spacing, and it's up to her to decide on the number. [. . .] Nobody in the whole world has the right to impose a certain number of children on a family, especially in our region. We are governed by our inner conscience, which is very much developed by our religious behavior."[55]

Jordan's contraceptive prevalence rate is quite low, with only 56 percent of married women using any contraception, and 41 percent using modern methods.[56] This is despite the fact that awareness of contraception is high; the average married woman can name ten contraceptive methods.[57] Commenting on the relative stagnation of the contraceptive prevalence rate in the past several years, Dr. Salwa Bitar Qteit mentions, "To me this means that we have reached the easy-to-reach group, and now we have to reach the others who are more difficult to reach."[58] Contraceptive use did in fact double in just twenty-five years, from 23 percent of the married population using it in 1976 to 52 percent in 2000.[59] Unlike in many developing countries, the government is not the main provider of contraceptive services in Jordan; 38 percent of family planning users obtain their contraception from the private sector, and another 20 percent go to clinics run by the Jordanian Association for Family Planning and Protection (JAFPP), which was founded in 1964 in Jerusalem, and in 1972 in Amman.[60]

The most common contraceptive method in Jordan is the IUD, with 62 percent of family planning users currently using one.[61] Withdrawal is a particularly popular method in Jordan, perhaps because it is documented that the Prophet Muhammad approved of its use.[62] The method also presents no risk of physical harm and there is no cost associated with it, though there is arguably psychological harm involved, as well as a high failure rate. The popularity of traditional methods has increased in recent years; today 45 percent of fifteen- to twenty-four-year-old contraceptive users choose a traditional method.[63] Sterilization is an unpopular method, used by only 3 percent of women and decreasing in prevalence, perhaps because of the increased availability of other modern contraceptives.[64] In a 2002 study, one out of five doctors reported that they would never recommend a tubal ligation to any woman.[65] Sterilization, like divorce, is "hated" in Islam, but not "forbidden"; the method is generally used only in cases for which it is medically indicated.[66] Less than 20 percent of the population has even heard of male sterilization, and 2001 studies found no reported cases of vasectomy in the country.[67] Though condom use doubled between 1997 and 2002, condoms remain unpopular—the method is used by just 3.4 percent of currently married couples—partly due to men's distaste for the method and their expense.[68] Emergency contraception is essentially unheard of in Jordan, even among health professionals.[69]

Studies have shown that service providers have strong biases when counseling women about family planning methods. Most are biased against modern methods, particularly injectables or Depo Provera. One study of female providers, conducted by Commercial Market Strategies, found that 70 percent of providers would advise a nulliparous (childless) woman to have a baby before using family planning.[70] Michael Bernhart of CMS explains that many providers tell their patients, "Don't do it—have that first child. Test yourself."[71] A majority of these providers also report that they only prescribe natural methods, such as withdrawal or periodic abstinence, to those nulliparous women who persist in requesting contraceptive protection. The survey discovered that these physicians believe many of the rumors circulating about oral contraceptives, Depo Provera, and Norplant.[72] Many rumors color women's perceptions of contraceptives, particularly those that claim the Pill or the IUD cause cancer and infertility. In a 2001 survey, only 30 percent of women report that they trust the Pill as "safe," and only 16 percent feel that injectables are safe.[73] Norplant is particularly mistrusted in Jordan; circulating rumors state that Norplant leads to heart disease, cancer, blood toxicity, and infertility. One study describes a woman who was afraid of the effects of Norplant on her heart, so she asked her provider to place the implants in her right arm, away from her heart. The provider acquiesced, without discussing her fear of heart problems.[74] Some women actually use Depo Provera *because* of the rumor that it causes infertility, since they do not want any more children.[75] The prevalence of myths surrounding contraception seems to have declined, however, perhaps as a result of an intense campaign that CMS and other concerned entities like the Jordan National Population Commission/General Secretariat conducted from 1997 to 2002 to increase contraceptive knowledge and to dispel such rumors.[76]

The side effects of many modern contraceptive methods present a sizable obstacle to women because of their religious beliefs; according to the teachings of Islam, a woman may not pray, fast, or have sexual relations if she is bleeding. The spotting and irregular bleeding sometimes associated with methods like the birth control pill or the IUD can create a serious disturbance in a woman's daily life.[77] The inadequate counseling most women receive at health centers contributes to a high discontinuation rate; women are often unaware that they may have side effects for a few weeks until their bodies adjust to the new hormone levels. Without this information, more women discontinue using the contraception as soon as side effects surface.[78] The 2002 Population and Family Health Survey found that 42 percent of women discontinue use of their modern contraceptive method within one year of beginning to use it.[79]

Jordan is a conservative Muslim society in which extramarital sexual relations are relatively rare. Bernhart makes clear, "It appears that in many, perhaps most, families it is necessary for a woman to demonstrate her virginity on her wedding night."[80] One interviewee referred to the burgeoning industry in hymen repair for women who were raped, lost their hymen in an accident, or were sexually active before marriage.[81] As Dana Khan Malhas of UNIFEM points out, "Honor is in this little piece of meat called the hymen."[82] It is illegal to provide contraception to unmarried women in Jordan, though some contraceptives, like condoms, are available over the counter in pharmacies.[83] Leila Hamarneh of Arab Women Organization believes the government should open clinics specifically for adolescents, but "nobody has the courage to say it," including the Jordanian Association for Family Planning and Protection.[84] In the meantime, AWO's two clinics must abide by the law prohibiting contraception for unmarried women to avoid being shut down. When asked whether she believes that premarital sexual relations are very common, Dr. Basma Khraisat answers, "Well, in the study we did, half of the STD cases were adolescents. Does that answer your question?"[85]

Religious Influences on Reproductive Health and Men's Attitudes

Many interviewees cite the attitudes of men—husbands, fathers, and brothers—as a substantial obstacle to women's use of family planning. A 1998–2000 study found that men are unclear about Islam's stance on contraception, and many do not realize that Islam allows contraception as long as it is not used to limit the total number of children.[86] Indeed, the Qu'ran calls for at least thirty months between births, yet over one-third of births in Jordan are spaced twenty-four or fewer months apart.[87] A recent study of nine Muslim countries, representing two-thirds of the world's Muslim population, finds no clear pattern in total fertility rate or contraceptive use. Socioeconomic levels and the strength of each country's family planning programs seem to be more important factors in determining the country's fertility levels. "Islam . . . seems to be neither a hindrance nor a stimulating factor in fertility decline, at the global level."[88] Although highly educated religious leaders agree that Islam permits the use of contraception, less-educated religious leaders found in many community mosques are often against family planning, according to Abdul Rahim Ma'ayta of the Higher Population Council General Secretariat. Many lower-level religious leaders do not discuss family planning or talk in their sermons about the national need to have smaller families.[89]

In an attempt to address the widespread misunderstanding of Islam's teachings on family planning, the Jordan National Population Commission/General Secretariat, with technical assistance from the Johns Hopkins University's Center for Communication Programs, asked prominent Islamic religious leaders, including the Mufti of Jordan, to write brochures on the very subject. These brochures highlighted Islam's stance on family planning, spousal communication about family planning, equity between male and female children, and family size. The brochures were then distributed to community leaders through discussion sessions led by triads of professionals: religious guides, physicians, and social workers. Over four thousand community leaders each distributed at least ten brochures of each topic to their friends, neighbors, and colleagues. These same brochures were distributed to the general public as newspaper inserts in the two prominent daily newspapers in Jordan. The project also borrowed popularity from the royal family, with photographs of King Abdullah II and Queen Rania prominently displayed.[90] This large-scale campaign succeeded in dispelling to a large extent myths about Islam's stance on contraception. For example, men who believed that the Pill is approved by Islam increased from 28 percent in 1996 to 51 percent in 2001, and religious leaders who advocated family planning increased from 36 percent in 1996 to 60 percent in 2001.[91] However, these impact evaluation figures reveal the need for additional awareness campaigns.

Asma Bishara believes that some of Jordan's family traditions are obstacles to women using contraception. Newlywed couples are usually under tremendous pressure from family and friends to begin reproducing immediately after getting married, and they are also generally not accustomed to thinking about contraception.[92] Commercial Market Strategies aired a television commercial that encouraged newlyweds to delay childbearing, and the backlash was so strong that CMS was temporarily kicked off the air.[93] Cultural traditions that emphasize lineage, power, and the influence of a tribe (measured by its number of male members) all contribute to a strong desire for large families.[94] Marriage within families is a common way to build up the family's power; a striking 43 percent of marriages in Jordan are consanguineous, often between first cousins.[95] "Here in Jordan, in our tradition, the more children you have, the more powerful you will be—not in money, but your children will give you power."[96] Additionally, there is a widespread belief that when a child enters the world, God will provide all the food and supplies that child needs: "Children come by God's will, so it's God's will [to have them]."[97]

Men tend to be ignorant about modern family planning methods and are reluctant to allow their wives to try them.[98] Spousal communication appears to be associated with family planning use; one study found that 80 percent of family planning users had discussed family planning with their husbands, compared to only 40 percent of nonusers.[99] Partly due to poor communication, women may erroneously assume that their husbands want large families.[100] Men's input in contraceptive decision-making is strong; in some areas of the country, women need their husband's permission to obtain family planning from a health clinic, and, nationally, a woman needs her husband's signature to obtain a tubal ligation.[101] Nouf Al-Omari, a nurse, relates the story of one patient who was referred to the hospital for a cesarean section. She and her husband had agreed to get a tubal ligation, but he was in the southern part of the country at the time. His authorization over the phone was not sufficient, so the physicians refused to perform the tubal ligation at the time of her c-section. She had to return later for a second surgery.[102]

Jordan is quite a traditional society, in which men still dominate the decision-making process. A 2000 study found that men are involved in the decision to adopt a contraceptive method but then recede in the process when deciding on which method to use.[103] Dr. Al-Zu'bi insists, however, that most men provide little resistance to family planning use. "They see the media coverage, and they witness the hard economic times, and they know it is better to have two children you can provide for than to have ten."[104]

Abortion

Jordan is among one of the most conservative countries in the Middle East when it comes to abortion; abortion is illegal in every case (including rape and incest) except to save the woman's life or health, or in the case of severe fetal anomaly.[105] Despite the near-total illegality of abortion in Jordan and the country's strict societal prohibitions of the practice, abortions do in fact occur, albeit less frequently than in many other countries. One-third of pregnancies in Jordan are unplanned.[106] Data from the 2002 Population and Family Health Survey suggest that 2.6 percent of all pregnancies end in induced abortion in Jordan.[107]

More than one interviewee cited the arrival of satellite television, which nearly half of Jordanian households enjoy, as a factor contributing to more liberal behavior, premarital sex, and illegal abortions.[108] Dr. Zuhair Al-Zu'bi recalls, "When I was in school, talking to a girl who is not your relative was frowned upon, like they would think I was flirting or a bad guy or something. But now [. . .] having a boyfriend or girlfriend is more accepted."[109] The absence of studies on abortion in Jordan makes the topic a difficult one to assess. Dr. Nisreen Haddadin Bitar laments, "We need someone courageous enough to do this! Nobody is talking about it."[110] Conducting a study on abortion is difficult for more than just political reasons; as Dr. Salwa Qteit points out, "A woman may tell you casually in a conversation that yes, I had an abortion—I could not have another child then—but in a general survey [she] will not tell you that."[111] One development worker in Amman, when asked if there are many illegal abortions in Jordan, responded without hesitation, "Yes." When asked why s/he believed that, the answer was "Because we have contact with the doctors who provide them." This person later confided that s/he has personally funded abortions for a few desperate women.

Although the scope of the problem is impossible to pinpoint, there seem to be few complications from abortions because they are generally done in the private sector by competent health professionals, though exceptions certainly exist.[112] The cost of an illegal abortion, however, is exorbitant, around US$500. Women who are unable to secure a doctor's assistance may take certain medicines or insert traditional herbs into the vagina in an attempt to start bleeding. The drug misoprostol, available from some pharmacies, also induces bleeding.[113] A woman in this situation can then go to any health center and receive treatment for a miscarriage.[114] Most of the complications seen from illegal abortions are among poor patients, Leila Hamarneh points out. Many private clinics, including those of the Arab Women Organization, want nothing to do with treating such patients because they do not want to be associated with abortion.[115] Despite the paucity of real data on complications from illegal abortion, it appears that the magnitude of the problem in Jordan is not as great as in many other developing countries.[116]

There is considerable controversy among Islamic scholars as to the position of the religion on abortion. One major trend in Islamic doctrine claims that abortion up to three months or 100 days into the pregnancy is acceptable.[117] Dr. Zuhair Al-Zu'bi explains that, before the time of urine pregnancy tests and ultrasounds, only an abortion after "quickening"—when the woman can feel the fetus move—was considered murder by Islamic teachings.[118] A study in Egypt found that "[m]ajor differences in Islamic religious opinions regarding the legitimacy of abortion create a climate of moral confusion for Egyptian women who face unwanted or risky pregnancies."[119] One interviewee expressed his surprise at how conservative Jordanian society is, as Islam's fundamental teachings are not nearly as strict.[120]

Advocacy to legalize abortion is essentially unheard of in Jordan. Dr. Salwa Qteit relates the story of an official in the Ministry of Social Development who recently suggested that the country adopt a more liberal abortion policy, modeled on Tunisia's. The idea sparked a strong, negative reaction from the public.[121] Women's rights organizations tend to feel that there is plenty of room for improvement in other areas of reproductive health in Jordan, such as increasing access to family planning and strengthening the counseling available. These activists will likely be more successful in addressing these relatively noncontroversial issues before tackling the issue of legalizing abortion.

According to nurse Nouf Al-Omari's experience, the majority of abortion patients are married and feel they cannot handle another child at that time.[122] But some number of abortion patients are unmarried, and numerous social strictures make it difficult to be an unwed pregnant woman. When a baby is born in the hospital, the name of the baby's father, as well as his birth certificate, must be presented to the hospital staff.[123] Hamarneh points out that this strict policy is even more conservative than in other Arab countries like Algeria and Tunisia. Perhaps most immediate in the mind of an unmarried pregnant woman is the possibility of an "honor killing."

"Honor Killings"

The phenomenon of "honor killings" has received considerable press coverage worldwide. In a country like Jordan, where the family's honor is held above nearly all else, both women and men have been killed for tainting the family's good name (though the vast majority of such victims are women and girls). Since 1986, honor crimes have accounted for nearly 30 percent of all murders in Jordan, and in 2000 alone, there were 718 honor crimes (including over 20 murders) reported, though estimates of the actual number are much higher.[124] The judicial system deals with perpetrators of honor crimes leniently; the jail sentence for killing a daughter or sister accused of adultery, for example, is only six months to three years.[125] Until recently, Article 340 of the penal code read, "He who discovers his wife or one of his female relatives committing adultery and kills, wounds, or injures one of them, is exempted from any penalty."[126] Many women's organizations, including the Jordanian National Committee for Women, lobbied the government to change this article and, in December 2001, Article 340 was amended to state that the perpetrator will have a "reduction of penalty" rather than exemption.[127] Not surprisingly, the number of honor killings reported in Jordan has not dropped since the amendment of Article 340. Not infrequently, honor crimes are actually cases of incest; murdering the pregnant girl can avert a shameful scandal.[128] Other times, an honor crime is committed based on rumors, and a physical examination of the woman after her death reveals that she was still a virgin.[129] In this context of honor crimes, it is not surprising that induced abortions occur.

When posed the question, "What would happen if a young woman became pregnant but she was not married?" numerous respondents gave the same answer: "Her family would kill her."[130] Though the family may move to another city or force the woman to marry her boyfriend, these options seem less common than an honor killing.[131] Abbaro points out that the effect of honor killings extends beyond the actual victims; the phenomenon also causes "young women [to] try to conform as much as possible to social needs."[132] In many cases, the woman will commit suicide in the name of saving her family's honor.[133]

Some women who are accused of adultery or another misdemeanor that would threaten their family's honor are kept in reformation centers. These centers are not meant to be like prisons, punishing women for committing a crime, but are instead designed to protect the women's lives. "The moment that they are released, they would instantly face death at the hands of their family members, with the pretext of defending the honour of the family, and 'washing shame.' "[134] However, in some places, such as the facilities at Juweideh, the reformation center and women's prison are one and the same, though the "protected" women and convicts do not mingle.[135]

Dr. Basma Khraisat calls attention to the fact that the original teachings of Islam are explicit about matters regarding sexuality, unlike many religions, and there is no basis for honor crimes. Even in a literal reading of the Qu'ran and the laws it sets forth in Shari'a, one finds that punishment for adultery is only legitimate when there are at least four witnesses, which is rarely the case.[136] The enforcement of social norms against adultery is also sexist, in that a man who has extramarital relations will not usually be killed, though his name will be tarnished.[137] Despite the work of multiple NGOs to tighten the laws related to honor crimes, little progress has so far been made.[138] Dr. Khraisat insists that a slow and careful approach must be taken—one that is culturally and re-ligiously sensitive, given the delicacy of the issue.[139] Criticism of honor crimes must come from *within* Jordan, to avoid the defensiveness so commonly seen when an attack is perceived as external or Western. Changes must occur not only on a legislative level, but in individual communities as well.

A similar strategy is needed to combat domestic violence, which is also a common, but seldom discussed, topic. The few studies conducted show that anywhere from 15 to 80 percent of women report being beaten in the last six months.[140] The most credible survey, according to Michael Bernhart, was conducted in Zarqa and reported that 38 percent of women were beaten in the past six months. Although the general laws against assault technically apply in these domestic disputes, the reality is that police and the courts do not want to get involved in such cases, and the affected individuals also try to avoid police involvement. Domestic violence is usually considered a private, family affair, and even the extended family often does not want to know about it. If the family involved does decide to take legal action, they may attempt to resolve the problem using their own tribal laws and authorities.[141]

Son Preference

Like in Vietnam, a strong preference for sons affects women's rights and drives up the fertility rate in Jordan. From the time a man is a child, people assume he will grow up to be a father of sons, so he lives with that expectation his entire life, according to Basem Abu Ra'ad, executive director of the Jordanian Association for Family Planning and Protection (JAFPP).[142] If a man's wife has two or three daughters, he will almost always insist on continuing reproduc-tion until they have one, or preferably two, sons.[143] In many cases, it is actu-ally the woman who insists on continuing childbearing; many women believe that their husbands will be happier if they have at least one son.[144] Although Lina Qardan and her colleagues at the Johns Hopkins University Center for Communication Programs specifically make equity between male and female children a main message in their campaigns, evaluations of the projects show little progress in changing people's preferences.[145] Son preference is a deep-rooted tradition in Jordan, as in most of the Arab world, even though it is not a part of Islam's teachings. In fact, Islam censures those who are displeased with having female children, and discrimination between male and female children is a punishable sin.[146]

STIs and HIV/AIDS in Jordan

Probably due in large part to Jordan's conservative Muslim society, the prevalence of sexually transmitted infections (STIs) is low.[147] Recognizing the tremendous stigma associated with STIs, health workers prefer the term "reproductive tract infection" (RTI), explaining to people that they are sexually transmitted.[148] Though Jordan does indeed have low STI rates, both the general population and the government appear to underestimate the true prevalence. "We did a study on RTIs among 1,200 women. [. . .] The results were really shocking news to the government—look! We have gonorrhea! That was a surprise."[149] In fact, the 2004 study Dr. Khraisat refers to was the first major study ever done on STIs in Jordan.[150] In the public sector, there are no STI clinics; STI care is integrated into the dermatology or obstetrics and gynecology clinics.[151] A recent survey found that practitioners are concerned about the problem of STIs, but in reality they rarely educate their patients about them.[152] Awareness of STIs among the general population is low; a 2001 survey found that less than half the population knows what syphilis or gonorrhea are, and even fewer people are familiar with chlamydia and genital herpes.[153]

Slowly entering the public consciousness is the issue of HIV/AIDS. Reports range from 132 to 300 current documented cases of HIV/AIDS in the country, though the real number is likely to be far higher.[154] The majority of Jordanians seem to be in denial about HIV/AIDS becoming a major problem in their country; the illness is still perceived to be an outside threat that foreigners bring into the country. While it is true that roughly two-thirds of the documented HIV/AIDS cases are foreigners, that likely stems from the fact that there is no surveillance system in place for regular Jordanian citizens. When a foreigner applies for residency in Jordan, he or she must be tested for HIV and hepatitis within one month.[155] No regular testing exists for Jordanian citizens, however—a fact that surely masks a higher prevalence than 300 cases. One interviewee, a businesswoman not affiliated with the health sector, demonstrates this bias: "As a matter of fact, these infections—we get them from outside, not from here. From laborers coming from outside—no, it's not much. It's not because a man is having an affair and then he brings it to his wife—no."[156] According to a large study in 2002, only 75 percent of women believe there is a way to prevent HIV/AIDS, and just 39 percent of women know two or more ways to avoid infection.[157] Fewer than half of the women know that a healthy-looking person could be HIV-positive.[158]

There are few NGOs who have the courage and funding to address the issue of HIV/AIDS, though the government has recently established a National AIDS Program.[159] Funding from international donors is difficult to come by, no doubt partly because of the much higher infection rates in other parts of the world, "but that's why this work is important here—we need to keep the infection rate low!" opines Dana Malhas.[160] Another development worker highlights the proximity of major HIV epidemics to the Middle East—in Africa, Eastern Europe, and India. HIV work is not considered a priority in the Middle East, but it should be, Dr. Khraisat argues, "because prevention is far cheaper than treatment. [. . .] We have to ask, 'Will the low prevalence countries remain low prevalence?' What happens five years from now?"[161] Because a discussion of HIV/AIDS requires open talk of sexuality, it is still a taboo subject.

HIV transmission through sex, contaminated blood products, IV drug use, and mother-to-child transmission during delivery are all known routes of exposure in Jordan. Sexual transmission accounts for 45 percent of HIV infections, though what portion is homosexual or heterosexual is unknown.[162] Homosexuality is extremely stigmatized in Jordan. A development worker from one organization told me, "We have done some peer education with [homosexuals], off the record—unofficially. No organization would openly say they are working with homosexuals." Stigma surrounding HIV/AIDS is also strong; Dr. Al-Zu'bi argues that campaigns need to get people to think of HIV-positive people as sick, rather than as a disease in and of themselves.[163]

To its credit, the government has established a National AIDS Committee, which is its own entity, not housed in the Ministry of Health.[164] Additionally, the Higher Youth Council has recently agreed to make STIs one of their priority areas—a major breakthrough.[165] Development organizations are neglecting to target other at-risk groups, however, such as truck drivers and prostitutes. Prostitution in Jordan is a very sensitive topic and one whose presence is denied by most Jordanians.[166]

Influence of Regional Politics
on Reproductive Health

One cannot ignore the role that regional politics has historically played in Jordanians' decisions regarding family planning. Although there are no official figures and it is a highly sensitive issue, estimates place the Palestinian population in Jordan anywhere from 40 to 70 percent.[167] In the early 1970s, when the Jordanian Association for Family Planning and Protection (JAFPP) was gearing up their work on family planning, they met much resistance from religious leaders and the media, who claimed they were trying to limit the number of children that are able to fight Israel in the future.[168] Dr. Zuhair Al-Zu'bi of UNRWA relates a similar experience; UNRWA did not officially start offering family planning until 1994, though they provided it prior to that if women specifically requested it. In 1994, when they went public with family planning services, the reaction was surprisingly positive. "People were happy—they were eager to use these services."[169] Jordan's 1994 peace treaty with Israel, coupled with the higher cost of living and increased education levels in recent years, may have contributed to an increase in family planning use. In surveys, many Palestinians agree that they need a larger population to fight the Israelis; however, Michael Bernhart of CMS reports, "In our extensive work in the camps and elsewhere—over 600,000 couples—it soon appeared that these sentiments meant *other* couples should add to the ranks of future fighters. The individual couple still made the decision on the usual bases: income, gender, family pressure, etc.—not regional politics."[170]

Political pressure for Palestinians to have many children continues today. According to Dr. Issa Al-Masarweh, "many in the country here [. . .] believe that family planning policies are foreign policies and they are imposed by [a] foreign agenda, and also they believe that we don't need such policies since we still have a struggle with the Israelis. They believe that population increase is one weapon in this struggle."[171] Politically motivated resistance to family planning extends to health professionals as well. Dr. Nisreen Haddadin Bitar relates,

> I can tell you from my personal experience that there were two times in the past two years when we had to cancel trainings we had scheduled with physicians in laparoscopic technique [sterilization] because of the Intifada—when the Intifada flared up. The physicians would even say, "We're not in a good position to do this training. They are killing our people, and you are talking about tubal ligations and family planning."[172]

Dana Khan Malhas of UNIFEM, however, maintains that Palestinians' desire to have more children is not driven by their intention to create more soldiers or suicide bombers. "They want more children for their identity, to express their right to live here, their right to exist. Having children is the simplest thing they can do to prove their existence, especially because everything else has failed."[173]

The role that the United States has played in the Israeli–Palestinian conflict is particularly troubling to many Jordanians. According to Dr. Nisreen Haddadin Bitar, people "feel the U.S. is hurting the country's privacy, that whatever the U.S. wants, they get."[174] Some Arabs believe there is an American scheme to control their culture and way of life. The fact that the United States Agency for International Development (USAID) is the prime donor for reproductive health and population activities in Jordan fuels conspiracy theories.[175] "USAID funds the procurement and shipment of all contraceptives to meet the supply needs of the government and NGO sectors."[176] Dr. Bitar believes most other organizations (excluding UNFPA) do not focus on reproductive health in Jordan because they have more limited funds and decide to funnel it to the countries in greater need, while the United States has greater political interest in funding Jordanian projects.[177] USAID actually pours far more money into economic opportunity programs and water resources management than into "family health and family planning," which comprised barely 10 percent of its 2001 budget.[178] Still, Dr. Bitar relates that anytime she works on a USAID project, she hears conspiracy theories of the United States' attempt to take over Jordanian culture. She puts it bluntly, "If you hate someone, you don't expect something good from them. And people here don't exactly see the U.S. as an angel, you know? They are suspicious of their motivations."[179] Although some people may be more open and understanding about U.S. assistance to Jordan now, Dr. Bitar points out that there are many influential people, such as leaders of the Obstetrics and Gynecology Society, who still mistrust the United States' motives.[180]

In response to such negativity toward the United States, Dr. Salwa Qteit of USAID emphasizes in conversations with Jordanians that USAID's work is supporting Jordan's own country strategies. Likewise, Dr. Bitar attempts to show the rationale for why the United States is working on these issues and why there is a local need for them. Since the royal family publicly came out in support of reproductive health in the recent past, it has been easier for USAID workers to convince the population of the benefit of their work.[181]

Influence of the ICPD

Prior to the 1994 International Conference on Population and Development (ICPD) in Cairo, the Jordanian government generally avoided the issue of family planning because of its sensitive nature. In the absence of any clear population or reproductive health policies, the government relied on vague socioeconomic policies to address the population issue.[182] In 1993 Jordan hosted the Arab preparatory meeting for the ICPD, which resulted in the Amman Declaration, detailing the general stance of the Arab countries on reproductive health issues.[183]

Jordan's participation in the ICPD was controversial; many civil society organizations, including the Islamic Brotherhood, came out against it. Dr. Issa Al-Masarweh remembers, "[Those of us participating] were accused of being Zionists, Israelis, traitors—every kind of description! It was very tough."[184] Her Royal Highness Princess Basma bint Talal managed, in a clever maneuver, to soothe the concerns of those opposed; she invited everyone to come together and talk about the upcoming conference and proceeded to convince them that the ICPD would be an opportunity for the Arab nations to express their views. Jordan would be under no obligation to accept anything presented there, and it would be better to participate than to hide.[185] The Islamists were also encouraged by the participation of the Vatican, knowing its staunch anti-abortion and generally anti–family planning stance.[186] The Jordanian delegation did attend and participate, and when they returned they incorporated the reproductive health concept into the country's first national population strategy.[187] As Seifeldin Abbaro of UNFPA points out, at any global conference there are bound to be differences of opinion on certain issues and practices. Jordan agreed with the ICPD's Program of Action as a whole, but with the reservation that the document "will be applied within the framework of Islamic Shari'a and our ethical values, as well as the laws that shape our behaviour."[188] The Jordanian delegation also decided to interpret the word "individuals" in the ICPD as meaning "married couples."

Today, many interviewees believe, the government is committed to reproductive health. The newly released Reproductive Health Action Plan (RHAP) is not a contraception plan veiled in reproductive health terminology; it is truly based in a more comprehensive, reproductive health approach.[189] The field of reproductive health has public support from several members of the royal family, including King Abdullah II, Queen Rania, and Princess Basma bint Talal (former King Hussein's sister), who is the host of the Higher Population Council/General Secretariat and the head of the Jordanian National Committee for Women.[190] The current prime minister has also been outspoken on reproductive health and population issues.[191] Even adolescent reproductive health is slowly gaining attention; King Abdullah II and Queen Rania have publicly expressed their support of the topic.[192] As a further gesture of support for more accessible family planning services, in 2001 the government abolished the duties, tariffs, and sales taxes previously levied on imported contraception.[193]

Nevertheless, some government documents on reproductive health still focus on set quotas and demographic targets, which run counter to the spirit of the ICPD. The Reproductive Health Action Plan, which is part of the National Population Strategy, specifies numeric targets for population growth, including reaching replacement fertility level (2.1 children per woman) by 2020.[194] The policy repeatedly refers to the need to "rationalize Jordan's population growth" and laments one of its "programmatic issues" as the "discordance between women's expressed family size and the government's expressed objectives."[195] The policy also stresses that "all persons must accept responsibility for assisting in stabilizing the growth of the nation's population."[196] Though goals for maternal and infant mortality are also outlined in this document, it is only the goal for the total fertility rate that is mentioned repeatedly throughout the policy. Still, the government's incorporation of many of the sentiments expressed in the ICPD is commendable, and the National Population Strategy even mentions the need to develop and implement programs to support a positive response to gender issues and reproductive rights.[197]

Feminism and the Women's Movement in Jordan

The first women's society in Jordan was established in 1944, with a focus on motherhood education and childcare. In 1954, a lawyer named Emily Bisharat formed the Jordanian Women's Alliance, whose slogan was "Equal rights, equal responsibilities, total Arab unity." The alliance was dissolved in 1957, along with all other opposition nationalist movements, and women's rights activists went underground until Bisharat's organization was reestablished in 1974 with a new name: the Women's Union. It wasn't until 1974 that women gained the right to vote, though women who held elementary education certificates were eligible to vote from 1955 on. In 1982, the government shut down the Women's Union again and established the General Federation of Jordanian Women. The country did not adopt its first National Strategy for Women until 1993; to quell any fears of radical feminism, the document made clear that "[t]he National Strategy for Women seeks to promote the cohesion and unity of the family as the basic social cell on which society as a whole is based."[198] In 1995 the

Jordanian National Forum for Women came into existence as a "state feminist structure." The Jordanian Women's Union was reestablished for the third time in 1990, and today it is the only women's rights organization that openly advocates for legalization of abortion.[199]

The women's movement in Jordan is fragmented and hard to recognize. Many women's rights activists have worked cautiously, beginning with children's rights activism and then sneaking in issues like domestic violence whenever possible.[200] Though there are many individual women's rights organizations in Jordan, they seldom collaborate; the overall movement is divided.[201] Dana Khan Malhas of UNIFEM observes, "There's rarely a spirit of people coming together or being united."[202] There is even competition between the various groups for funding and for credit for any positive changes.[203] Similar to Vietnam, the Jordanian government has strict control over nongovernmental organizations. All NGOs must be members of the General Union of Voluntary Societies, through which they receive a stipend from the government. A 1966 law that still applies today prohibits NGOs from trying to achieve "political goals."[204]

The rather large degree of homogeneity among women's rights activists in Jordan further limits their ability to broaden the movement. "They only represent a specific class of Jordanian women, and they don't touch base with the grassroots women," Malhas claims.[205] Dr. Bitar concurs, arguing that the movement needs to bring in a more diverse set of women.[206] Kholoud Abu-Zaid, formerly of Save the Children, points out that the majority of women's rights activists are far from "ordinary women" in terms of socioeconomic and educational backgrounds.[207] She believes that most activists speak in terms of abstract theories and approach women's issues from a perspective that emphasizes individuality and personal freedom. In her projects at Save the Children, AbuZaid attempted to convey the message that their work does not advocate "for women to start making their own decisions by themselves." AbuZaid continues,

> The family is the nucleus of the whole world, so we are trying to build the capacity of the families, bring the women and men together, not to separate them by empowering women with a few slogans that would really destroy her house, because by the end of the day, you go back to your house, and you live with your family. You love your husband and you love your kids. This is life. This is what we want—we don't want to empower women to start making their *own* decisions, *by themselves*, away from the family. It's not—for me it's not right, because I'm not looking at the woman by herself, I'm looking at the Arab woman as part of the

community, as part of raising the next generation. The family is a unit—a whole unit.

AbuZaid's approach to women's rights may be more culturally acceptable than one that emphasizes individual freedom. She believes that many women's rights organizations have alienated women from their work by adopting the latter approach. AbuZaid notes that, as soon as people sense that they are being patronized or spoken down to, they stop listening. "And if [. . .] you're talking about something that is really, really far away from their knowledge or culture or education, you [won't] be fully accepted."[208] AbuZaid insists that the most appropriate way to proceed with women's rights work is to adapt Western methodologies to each country's culture, rather than accepting them wholesale. "So this way, when you talk people's language and you talk about their customs, habits, traditions, and let them buy into the new methodologies—that is the way you can get their support."[209]

Perhaps another obstacle is the unwillingness of some members of Jordan's women's rights movement to share their power with younger activists. Dana Khan Malhas mentions, "The people we work with are much older—they are our mothers' generation! And it's difficult, it's impolite, to tell an older woman she's wrong!"[210] Although activists who have been in the field for thirty years have undeniably valuable experience, Malhas bemoans the fact that many are set in their ways and refuse to look at the situation in a new light, refuse to let younger activists take leadership positions.

One of the difficulties that the Jordanian women's movement faces is the dearth of *Arab* women's rights experts and the resulting insufficiency of references in Arabic about women's rights. Though some translations of feminist material from English do exist, these works are not specific to the region or culture. In an attempt to rectify this gap, UNIFEM's human rights department has developed a manual with nine chapters on women's topics, including reproductive rights.[211] The manual, published in Arabic, will soon be available in several Arab countries.

Not surprisingly, many women's rights activists are accused of advocating a Western importation of feminism that is in direct conflict with their own Arabic culture. In these cases, activists strive to demonstrate how feminist principles are rooted in Arabic culture and history. In 1999, UNIFEM held a roundtable discussion with proponents of CEDAW (the Convention on the Elimination of All Forms of Discrimination against Women) and Shari'a (Islamic law). The exercise was a success in terms of showing that women's rights are not alien to Islam nor is the concept a Western importation. The discussion also served to highlight that Islam calls for equal rights for men and women alike.[212] One of the Prophet Muhammad's wives, Umm Salama, once asked him why men are mentioned in the Qu'ran and not women. A few days later, Muhammad replied (with Allah speaking through him) that the two sexes are completely equal when it comes to being believers and members of the community. In fact, the Prophet Muhammad's opinions about equality between the sexes sparked fierce debate in his day. "It is a debate that fifteen centuries later politicians are calling alien to the culture, alien to the Sunna, the Prophet's tradition."[213] The fact that Jordan has signed and ratified CEDAW helps activists convince citizens that such concepts are not completely foreign to the country. Dialogue about women's rights is difficult to translate in some cases, however; there is no word for "gender" in Arabic, for example. Two Arabic words have been coined to describe "gender" across the region: *Al naw' al ijtimai*, which literally translates to "social type."[214]

Leila Hamarneh's story of her organization's experience is a particularly telling example of the tension surrounding women's rights as a Western versus Arab construct. In 1999, a media campaign claimed the Arab Women Organization (AWO) introduced the Western way of thinking and Western contraceptive methods, and even that they were working for the CIA to decrease the number of Palestinians by pushing contraception on women. The Jordanian press also accused AWO of distributing contraceptives that were carcinogenic. In response, the Ministry of Health launched a full-scale investigation that lasted nine months, during which time AWO's clinics were ordered to close. In the end, the investigation concluded that all of AWO's contraceptives came directly from the Ministry of Health, and the clinics were given official letters reinstating their practice as legitimate and legal. The tabloids refused to publish the results of the investigation, and AWO clinics retained a tarnished name. AWO then started their outreach campaign to regain the trust and confidence of people in the areas where they work. The original media slur campaign was headed by a group of fundamentalists, including officials from the Ministry of Social Development.[215] Whether or not the attack came because AWO is a reproductive rights organization is difficult to ascertain.[216]

Advocating for women's reproductive rights is difficult in a country where the concept of individual human rights is generally not well accepted. Openly speaking about reproductive rights or sexual orientation is taboo and is likely to be met with people saying, "This is against our religion. This is against our traditions. This is against all the norms of our society."[217] Leila Hamarneh mentions pressure from officials to only speak about less controversial topics; they tell her, "Your reproductive health services are okay, but why mention the sexual orientation or [. . .] reproductive rights?"[218] Particularly now, in the midst of a revival of traditional understandings of gender roles, it is nearly impossible to speak about reproductive rights without provoking negative backlash. On a short-term basis, Leila Hamarneh believes, Jordan is slipping backward in terms of gender equality as the country experiences a swing towards more conservatism.[219] Dr. Nisreen Haddadin Bitar believes that most women do not know their rights and do not ask for them.[220]

As Asma Bishara explains, "We have powerful women here, but the traditions are very strong."[221] Women are generally subordinate to men in this male-dominated society, and womanhood is often equated with motherhood.[222] "The Jordanian society is one that considers the man as the rightful master of the family, having complete control over its members, especially the female members of the household."[223] Despite the recent backslide with women's rights, Asma Bishara believes that overall the situation for women has improved in the past twenty years, largely because of greater educational and work opportunities, as well as the existence of a national women's forum to advocate for their rights.[224] In 1996, the Arab Forum for Women outlined three priorities for their movement: increasing the number of women in decision-making positions, addressing poverty and its impact on women, and reassessing the role of women in the family.[225]

Various women's organizations are working with the Ministry of Education to change the portrayal of women in school textbooks, with some success. "It used to be that in Primary One, the very first book you have, on the first page, there is a picture of the mother cooking and the father reading. So this boy grows up thinking that mother cooks and father reads," Salwa Nasser notes.[226] Men are often portrayed in textbooks to be involved in history, science, and math, while women are confined to social studies and Arabic language.[227] Several women's rights activists mentioned the need for gender awareness to start early, when children are still young, particularly in shaping their perception of women's role in the family.[228]

Kholoud AbuZaid emphasizes the need to "let people depend on themselves," while providing them with access to knowledge and information. Though this concept is widely embraced by women's organizations in theory, AbuZaid argues that it rarely trickles down to the implementation level. There are many human resources and people of high caliber on the ground, but they are not always given a chance to rise to their full potential.[229] Illiteracy remains a major problem for women; 16.5 percent of women are illiterate, compared to 5.7 percent of men.[230]

One group has taken a creative approach to increase people's access to reproductive health information; the Jordan National Population Commission/ General Secretariat (JNPC/GS), with technical assistance from Johns Hopkins University/Center for Communication Programs (JHU/CCP) and funding from USAID, designed an entertainment-education program for youth. The program comprised fifteen episodes of a one-hour television variety show for young people. Segments included a mini-drama concentrating on reproductive health subjects, live discussion between young audiences, a guest with specialized knowledge on the subject, a song, and a quiz positioned at the end of each episode to test the audience's knowledge. A radio talk-show program that further discussed the topics raised in that week's episode accompanied the show. Lastly, the project included a contest for youth. Participants read a paragraph on one of the selected topics and then had to answer basic questions about it, sending in their response to be entered in a drawing. Two famous Jordanian singers contributed to the program, and the private sector donated prizes, like a car, for the contest. In the end, the National Youth Contest had 631,000 participants, representing 63 percent of the Jordanian youth ages fifteen to twenty-four. An impressive 85 percent of the answers sent in for the contest were correct.[231] By making ads on television, in newspapers, and on the Internet, JNPC/GS and JHU/CCP succeeded in reaching two-thirds of the Jordanian population with their reproductive health messages.

In another attempt to give the population more access to information, JHU collaborated with the Ministry of Islamic Affairs to build units for reproductive health and population issues in thirty-five of their major libraries, which are located in public and private mosques and Islamic centers across the country. These libraries serve as a valuable resource to anyone desiring information about reproductive health, youth, or gender.[232]

Using another approach to improving women's position in society, many NGOs recognize the fact that "[w]hen a woman is economically independent, [. . .] she becomes a leader at home first, and then she becomes a decision-maker in her community."[233] Only 18 percent of women are economically active in Jordan, and those women earn just 80 percent of what men with the same education earn.[234] The Jordan Forum for Business and Professional Women (JFBPW), established in 1976, strives to assist women in becoming economically independent; the JFBPW currently has 170 members—women who have started their own small businesses. Bringing in her own income gives a woman more leverage when it comes to health care and educational decisions, as Salwa Nasser, JFBPW's executive director, points out: "The father might be inclined to send [only] the boys to school, and they will say so because the boy will carry the name of the family, and he will be the breadwinner, but the girl will get married and she will have a husband. Now, if the woman is economically independent, she will say, 'No—let the girl go to school. I will pay for her books. I will pay for her uniform.' "[235]

Women's organizations also recognize the importance of getting men involved in reproductive health and women's rights issues. In one of Save the Children's outreach programs to women about reproductive health, the participants' request at the end of the workshop was that the organization hold similar sessions for men. AbuZaid observes that most talk of designing reproductive health programs for men has not materialized yet, with a couple notable exceptions.[236] The Center for Communication Programs at JHU conducted the first-ever Jordanian assessment of men's knowledge, attitudes, and practices (KAP) in relation to reproductive health, and the results were used to tailor their health communication campaigns accordingly.[237] The Arab Women Organization approached male participation in a unique way. Starting in 2003, AWO invited men to come and sit together to discuss reproductive health issues. They offered men a space where they could meet and provided them with a male physician to facilitate the discussion. The men were attracted to the idea of having an opportunity to ask a doctor questions, not all of which were reproductive health-related. In this setting the men could discuss reproductive health issues freely and in the presence of a specialist who could provide them with accurate answers to their questions. Sometimes these sessions are scheduled specifically for male adolescents, too, so they can have the opportunity to learn about reproductive health in an appropriate setting and in the absence of their parents.[238]

There are a number of crucial issues that the women's movement needs to address beyond increasing educational and job opportunities and improving women's reproductive health and rights. Women currently are required to obtain written permission from their male guardian (husband or father) to apply for a passport, even if the woman is foreign but married to a Jordanian man.[239] Securing the right for citizenship to be passed through women to their foreign husbands or children is important, as is addressing the issue of honor killings.[240] Rape is currently only a misdemeanor, in the same class as molestation, incest, adultery, and possession of pornography.[241] Raising awareness of violence against women and providing support services for abused women is of utmost importance, since support and rehabilitation services for such women are practically nonexistent.[242]

Women in Jordan do have some solid ground to stand on; they have the right to be lawyers and judges, to own property, and to own and manage their own businesses.[243] Just 1.4 percent of judges are women, and 2.5 percent of parliamentarians, but those numbers are greater than previously seen.[244] Women have also been ministers, in the Ministry of Social Development and the Ministry of Post and Telecommunications.[245] In 1999, a woman became the first minister of planning, and went on to become the deputy prime minister— the highest rank that a woman has ever reached in any executive body in the Arab world.[246] Furthermore, a full 51 percent of students in higher education today are women, though they remain a minority in Ph.D. programs.[247] Jordan's government also shows signs of commitment to women's rights; Jordan signed CEDAW in 1980 and ratified it in 1992.[248]

Conclusion

Jordan is unique in that, despite an urbanized population, high levels of education for women, and its status as a middle-income country, fertility levels remain high and family planning use very low. Cultural taboos against discussing reproductive rights and sexual health impede women's ability to learn about their bodies and how to control their own fertility. Jordan is a male-dominated society, in which preference for sons plays a key role in driving up fertility rates and negatively affects female children, who do not have equal access to job opportunities. Illegal, and sometimes unsafe, abortion is a nearly silent problem in this country where an unwed woman found to be pregnant may be killed in order to save the honor of her family. Yet women's rights activists point to many achievements for sources of hope; women today are entering the workforce and holding political positions in greater numbers than before, and sex education is slowly being incorporated into formal schooling. Reproductive health-related activities of nongovernmental organizations have increased substantially in the past decade alone, as the social climate changed and dialogue about family planning slowly became more acceptable. Having the public support of key influential figures in Jordan, such as the royal family and prime minister, has also granted women's health groups legitimacy in their work. Despite a recent turn toward more fundamentalism, the direction of Jordanian society is overall moving in a direction of greater rights and freedom for women and greater involvement of men in their wives' and their own reproductive health.

Conclusion

Commonalities across Borders

As evidenced by the stories and statistics detailed in this book, women across the globe are struggling to gain greater reproductive freedom, despite the multiple and daunting obstacles they face. A similar study of women's reproductive rights internationally concludes, "Women respondents [. . .] aspire to control their own fertility, childbearing and contraceptive use, although social, institutional and legal barriers may prevent them from succeeding."[1] In few countries do women enjoy an appreciable degree of reproductive autonomy. Absent or inadequate sex education programs, poor access to contraception and other health services, and, frequently, strict abortion laws all contribute to the lack of power many women experience in regard to controlling their fertility. Perhaps even more importantly, women in most of the countries highlighted in this book expressed frustration with unequal educational and economic opportunities, resulting in dependence on men for their livelihood. Millions of women truly have limited power to negotiate the terms of their sexual relationships and are thus made vulnerable to unwanted pregnancy and sexually transmitted infections, including HIV/AIDS.

In all seven countries in this book one encounters reproductive rights activists, even if the focus of their work varies considerably from country to country. Referring to reproductive rights organizations that represent various ethnic groups in the United States, Silliman et al. note,

> Each group had to address its particular history of reproductive
> oppression and to articulate its particular positive vision and agenda
> for reproductive freedom, which included demanding the right to have
> children free from coercion, either by the state or through community
> pressure. Claiming reproductive rights in a culturally specific and
> meaningful way was essential to developing a political agenda and a
> constituency base.[2]

197

The notion of reproductive rights is often met with skepticism and charges of Western imperialism in many developing countries; to counteract such accusations, it is imperative for activists to adapt reproductive rights principles to their local environment. In many countries, such as Jordan or Uganda, for example, the most useful strategy may be to tackle the least controversial issues first, such as increased access to family planning and education, rather than alienating potential supporters by advocating for the legalization of abortion. Any reproductive rights movement will be most effective if it is grassroots-driven, compatible with the local culture, and relevant to average people's lives.

Influences on Reproductive Rights: The Need for Sweeping Changes

A theme that repeatedly surfaced in each of these countries is the need for broader societal changes to take place in order for women to truly enjoy reproductive freedom. Since the International Conference on Population and Development (ICPD) in Cairo, dialogue on reproductive health has shifted to include talk of women's empowerment rather than strict demographic targets. Efforts to "empower" women solely through increased access to contraceptives drastically fall short of what is needed. If the newly adopted language of improving women's reproductive health is to be taken seriously, then governments and donors alike need to address barriers to women's reproductive rights both within the health care system and external to it. Women will have difficulty claiming power over their bodies and health care decisions until such fundamental changes occur.

Petchesky et al. report from their study, "With great consistency, respondents in all country settings complained about the poor quality, inaccessibility, and high cost of reproductive health and family planning services; above all they resented the disrespectful and abusive treatment they received from medical providers."[3] Substantial changes need to occur in the health care systems highlighted in this book to make services friendlier and more accessible.

Women have a right to comprehensive health services and not merely services aimed at reducing their fertility. In order to offer solid primary health care, health centers need to be adequately equipped with essential supplies like gloves and drugs (particularly antibiotics), in addition to basic amenities like running water and electricity. Health centers should be committed to providing a wide range of health services and not only those related to controlling women's fertility. Despite limitations on health care systems in most countries, women's health advocates point out that governments and donors have provided wide-scale contraceptive services to women in the past, even in poor and remote areas, and so there is little evidence to back up claims that the capacity for health service provision does not exist. Roberts notes, "It is amazing how effective governments—especially our own—are at making sterilization and contraception available to women of color, despite their inability to reach these women with prenatal care, drug treatment, and other health services."[4] Commenting on the abundance of funding for Norplant insertions during a time of deep welfare cuts in the United States, Roberts continues, "This willingness to pay for poor women's birth control but not for their basic needs is strong evidence that the government is more interested in population control than in furthering poor women's welfare."[5]

Within family planning services, women have a right to truly "informed choice" of a full range of contraceptives, including user-controlled, non-hormonal methods. Considering the great number of women who utilize traditional family planning methods like withdrawal and the rhythm method, proper counseling about such methods should be integrated in family planning clinics to maximize the methods' efficacy. Rather than treating traditional methods as inferior to modern methods, health professionals should recognize that many women will continue to prefer traditional methods for health and religious reasons, even after they have information about and access to modern methods. Dr. Zuhair Al-Zu'bi in Jordan points out that contraceptive use requires initiation and continuation, and most countries are lacking in their attention to the latter; when women receive inadequate contraceptive counseling, they are far more likely to become dissatisfied with the method and discontinue use.[6]

Beyond the health care system, in some countries, like Uganda and Peru, improvements in infrastructure such as roads and communication lines would directly benefit women's health. There is need to address these issues in every country; even in developed countries, there are pockets of "the South within the North," where mortality rates are much higher than the national average and women's ability to remain healthy is limited. Likewise, increasing women's access to financial resources would ease their dependence on men when it comes to making health-related decisions. Officials must recognize that, given better educational and employment opportunities, most people *choose* to limit their family size. This choice is empowering to the family and ultimately beneficial to society, but it cannot easily occur in a context of extreme poverty, entrenched patriarchy, and poor health services. Petchesky et al. conclude, "All participants agreed that, especially for the majority of women who are poor and marginalized, achieving reproductive self-determination would ultimately require fundamental changes, not only in the quality and availability of services, but also in the structural conditions and state policies that support an unjust economic and social order."[7]

Reproductive rights activists themselves have often neglected to address the larger socioeconomic inequities in society that have an impact on poor women's health. In the United States in particular, feminist activists must keep in mind a broad vision of reproductive rights. As Roberts articulates,

> Reproductive liberty must encompass more than the protection of an individual woman's choice to end her pregnancy. It must encompass the full range of procreative activities, including the ability to bear a child, and it must acknowledge that we make reproductive decisions within a social context, including inequalities of wealth and power. *Reproductive freedom is a matter of social justice,* not individual choice.[8]

Respondents in most of the countries highlighted in this book voiced the sentiment that women's movements are disproportionately comprised of privileged women. Addressing greater social inequities would make these movements much stronger and more inclusive—a critical point in the face of organized opposition to feminist activism.

Conservative Forces and the Struggle to Advance

In each of these countries, people working for improved women's health and well-being also encountered conservative forces that made progress difficult. Particularly with the upswing in religious fundamentalism in some areas of the world, such as the United States, Peru, and Jordan, achieving substantive progress in women's reproductive health is a challenge. As conservative political factions effectively restrict access to sex education, contraception, and abortion, proponents of the Cairo agenda grow frustrated. Trixsi Vargas, in Peru, comments indignantly, "How ridiculous that people say, 'I am against abortion, but I am also against contraception, and I'm not going to give you any information.' What are we talking about here?"[9] A common experience in many countries is the preponderance of misinformation, particularly in relation to abortion. Pregnancy resource centers in the United States, some health providers in South Africa, and politicians in Peru have all distributed antichoice propaganda in an attempt to stop women from having abortions.

History provides convincing evidence, however, that there will always be women desperate enough to end an unwanted pregnancy, even though they may believe that abortion is a sin, that their families will shun them, that they may lose their lives. Estimates based on figures from 2000 indicate that nineteen million unsafe abortions take place each year; approximately one in ten pregnancies end in unsafe abortion, giving a ratio of one unsafe abortion to about seven live births.[10] Of the nearly six hundred thousand pregnancy-related deaths each year, one-eighth of them are thought to be from abortion.[11] A study by the Alan Guttmacher Institute reveals that the legal status of abortion worldwide is not strongly correlated to abortion rates, though it is correlated to abortion safety.[12] Attacks on sex education and access to contraception, among other reproductive health services, will only drive up the number of abortions. Reproductive rights activists must contend with oftentimes powerful conservative factions in their efforts to improve women's health.

Motivation of Reproductive Rights Workers

The reproductive rights activists interviewed for this book come from a variety of backgrounds, yet all voice similar motivations for doing this work. For one doctor, his concern for women's and children's health keeps him working: "Family planning is not just about population control, it's about preventing abortions by decreasing unwanted pregnancies, it's about better spacing children to help the brothers and sisters, it is to keep women healthier so they are not constantly pregnant."[13] Many respondents, such as Rossina Guerrero of Flora Tristán in Peru, expressed their personal investment in this line of work:

> The fight for abortion is not only during these eight hours that you are sitting here, your fight for abortion is when you are talking with your friends, when you meet with your relatives, when you are explaining things, speaking to people. Because in reality, it's not just a fight for abortion, no? It's the fight for democracy, for the freedom to speak, to express yourself, to improve your life. . . . What gives me motivation, then, is that this is important to me personally, not just work.[14]

Some respondents saw the clear connection between information and power. Trixsi Vargas puts it simply, "If you have knowledge, you have freedom. If you don't have information, you are restricted in your freedom. When they ask me, 'Why do you talk about sexuality?' I say, 'So that people know about it.' People are scared, they don't talk about it."[15]

The ability to work for a healthier society motivates many reproductive health workers. Nestor Owomuhangi of UNFPA in Uganda explains, "Well, I enjoy it because you measure your achievement with time, you see your contributions. [. . .] And again, it is challenging, it's not like you are done—it keeps you moving—you never get bored, you never say, 'Okay, I am finished, now I can go to sleep.' "[16] Dr. Salwa Bitar Qteit in Jordan relates, "It's a very gratifying job. [. . .] You feel like you are affecting the whole nation. Not changing one life, but changing many lives."[17]

Still others are motivated by the pain and suffering they personally witnessed. Dr. Daniel Gho Aspilcueta remembers how he became involved in reproductive rights work:

I was a medical student and I worked in the emergency room, working with children, and I had a mentor who gave me a new perspective, explaining to me about "insufficient mothers." We worked with children, with babies, who were brought to the emergency room in the middle of the night to die. They were usually very small babies who arrived after many days of not eating, with diarrhea, with various complications— they were dying. And the mother inevitably did not want the baby, did not want to be pregnant in the first place, and she did not buy the medications. The mothers did not cry. It was like a relief to them that their babies died. But I had a friend who worked in the pharmacy and so I had access to those medications, and when these people arrived with their dying babies, I would treat the babies. A friend of mine and I would not allow them to just die alone like that. The doctors there would criticize us and say, "No, you are young, you do not understand. These babies are brought here to die." But we didn't care. And I started to look at what type of mother this was, and she was almost always young—they were almost always abandoned adolescent mothers with no partner. Their babies got sick and they didn't want these babies to die in their hands, so they brought the babies to the hospital to die in our hands—that would be better looked upon by society, no? They brought the babies to the hospital, but in the background they really wanted the babies to die. This called my attention very much, and I started to wonder why. I discovered the phenomenon of unwanted babies, and realized this was the problem. So through this I came to family planning and focused on prevention, trying to prevent these babies from being born to mothers who didn't want them. . . . [18]

Others, recognizing the complexities of working in abortion care, have decided to do their best to ease the pain attendant to the experience. Dr. Tersia Cruywagen in South Africa, speaking of her staff, elaborates, "We tell people, 'We don't know if abortion is right or wrong.' We don't, really. But what we do know is that we deal with a lot of patients in disastrous situations and a lot of emotional pain, and that is what we want to do—assist them through a very traumatic experience . . . and make it less traumatic. And that's very nice if our patients tell us, 'It wasn't that bad. It wasn't as bad as I thought.' "[19]

One respondent, Dr. Janet Cole, adopted a practical view of abortion, accepting that abortions will happen and attempting to minimize the damage done from one:

> I've always been very prochoice and right from when I was a resident
> I was willing to provide whatever services I could. . . . I am quite a
> practical person and they need to be done. There's no doubt about it. I
> won't even debate the ethics of abortion; I won't even debate when does
> life begin and all the rest of it. [. . .] For me, it's a completely pragmatic
> thing. As a health care professional with a particular interest in women's
> health, it is essential.[20]

Access to sensitive services like abortion could be drastically improved if more health providers felt the obligation Dr. Cole expresses to contribute to women's health in that particular way, either directly providing services or being an advocate for the liberalization of abortion laws.

Despite the many setbacks and slow pace of progress, some activists, like lawyer Tammy Quintanilla, feel a personal responsibility to contribute to a feminist cause because of their own benefit from the women's movement:

> [W]hen I look to when I started, in 1990, I can see how much change
> has taken place—how many advances, and this is what motivates me
> to continue. You can't feel that you have a useless career, because
> you realize that things are changing, just slowly. Looking at the years
> ahead, I can visualize a better society, with better access and healthier
> communities. I think that if we don't do this work—the feminists—then
> no one is going to do it! If it weren't for the feminist movement, maybe
> I wouldn't even be here! [. . .] Because in another time, I wouldn't be
> able to study. It's thanks to the feminist movement that I can do this, so I
> want to make sure it is the same for women in the future.[21]

Dr. Joy Kyeyune of the Association of Uganda Women Medical Doctors expresses a similar sentiment: "Because we are women, as women doctors, and we are a professional women's organization, we really need to give back to fellow women. Women suffer a lot, with the husbands or whatever, and women's issues are always brushed away. [. . .] So we realize that since we are privileged—we are doctors—we could help women, give something back."[22]

The extent to which women in these countries will be able to exercise their reproductive freedom in the future largely rests on the degree of success these reproductive rights activists and health professionals manage in their work to improve women's health and to expand their rights.

Appendix 1

Figures and Graphs

Total Fertility Rate

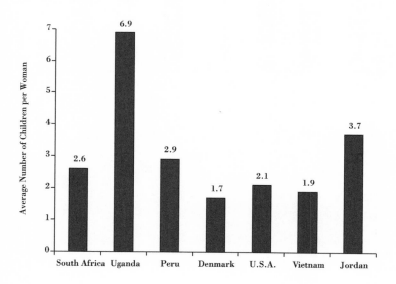

Contraceptive Prevalence Rate
(Percentage of Currently Married Women Using Contraception)

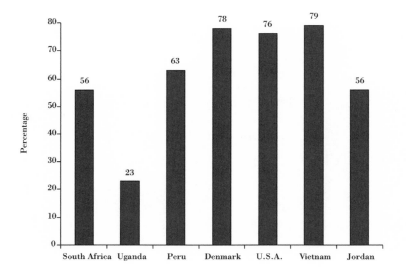

Maternal Mortality Rate

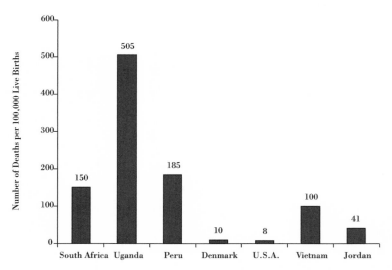

*Maternal mortality rates are the official rates reported by each government, rather than estimates from UNICEF and the World Health Organization, whose numbers tend to be much higher.

Gross Domestic Product per Capita in U.S. Dollars

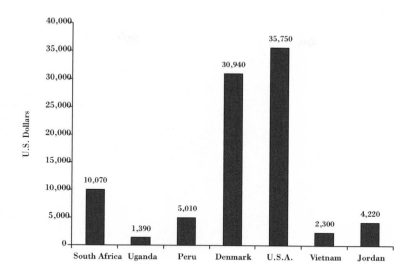

References

Denmark StatisticBank. "Fertility rates by age, region, and time." www.statbank.dk/stat-bank5a/default.asp?w=1024

Hashemite Kingdom of Jordan, Department of Statistics [DOS], ORC Macro. *Jordan Population and Family Health Survey 2002*. Calverton, Maryland, USA: ORC Macro, 2003. (2002 data)

República del Perú. *Encuesta Demográfica y de Salud Familiar, 2000*. Lima: USAID, UNICEF, Measure/DHS+, Macro International, 2001.

Socialist Republic of Vietnam, Committee for Population, Family and Children (CPFC). "Viet Nam 2002 Demographic and Health Survey: Major Findings."

Uganda Bureau of Statistics (UBOS) and ORC Macros, *Uganda Demographic and Health Survey 2000-2001*. Calverton, Maryland, USA: UBOS and ORC Macro, 2001.

United Nations Development Fund for Women (UNIFEM), Arab State Regional Office. "Paving the road towards empowerment: Egypt, Jordan, Lebanon, Palestine, Syria, the United Arab Emirates and Yemen." Amman: UNIFEM, 2002.

United Nations Development Program (UNDP). *Human Development Report 2004*. New York: UNDP, 2004.

United Nations Population Fund (UNFPA). *State of World Population 2003*. New York: UN, 2003.

Appendix 2

Country-Specific Contact Lists

South Africa

Groote Schuur Hospital
1445, Old Main Building
    Observatory 7925
Cape Town, South Africa
Tel: (021) 404-4333
Fax: (021) 448-6921

Marie Stopes Clinic
320 Fountain Medical Centre
Cape Town, South Africa
Tel: (021) 418-0560

Hillcare Women's Clinic
PO Box 23709
Johannesburg, South Africa
Tel: (011) 331-2348
Fax: (011) 331-0839

Johannesburg Hospital
10 George Weimer Street
Eldorado Park Ext. 6, 1813
Johannesburg, South Africa

Planned Parenthood
    Association of South Africa
PO Box 1008
Melville, 2109
Johannesburg, South Africa
Tel: (011) 482-4601, 482-4661,
Fax: (011) 482-4602
ceo@ppasa.org.za

Planned Parenthood
    Association of Western Cape
12 Anson Rd.
Observatory 7795
Cape Town, South Africa
Tel: (021) 448-7312
Fax: (021) 448-7320
ppawc@ppawc.co.za

Reproductive Choices
PO Box 31301 Totiusdal, 0134
Johannesburg, South Africa
Tel: (011) 315-6303, 315-6304
Fax: (011) 315-6305
choices@global.co.za

Reproductive Health Research Unit
PO Bertsham, 2013
Johannesburg, South Africa
Tel: (011) 933-1228
Fax: (011) 933-1227

Western Cape Department
    of Health and Social Services
PO Box 2060
Cape Town, South Africa 8000
Tel: (021) 483-2684
Fax: (021) 483-2264

Women's Health Project
University of Witwatersrand
PO Box 1038
Johannesburg 2000, South Africa
Tel: (011) 489-9917, 489-9905
Fax: (011) 489-9922

Uganda

Association of Uganda
    Women Medical Doctors
PO Box 10035; Kampala, Uganda
Tel: (041) 251333, 566820
Fax: (041) 230262
auwmd@uol.co.ug

Makerere Institute of Social Research
PO Box 16022
Kampala, Uganda
Tel: (041) 554582
Fax: (041) 532821
misrlib@imul.com

Marie Stopes Uganda
PO Box 10431
Kampala, Uganda
Tel: (041) 531255, 342247
msu@infocom.co.ug

Ministry of Health
Reproductive Health Division
PO Box 7272
Kampala, Uganda
Tel: (041) 230358, 340874
rhp@infocom.co.ug

Mulago Hospital Family Planning Clinic
PO Box 7051
Kampala, Uganda

Population Secretariat
PO Box 2666
Kampala, Uganda
Tel: (041) 343356, 342292, 343378
Fax: (041) 343116
popsec@imul.com
www.uganda.co.ug/population

Uganda Private Midwives Association
PO Box 30962
Kampala, Uganda
Tel: (041) 273943

UNFPA-Uganda
Plot 2 Katego Rd., off Kira Rd.
PO Box 10746
Kampala, Uganda
Tel: (041) 540658, 540665
Fax: (041) 540657
fpau@africaonline.co.ug

Commercial Market Strategies
PO Box 27659
Kampala, Uganda
Tel: (041) 230080, 232905, 230283
Fax: (041) 258678

Peru

Apoyo a Programas de
    Poblacion (APROPO)
Los Lirios 192; Lima 27, Peru
Tel: (51-1) 442-7440, 441-0155
Fax: (51-1) 442-2111
apropo@terra.com.pe
www.apropo-ong.com

Centro de la Mujer Peruana Flora Tristán
Programa de Derechos Sexuales
    y Ciudadania en Salud
Parque Hernan Velarde #42
Lima 1, Peru
Tel: (51-1) 433-2765, 433-1457
Fax: (51-1) 433-9500
www.flora.org.pe

Centro Documentacion Sobre la
    Mujer (CENDOC—Mujer)
Avenida Mcal. La Mar 170
Miraflores, Lima, Peru
Gladys Camere, Technical Director
Tel: (51-1) 447-2355, 242-9206
Fax: (51-1) 241-3688
postmast@lechuza.org.pe
www.cendoc-mujer.org.pe

Comite de America Latina y el
   Caribe para la Defensa de los
   Derechos de la Mujer—CLADEM
   Apartado Postal 11-0470, Lima
Jr. Estados Unidos 1295, oficina 702
Lima 11, Peru
Tel: (51-1) 463-9237
Fax: (51-1) 463-5898
oficina@cladem.org
www.cladem.org

Defensoria del Pueblo
Jr. Ucayali 388
Lima 1, Peru
Tel: (51-1)426-7800 ext. 285
Fax: (51-1) 426-7889
www.ombudsman.gob.pe

Development Studies and
   Promotion Center
www.desco.org.pe

DEMUS—Estudio para la Defensa
   de los Derechos de la Mujer
Jr. Caracas 2624
Jesus Maria, Lima, Peru
Tel: (51-1) 463-1236, 463-8515
www.demus.org.pe

Inppares—Instituto Peruano de
   Paternidad Responsable
Gregorio Escobedo 115
Jesus Maria, Lima, Peru
Tel: (51-1) 463-5778/5965/3152

Instituto de Educacion y Salud
Calle Chile 641
Lima, Peru
Tel: (51-1) 433-6314
www.ies.org.pe

Ministerio de la Mujer y
   Desarrollo Social
Camana 616
Lima 1, Peru
www.mimdes.gob.pe

Ministerio de Salud
Av. Salaverry, cdra. 8 s/n
Jesus Maria, Lima, Peru
www.minsa.gob.pe

Movimiento El Pozo (anti-prostitution)
Republica del Portugal 492
Breña, Lima, Peru
Tel: (51-1) 423-5852
creapozo@terra.com.pe
www.creapozo.com

Movimiento Manuela Ramos
Av. Juan Pablo Fernandini 1550
Lima 21, Peru
Tel: (51-1) 423-8840, ext. 306
Fax: (51-1) 431-4412, 332-1280
www.manuela.org.pe

Pathfinder International
Alameda La Floresta #285
Lima 41, Peru
Tel: (51-1) 372-5799/5073/5999
Fax: (51-1) 372-3992

Population Concern
Av. Pedro de Osma 306, oficina 301
Lima 4, Peru
Tel: (51-1) 252-1593

Population Council
Paseo Padre Constancio Bollar 225
El Olivar, Lima 27, Peru
Tel: (51-1) 442-0448
Fax: (51-1) 440-0635
www.popcouncil.org

Sociedad Peruana de
   Medicina Reproductiva
Tel: (51-1) 225-7708
Fax: (51-1) 225-7097

Sociedad Peruana de
   Obstetricia y Ginecologia
Av. Aramburu 321, oficina 4
San Isidro, Lima, Peru

Unidad de Sexualidad y
   Salud Reproductiva
Universidad Nacional Cayetano Heredia
Av. Honorio Delgado 430
Lima 31, Peru
Tel: (51-1) 319-0041/382-0320
   (ext. 2538)
Fax: (51-1) 381-9072

Denmark

Center For Kvinde- Og Kønsforskning
   (Center for Feminist Research
   and Women's Studies)
Københavns Universitet
   Amager, Njalsgade 80
2300 København S, Denmark
Tel: (45) 35 32 88 11, 35 32 83 43
Fax: (45) 35 32 83 77

Danish Association of Midwives
   (Den Almindelige Danske
   Jordemoderforening)
Norre Voldgade 90DK-1358
Copenhagen, Denmark
Tel: (45) 33 13 82 11
Fax: (45) 33 93 82 14

Foreningen Sex og Samfund
   (Danish Family Planning
   Association)
Skindergade 28A, 1
DK-1159 Copenhagen K, Denmark
Tel: (45) 33 93 10 10
Fax: (45) 33 93 10 09
Danish-fpa@sexogsamfund.dk

Frederiksberg Hospital, OB-GYN clinic
Nordre Fasanvej 57
2000 Frederiksberg, Denmark
Tel: (45) 38 16 34 27
Fax: (45) 38 16 34 09
cwj@dadlnet.dk

Institute of Public Health—
   Panum 42, Room 34
Panum Institute; Blegdamsvej 3
DK-2200 Copenhagen N, Denmark
Fax: (45) 35 32 76 29

Kvinfo, om kvinde- og kønsforskning
   (Kvinfo, Danish Centre for
   Information on Women and Gender)
Christians Brygge 3
DK-1219 Copenhagen, Denmark
Tel: (45) 33 13 50 88
Fax: (45) 33 14 11 56
kvinfo@kvinfo.dk
   or kvinfo@inet.uni-c.dk
www.kvinfo.dk or www.kulturnet.
   dk/homes/kvinfo/kvinfoe.htm

Ministry of Health
Holbergsgade 6
1057 Copenhagen K, Denmark
Tel.: (45) 33 92 33 60
Fax: (45) 33 93 15 63
sum@sum.dk
www.sum.dk

University of Copenhagen
Center for Women & Gender Studies
Lejrevej 20; 3650 Olstykke, Denmark

World Health Organization
Scherfigsvej 8; DK-2100 Copenhagen O
Tel: (45) 39 17 13 41

United States
   (clinic addresses have been
   omitted for security reasons)

Abortion Access Project
552 Massachusetts Avenue, Suite 215
Cambridge, MA 02139
Tel: (617) 661-1161
Fax: (617) 492-1915
www.abortionaccess.org

Advocates for Youth
2000 M St. NW, Suite 750
Washington, DC 20036
Tel: (202) 419-3420
Fax: (202) 419-1448
www.advocatesforyouth.org

The Alan Guttmacher Institute
1301 Connecticut Avenue
    N.W., Suite 700
Washington, D.C. 20036
Tel: (202) 296-4012
Fax: (202) 223-5756
www.agi-usa.org

American College of Obstetricians
    and Gynecologists
409 12th St., S.W., PO Box 96920
Washington, D.C. 20090-6920
Tel: (202) 638-5577
www.acog.org

Catholics for a Free Choice (CFFC)
1436 U Street NW, Suite 301
Washington, DC 20009-3997
Tel: (202) 986-6093
Fax: (202) 332-7995
cffc@catholicsforchoice.org
www.catholicsforchoice.org

The Center for Reproductive Rights
120 Wall St., New York, NY 10005
Tel: (917) 637-3600
Fax: (917) 637-3666
info@reprorights.org
www.crlp.org

Choice USA
1010 Wisconsin Ave. NW, Suite 410
Washington, DC 20007
Toll-free: (888) 784-4494
Tel: (202) 965-7700
Fax: (202) 965-7701
info@choiceusa.org
www.choiceusa.org

Kaiser Family Foundation
Washington, D.C. Office/
    Public Affairs Center
1330 G Street, NW
Washington, DC 20005
Tel: (202) 347-5270
Fax: (202) 347-5274
www.kff.org

Medical Students for Choice (MS4C)
P.O. Box 70190, Oakland, CA 94612
Tel: (510) 238-5210
Fax: (510) 238-5213
www.ms4c.org

NARAL Pro-Choice America
1156 15th Street, NW, Suite 700
Washington, DC 20005
Tel: (202) 973-3000
Fax: (202) 973-3096
www.naral.org

National Abortion Federation
1755 Massachusetts Avenue,
    NW, Suite 600
Washington, DC 20036
Tel: (202) 667-5881
Fax: (202) 667-5890
naf@prochoice.org
www.prochoice.org

National Association for the
    Advancement of Colored
    People (NAACP)
NAACP National Headquarters
4805 Mt. Hope Drive
Baltimore, MD 21215
Toll Free: (877) NAACP-98
Tel: (410) 521-4939
www.naacp.org

National Latina Institute for
Reproductive Health
50 Broad Street, Suite 1825
New York, NY 10004
Tel: (212) 422-2553
Fax: (212) 422-2556
nlirh@latinainstitute.org
www.latinainstitute.org

National Women's Health Network
514 10th Street NW, Suite 400
Washington, DC 20004
Tel: (202) 347-1140
Fax: (202) 347-1168
nwhn@nwhn.org
www.womenshealthnetwork.org

National Women's Law Center
11 Dupont Circle, NW, #800
Washington, DC 20036
Tel: (202) 588-5180
Fax: (202) 588-5185
www.nwlc.org

Planned Parenthood
Federation of America
434 West 33rd Street
New York, NY 10001
www.ppfa.org

The Religious Coalition for
Reproductive Choice (RCRC)
1025 Vermont Ave. NW, Suite 1130
Washington, DC 20005
Tel: (202) 628-7700
Fax: (202) 628-7716
info@rcrc.org
www.rcrc.org

SisterSong: Women of Color
Reproductive Health Collective
PO Box 311020
Atlanta, GA 31131
Tel: (404) 344-9629
Fax: (404) 346-7517
info@sistersong.net
www.sistersong.net

The Young Men's Clinic
21 Audubon Avenue
New York, NY 10032
Tel: (212) 342-3201

Vietnam

Action Aid Vietnam (AAV)
(To chuc Hanh dong Vien tro Anh)
Room 206, 521 Kim Ma Street
Ba Dinh; Hanoi, Vietnam
Tel: (84-4) 771-7692, 846-2748,
846-2749

Care International
25 Hang Bun St.
Ba Dinh, Hanoi, Vietnam
Tel: (84-4) 716-1930

Center for Family and Women's Studies
6 Dinh Cong
Trang, Hanoi, Vietnam

Centre for Population Studies and
Information (CPSI, with NCPFP)
12 Ngo Tat To Street
Dong Da, Hanoi, Vietnam
Tel: (84-4) 823-7698

Center for Reproductive
and Family Health.
No. 63, Lane 35 Cat Linh
Hanoi, Vietnam
Tel: (84-4) 733-3613
Fax: (84-4) 823-4288
rafh@hn.vnn.vn
www.rafh-vie.org

Family Health International
30 Nguyen Du, Suite 201
Hanoi, Vietnam
Tel: (84-4) 942-2667/0737, 943-1828

Ford Foundation, Sexuality and
   Reproductive Health
Vietcombank Tower, 15th Floor
198 Tran Quang Khai St.
Hanoi, Vietnam
Tel: (84-4) 934-9766/7/8/9
Fax: (84-4) 934-9765

General Statistics Office of Vietnam
2 Hoang Van Thu Street
Hanoi, Vietnam

Ipas Organization
Room 203, Van Phuc Bldg.,
   #2 Nui Truc St.
Hanoi, Vietnam
Tel: (84-4) 726-0548
www.ipas.org

Marie Stopes International Vietnam.
Room 104, 521 Kim Ma
Hanoi, Vietnam
Tel: (84-4) 771-7728/30
Fax: (84-4) 771-7713
www.mariestopes.org.vn

National Committee for the
   Advancement of Women in Vietnam
39 Hang Chuoi
Hanoi, Vietnam
Tel: (84-4) 821-0068, 971-1349
ncfaw@hn.vnn.vn
www.ubqgphunu.gov.vn

NGO Resource Center
Khach san La Thanh at 218
   Doi Can Street
Hanoi, Vietnam
Tel: (84-4) 832-8570
www.ngocentre.netnam.vn/
   directory2002-2003

PATH Canada
23-25 Dang Tien Dong
Hanoi, Vietnam
Tel: (84-4) 823-6360, 857-1193
pathCan@netnam.org.vn

Pathfinder International
Room 205, B4b Giang Vo Building
269 Kim Ma Street
Hanoi, Vietnam
Tel: (84-4) 846-0807
Fax: (84-4) 846-0806

Plan International—Vietnam (PIVN)
CI-2 Phuong Liet
Giai Phong Rd.
Dong Da
PO Box 117
Hanoi, Vietnam
Tel: (84-4) 692100, Fax: (84-4) 692769
www.plan-international.org

Population Council.
2 Dang Dung St.
Hanoi, Vietnam
Tel: (84-4) 716-1716/7/8/9
Fax: (84-4) 716-1707
www.popcouncil.org

Population Development International
7th Floor, 42 Lo Duc
Hanoi, Vietnam
Tel: (84-4) 978-2514/5
Fax: (84-4) 978-2506
pdihanoi@fpt.vn

Research Center for Gender,
   Family and Environment in
   Development (CGFED)
19-A26 Nghia Tan, Cau Giay
Hanoi, Vietnam
Tel: (84-4) 756-5929
Fax: (84-4) 756-5874
cgfed@hn.vnn.vn

UNAIDS
44B Ly Thuong Kiet, Hanoi
Tel: 934-3416/7
www.unaids.org.vn

UNDP
29 Phan Boi Chau
Hanoi, Vietnam
Tel: 04-825-7495
www.undp.org.vn

UNFPA—RH Initiative for
    Youth in Asia.
1st Floor, UN Apartment Building,
    2E Van Phuc Compound
Hanoi, Vietnam
Tel: (84-4) 823-6632
Fax: (84-4) 823-2822

USAID
Rose Garden, 3rd Floor, 6
    Ngoc Khanh St.
Hanoi, Vietnam
Tel: (84-4) 831-4580
Fax: (84-4) 772-1092

Vietnam Family Planning
    Association (VINAFPA)
138A Giang Vo St.
Hanoi, Vietnam
Tel: (84-4) 846-1143
Fax: (84-4) 844-7232
vinafpa@netnam.org.vn

Vietnam Women's Union
39 Hang Chuoi
Hanoi, Vietnam
Tel: (84-4) 972-0056
Fax: (84-4) 971-3141
cssk@hn.vnn.vn

WHO
63 Tran Hung Dao St. PO Box 52
Hanoi, Vietnam
Tel: 943-3737
Fax: 943-3740
who@vtn.wpro.who.int

Jordan

Arab Women Organization of Jordan
PO Box 6864
Amman 11118, Jordan
Tel: (962) 6-465-0414
Fax: (962) 6-438-5478
awo@nets.com.jo

Commercial Market Strategies
33 Sulayman Bilbeisi St., Abdoun
PO Box 940899
Amman 11194, Jordan
Tel: (962) 6-592-1653
Fax: (962) 6-593-1945

Higher Population Council
    General Secretariat
PO Box 5118, Amman 11183, Jordan
Tel: (962) 6-556-0741
Fax: (962) 6-551-9210
hpc@johud.org.jo
www.hpc.org.jo

Impact Project, Family
    Health International
PO Box 510648, Amman 11151, Jordan
Tel: (962) 6-462-8077
www.fhi.org

Johns Hopkins University
Center for Communication Programs
PO Box 942143, Amman 11194, Jordan
Tel: (962) 6-566-9931

Jordan Forum for Business &
    Professional Women (JFBPW)
PO Box 910415, Amman 11191, Jordan
Tel: (962) 6-551-4592
Fax: (962) 6-551-4591
jfbpw@nets.com.jo
www.bpwa.org.jo

Jordanian Association for Family
    Planning and Protection (JAFPP).
PO Box 8066, Amman, Jordan
Tel: (962) 6-516-0999
Fax: (962) 6-516-1020
jafpp@nol.com.jo

National Commission for Women
    (in same building as JOHUD,
    off Al-Madeena)
PO Box 5118, Amman 11183, Jordan
Tel: (962) 6-582-5241
Fax: (962) 6-582-7350
jncw@nets.com.jo
www.jncw.jo

POLICY Project
33 Sulayman Bilbeisi St.,
    Abdoun, Amman, Jordan

Primary Health Care Initiatives
Al-Tahajud St., Al-Nissir
    International No. 10
PO Box 851275, Amman 11185, Jordan
Tel: (962) 6-586-6501, 586-6502,
    586-6503, 586-6504
Fax: (962) 6-586-6508

Queen Zein Al Sharaf Institute
    for Development-ZENID
Princess Basma Women's
    Resource Centre (PBWRC)
P.O. Box 230511, 11123 Amman Jordan
Tel: (962) 6-505 2431
Fax: (962) 6 505 8199
pbwrc@amra.nic.gov.jo or
    info@zenid.org.jo
www.nic.gov.jo/jmaw or www.zenid.org.jo

UNFPA
UN Building, PO Box 941631,
    Amman 11194, Jordan
Tel: (962) 6-569-3601, 569-3602,
    566-8171
Fax: (962) 6-569-3603

UNIFEM
PO Box 830896, Amman 11183, Jordan
Tel: (962) 6-567-8586, 567-8587
Fax: (962) 6-567-8594

UNRWA
PO Box 484, Amman 11118, Jordan
Tel: (962) 6-560-7194, ext. 450,
    560-9100
Fax: (962) 6-585-0717

USAID, Office of Population
    and Family Health
PO Box 354, Amman, Jordan
Tel: (962) 6-590-6000

WHO
PO Box 811547, Alal Al Fasi St.
Shmaisani, Amman, Jordan
Tel: (962) 6-568-4651, 567-
    7532, 560-5027

Notes

Preface

1. Rosalind P. Petchesky, Introduction,"
in *Negotiating Reproductive Rights:
Perspectives across Countries and Cultures*,
ed. Rosalind P. Petschesy and Karen Judd
(London: Zed Books, 1998), 25.

2. Dorothy Roberts, *Killing the Black
Body: Race, Reproduction, and the
Meaning of Liberty* (New York: Vintage
Books, 1997), 6. Emphasis in original.

3. Devon A. Mihesuah, "Commonality
of Difference: American Indian Women
and History," *American Indian Quarterly*
20, no. 1 (Winter 1996): 17–18.

Introduction

1. World Health Organization, Department of Reproductive Health and Research,
"Improving Reproductive Health—A
Global Imperative," biennial report,
2002–2003 (Geneva: WHO, 2004), 11.

2. United Nations, "Program of
Action of the International Conference
on Population and Development," www.
un.org/popin/icpd/conference/offeng/poa.
html (accessed April 7, 2003).

3. Alan Guttmacher Institute, *Sharing
Responsibility: Women, Society, and
Abortion Worldwide* (New York: Alan
Guttmacher Institute, 1999), 26–27.

4. Ibid.; Alan Guttmacher Institute,
"Abortion in Context: United States and

Worldwide." Issues in Brief, Series 1 (New
York: Alan Guttmacher Institute, 1999), 2.

5. Paul Ehrlich, *The Population Bomb*
(New York: Ballantine Books, 1968),
148–49.

6. Betsy Hartmann, *Reproductive
Rights and Wrongs: The Global Politics
of Population Control and Contraceptive
Choice.* (New York: Harper & Row, 1987),
13; Thomas Malthus, *On Population*
(London: unknown press, 1798; reprint,
New York: Random House, 1960), 9.

7. Malthus, *On Population*, 9.

8. Ibid.; Hartmann, *Reproductive Rights
and Wrongs*, 13.

9. Ehrlich, *Population Bomb*, 6.

10. Ibid.

11. Ibid., 80.

12. Ibid., 122.

13. Claudia Garcia-Moreno and
Amparo Claro, "Challenges from the
Women's Health Movement: Women's
Rights versus Population Control," www.
hsph.harvard.edu/rt21/globalism/CLARO.
html (accessed March 3, 2002).

14. Alaka M. Basu, "The New
International Population Movement: A
Framework for a Constructive Critique,"
Health Transition Review 7, supp. 4 (1997):
7–31. www.nceph.anu.edu.au/htc/html/
htrV7.htm (accessed March 9, 2002).

15. Lisa Ann Richey, "Does Economic
Policy Conflict with Population Policy?
A Case Study of Reproductive Health
in Tanzania." Working paper, Centre for

Development Research. Copenhagen, Denmark, 2001, 2, 4, 7, 9. Interestingly, the World Bank's decision to disburse SAP loans only after a given country has adopted a population policy is even more extreme than what many of the population alarmists of the '60s advocated. In 1963, Frank Lorimer wrote, "Any attempt to coerce other governments as, for example, by making aid contingent on the adoption of a family limitation program (as has been rashly suggested by some enthusiasts), would obviously be resented. No responsible statesman endorses any such idea." Frank Lorimer, "Issues of Population Policy," in *The Population Dilemma*, ed. American Assembly, Columbia University (Englewood Cliffs, NJ: Prentice Hall, 1963), 153.

16. Richey, "Does Economic Policy Conflict," 7.

17. World Bank, "Population and Development: Implications for the World Bank," 1994. www.worldbank.org/html/extdr/hnp/population/pop_dev.htm (accessed March 17, 2002).

18. Soheir A. Morsy, "Deadly Reproduction among Egyptian Women: Maternal Mortality and the Medicalization of Population Control," in *Conceiving the New World Order*, ed. Faye D. Ginsburg and Rayna Rapp (Berkeley and Los Angeles: University of California Press, 1995), 163.

19. Lori S. Ashford, "New Population Policies: Advancing Women's Health and Rights." *Population Bulletin* 56, no. 1 (March 2001). www.prb.org (accessed March 16, 2002).

20. Richey, "Does Economic Policy Conflict," 10.

21. Ibid.

22. Hartmann, *Reproductive Rights and Wrongs*, 32.

23. Ashford, "New Population Policies."

24. Ibid.

25. Edward K. Kirumira, "Developing a Population Policy for Uganda," in *Developing Uganda*, ed. Holger Bernt Hansen and Michael Twaddle (Kampala: Fountain Publishers, 1998), 186.

26. Ashford, "New Population Policies."

27. Ibid.

28. United Nations, "Program of Action"; Fred T. Sai, "The ICPD Program of Action: Pious Hope or a Workable Guide?" *Health Transition Review* 7, supp. 4 (1997): 1. www.nceph.anu.edu.au/htc/html/htrV7.htm (accessed March 9, 2002).

29. United Nations, "Program of Action."

30. Susan Cotts Watkins and Dennis Hodgson, "Feminists and Neo-Malthusians: Past and Present Alliances," *Population and Development Review* 23, no. 3 (September 1997): 469–523.

31. Ashford, "New Population Policies"; Sai, "The ICPD Program of Action," 1.

32. United Nations, "Program of Action."

33. Marianne Haslegrave, "Implementing the ICPD Program of Action: What a Difference a Decade Makes," *Reproductive Health Matters* 12, no. 23 (2004): 14.

34. Haselgrave, "Implementing the ICPD," 14, 15.

35. The Corner House, "A Decade after Cairo: Women's Health in a Free Market Economy," Briefing 31, The Corner House, June 2004, 9, 10.

36. Ibid., 10.

37. Ibid., 14.

38. Ibid., 15.

39. Garcia-Moreno and Claro, "Challenges from the Women's Health Movement."

40. Hartmann, *Reproductive Rights and Wrongs*.

41. Lisa Ann Richey, "Is Over-population Still the Problem? Global

Discourse and Reproductive Health Challenges in the Time of HIV/AIDS," Working paper, Centre for Development Research, Copenhagen, Denmark, 2002, 14.

42. Rajani Bhatia, "Ten Years after Cairo: The Resurgence of Coercive Population Control in India," *DifferenTakes*, no. 31 (Spring 2005).

43. Richey, "Does Economic Policy Conflict," 14.

44. Ibid., 15.

45. Ibid., 16.

46. Ibid., 4.

47. Corner House, "A Decade after Cairo," 2, 8, 9.

48. United States Government, Office of President George W. Bush, "Memorandum of March 28, 2001: Restoration of the Mexico City Policy," *Federal Register* 66, no. 61 (March 29, 2001): 17303–13.

49. Center for Reproductive Rights, *Breaking the Silence: The Global Gag Rule's Impact on Unsafe Abortion* (New York: Center for Reproductive Rights, 2003), 39.

50. Haslegrave, "Implementing the ICPD," 17–18.

1. South Africa

1. Republic of South Africa, Statistics South Africa, "Census 2001," www.statssa.gov.za/census01/html/default.asp (accessed January 15, 2005).

2. Republic of South Africa, Department of Health, *South Africa Demographic and Health Survey 1998: Full Report* (Johannesburg: Department of Health, 1998), 34.

3. All of the information in this paragraph is taken from V. Goosen and B. Klugman, eds., Women's Health Project, *The South African Women's Health Book* (Cape Town: Oxford University Press, 1996), 283.

4. Ibid., 337.

5. Ibid.

6. Ibid., 286.

7. Center for Reproductive Law and Policy, International Federation of Women Lawyers (Kenya chapter), *Women of the World: Laws and Policies Affecting Their Reproductive Lives (Anglophone Africa)* (New York: Center for Reproductive Law and Policy, 1997), 95; Barbara Klugman, Marion Stevens, Alex van den Heever, and Meryl Federl, *From Words to Action: Sexual and Reproductive Rights, Health Policies, and Programming in South Africa, 1994–1998* (Johannesburg: Women's Health Project, 1998), 4.

8. Klugman, et al., *From Words to Action*, 4, 15.

9. Ibid., 4.

10. Ibid., 75.

11. Goosen and Klugman, *South African Women's Health Book*, 334–35.

12. Khin San Tint, senior researcher, Department of Community Health, University of Witwatersrand. Interview May 24, 2000, Johannesburg, South Africa.

13. Kim Dickson-Tetteh and Helen Rees, "Efforts to Reduce Abortion-Related Mortality in South Africa," in *Safe Motherhood Initiatives: Critical Issues*, ed. Marge Berer and T. K. Ravindran (Oxford: Blackwell Science, 1999), 191.

14. Goosen and Klugman, *The South African Women's Health Book*, 334–35.

15. Ibid., 337.

16. Center for Reproductive Law and Policy, *Women of the World*, 92. South Africa is the only country in the world to include "sexual orientation" in this clause in its original constitution. The 1994 constitution also outlaws the death penalty. (Senne Motsomi, Chief Executive Officer, Planned Parenthood Association of South Africa. Interview May 19, 2000, Johannesburg, South Africa.)

17. Center for Reproductive Law and Policy, *Women of the World*, 92.

18. Marie Adamo, deputy director of reproductive health for the provincial administration, Western Cape; Department

of Health and Social Services. Personal communication, June 15, 2005.

19. Klugman, et al., *From Words to Action*, 3; Center for Reproductive Law and Policy, *Women of the World*, 90–91.

20. Senne, interview; Janet Cole, personal communication, March 30, 2005.

21. Claudia Mogale, head nurse, Family Planning Clinic, Johannesburg Hospital. Interview May 22, 2000, Johannesburg, South Africa.

22. Senne, interview.

23. Republic of South Africa, *Sterilization Act 44 of 1998*.

24. Center for Reproductive Law and Policy, *Women of the World*, 90.

25. Ibid.

26. Mogale, interview; Adamo, personal communication, June 15, 2005.

27. Adamo, personal communication, June 15, 2005.

28. Janet Cole, head of Termination of Pregnancy Services, Gynaecological Oncology Unit, Groote Schuur Hospital. Interview April 18, 2000, Cape Town, South Africa.

29. Mandy Ewan, clinic worker/administrator, Marie Stopes clinic. Interview April 19, 2000, Cape Town, South Africa.

30. Cole, interview.

31. Margaret Moss, head of Contraceptive and Sexual Health Services, Department of Obstetrics and Gynaecology, Groote Schuur Hospital. Interview April 17, 2000, Cape Town, South Africa.

32. Ibid.

33. Center for Reproductive Law and Policy, *Women of the World*, 91; Adamo, personal communication, June 15, 2005.

34. Republic of South Africa, *South Africa Demographic*, 42.

35. Goosen and Klugman, *South African Women's Health Book*, 222.

36. Klugman, et al., *From Words to Action*, 43.

37. Goosen and Klugman, *South African Women's Health Book*, 239.

38. Senne, interview.

39. Center for Reproductive Law and Policy, *Women of the World*, 106; Klugman, et al., *From Words to Action*, 47.

40. Adamo, personal communication, June 15, 2005.

41. LoveLife, "Young People Flock to Trendy loveLife Clinics," June 19, 2002, www.lovelife.org.za/corporate/media_room/article.php?uid=124 (accessed August 11, 2005).

42. Senne, interview.

43. Antoinette Ntuli, Solani Khosa, and David McCoy, *The Equity Gauge* (Durban: Health Systems Trust, 1999), 44.

44. Klugman, et al., *From Words to Action*, 25.

45. Moss, interview.

46. Ntuli, et al., *Equity Gauge*, 40.

47. Center for Reproductive Law and Policy, *Women of the World*, 90; Ntuli, et al., *Equity Gauge*, 41.

48. Moss, interview.

49. Adamo, personal communication, June 15, 2005.

50. Gloria Mokoena, head nurse-midwife, Hillcare Women's Clinic. Interview May 16, 2000, Johannesburg, South Africa; Senne, Interview.

51. Ntuli, et al., *Equity Gauge*, 44.

52. Ewan, interview.

53. Cole, interview.

54. Sanjani Jane Varkey, Sharon Fonn, and Mpefe Ketlhapile, "The Role of Advocacy in Implementing the South African Abortion Law," *Reproductive Health Matters* 8 (November 2000): 106.

55. Tersia Cruywagen, clinic owner, Reproductive Choices. Interview May 19, 2000, Johannesburg, South Africa.

56. Cole, interview.

57. Center for Reproductive Law and Policy, *Women of the World*, 106–7.

58. Moss, interview.

59. Cruywagen, interview.

60. Cole, interview.

61. Ibid.; Adamo, personal communication, June 15, 2005.

62. Senne, interview.

63. Varkey, et al., "Role of Advocacy," 106.

64. Adamo, personal communication, June 15, 2005.

65. Mokoena, interview.

66. Goosen and Klugman, *South African Women's Health Book*, 239.

67. Klugman, et al., *From Words to Action*, 73.

68. Kim Dickson-Tetteh, clinical director, Reproductive Health Research Unit, Department of Obstetrics and Gynaecology, Chris Baragwanath Hospital. Interview May 24, 2000, Soweto, South Africa.

69. Republic of South Africa, *South Africa Demographic*, 45.

70. Center for Reproductive Law and Policy, *Women of the World*, 91.

71. Moss, interview.

72. Mokoena, interview.

73. Moss, interview.

74. Dickson-Tetteh, interview.

75. Republic of South Africa, *South Africa Demographic*, 50.

76. Ibid.; Klugman, et al., *From Words to Action*, 70.

77. Moss, interview.

78. Mogale, interview.

79. Varkey, et al., "Role of Advocacy," 104–5.

80. Ibid.

81. Center for Reproductive Law and Policy, *Women of the World*, 103.

82. Senne, interview.

83. Moss, interview.

84. Cole, interview.

85. Senne, interview.

86. Klugman, et al., *From Words to Action*, 49.

87. Goosen and Klugman, *South African Women's Health Book*, 222.

88. Ibid., 334–35.

89. Republic of South Africa, National Committee on Confidential Enquiries into Maternal Deaths (NCCEMD), "Shortfall in Provision of Abortion Services Has Serious Consequences," 1998; Dickson-Tetteh and Rees, "Efforts to Reduce," 192.

90. Dickson-Tetteh and Rees, "Efforts to Reduce," 190.

91. Republic of South Africa, President's Office, *Choice on Termination of Pregnancy Act, 1996,* no. 1891.22, November 1996.

92. Ibid.

93. Dickson-Tetteh and Rees, "Efforts to Reduce," 192.

94. Laurice Taitz, "Medics Refuse to Perform Abortions," *Sunday Times,* June 4, 2000.

95. Varkey, et al., "The Role of Advocacy," 103.

96. Dickson-Tetteh and Rees, "Efforts to Reduce," 193.

97. Mogale, interview.

98. Senne, interview.

99. Dickson-Tetteh, interview.

100. Phindile Ngubane, "Stigma of Abortion Leaves Facilities Unused," *Star,* April 20. 2000.

101. Dickson-Tetteh and Rees, "Efforts to Reduce,"194.

102. Dickson-Tetteh and Rees, "Efforts to Reduce," 195.

103. Varkey, et al., "The Role of Advocacy," 104.

104. Klugman, et al., *From Words to Action*, 60; Varkey, et al., "The Role of Advocacy," 104.

105. Cole, interview.

106. Sanjani Jane Varkey and Sharon Fonn, "Termination of Pregnancy," in *South African Health Review: 1999* (Durban: Health Systems Trust, 1999), 360.

107. Klugman, et al., *From Words to Action*, 67.

108. Cruywagen, interview.

109. Republic of South Africa, Statistics South Africa, "Earning and Spending in South Africa: Selected Findings and Comparisons from the Income and Expenditure Surveys of October 1995 and October 2000" (Pretoria: Statistics South Africa, 2002), 27.

110. Cruywagen, interview.

111. Adamo, personal communication, June 15, 2005.

112. Cruywagen, interview.

113. Cole, interview.

114. Ibid.

115. Rachel Ramphora, head nurse, Termination of Pregnancy Services, Johannesburg Hospital. Interview May 22, 2000, Johannesburg, South Africa.

116. Moss, interview.

117. Ibid.

118. Senne, interview.

119. Goosen and Klugman, *South African Women's Health Book*, 328.

120. Klugman, et al., *From Words to Action*, 65–66.

121. Varkey, et al., "Role of Advocacy," 105–6.

122. Klugman, et al., *From Words to Action*, 656.

123. Varkey and Fonn, "Termination of Pregnancy," 363.

124. Varkey, et al., "Role of Advocacy," 106–7.

125. Ibid.

126. Taitz, "Medics Refuse."

127. Cruywagen, interview.

128. Ibid.

129. Moss, interview.

130. Cole, interview; Republic of South Africa, *Choice on Termination of Pregnancy Act, 1996.*

131. E. M. H. Mitchell, K. A. Trueman, M. C. Gabriel, A. Fine, and N. Manentsa, "Accelerating the Pace of Progress in South Africa: An Evaluation of the Impact of Values Clarification Workshops on Termination of Pregnancy Access in Limpopo Province" (Johannesburg, South Africa: Ipas, 2004).

132. Varkey and Fonn, "Termination of Pregnancy," 362.

133. Tint, interview.

134. Mitchell, et al., "Accelerating the Pace of Progress" 11, 19.

135. Varkey, et al., "Role of Advocacy," 106.

136. Cole, personal communication, March 30, 2005.

137. Varkey, et al., "Role of Advocacy," 105–6.

138. Cruywagen, interview.

139. Ibid.

140. Republic of South Africa, *Choice on Termination of Pregnancy Act, 1996.*

141. Cruywagen, interview.

142. Republic of South Africa, *Choice on Termination of Pregnancy Act, 1996.*

143. Kim Dickson-Tetteh and Deborah L. Billings, "Abortion Care Services Provided by Registered Midwives in South Africa," *International Family Planning Perspectives* 28, no. 3 (2002): 145.

144. Ibid.

145. Dickson-Tetteh and Rees, "Efforts to Reduce," 195.

146. Ibid.

147. Dickson-Tetteh and Billings, "Abortion Care Services," 149.

148. Dickson-Tetteh and Rees, "Efforts to Reduce," 196; Barbara Klugman, program officer in Sexuality and Reproductive Health, Ford Foundation. Personal communication April 25, 2005; Women's Legal Centre, "South Africa: Reflection on 10 Years after Cairo," 2004, www.wlce.co.za/advocacy/article1.php (accessed June 15, 2005).

149. Ewan, interview.

150. Mogale, interview.

151. Ntuthu Manjezi, project manager, Community-Based Reproductive Health Services, Planned Parenthood of South Africa—Western Cape. Interview April 17, 2000, Cape Town, South Africa; Moss, Interview.

152. Cruywagen, interview.

153. Senne, interview.

154. Republic of South Africa, Department of Health, "HIV/AIDS/STD Strategic Plan for South Africa, 2000–2005" (Pretoria: Department of Health, 2000), 9.

155. Klugman, et al., *From Words to Action*, 76.

156. Steve Berry, "HIV & AIDS in South Africa," July 2005, www.avert.org/aidssouthafrica.htm (accessed August 15, 2005); UNAIDS, *2004 Report on the Global AIDS Epidemic* (Geneva: UNAIDS, June 2004).

157. Center for Reproductive Law and Policy, *Women of the World*, 99.

158. UNAIDS, *2004 Report on the Global AIDS Epidemic*.

159. Ibid., 6.

160. Berry, "HIV & AIDS in South Africa."

161. Ibid.

162. Ibid.

163. Barnaby Phillips, "Ministry Attacks Mbeki Aids Stance," BBC News. September 21, 2001, news.bbc.co.uk/1/hi/world/africa/1556715.stm (accessed August 15, 2005).

164. Phillips, "Ministry Attacks Mbeke Aids Stance.".

165. Cole, personal communication, March 30, 2005.

166. Berry, "HIV & AIDS in South Africa."

167. Women's Legal Centre, "South Africa: Reflection on 10 Years after Cairo."

168. Berry, "HIV & AIDS in South Africa."

169. Ibid.

170. UNAIDS, *2004 Report on the Global AIDS Epidemic*.

171. Rita Sonko, David McCoy, Eva Gosa, et al., "Sexually Transmitted Infections: An Overview of Issues on STI Management and Control in South Africa" (Durban: Health Systems Trust, March 2003), 11.

172. Sonko, et al., "Sexually Transmitted Infections," 21.

173. Ibid., 11.

174. Republic of South Africa, *South Africa Demographic and Health Survey 1998*, 16.

175. Ibid., 27.

176. Manjezi, interview.

177. Quoted in Goosen and Klugman, *South African Women's Health Book*, 432.

178. Cole, interview.

179. Dickson-Tetteh, interview.

180. Moss, interview.

181. Barbara Klugman, Marion Stevens, and Alex van den Heever, "South Africa," in *Promoting Reproductive Health: Investing in Health for Development*, ed. Shepard Formand and Remita Ghosh (Boulder: Lynne Rienner Publishers, 2000), 152.

182. Klugman, et al., "South Africa," 149.

183. Ibid.

184. Marianne Haslegrave, "Implementing the ICPD Program of Action: What a Difference a Decade Makes," *Reproductive Health Matters* 12, no. 23 (2004): 14–15.

185. Barbara Klugman, program officer in Sexuality and Reproductive Health, Ford Foundation. Personal communication April 25, 2005.

186. Klugman, personal communication, April 25, 2005.

187. Republic of South Africa, *Constitution of the Republic of South Africa, 1996*. Act 108 of 1996.

188. Center for Reproductive Law and Policy, *Women of the World*, 90.

189. Senne, interview.

190. Moss, interview.

191. Manjezi, interview.

192. Dickson-Tetteh, interview.

2. Uganda

1. Sylvia Tamale, When Hens Begin to Crow: Gender and Parliamentary Politics in Uganda (Kampala: Fountain Publishers, 1999), 150.

2. Republic of Uganda, "Some Salient Population and Development Indicators for Uganda" (Kampala: Population Secretariat, Ministry of Planning and Economic Development, based on

1991 census); Justus Mugaju, "District Rural Health Systems: Case Studies of Bushenyi, Kisoro, and Sembabule," in Rural Health Providers in South-West Uganda, ed. Mohammad Kisubi and Justus Mugaju (Kampala: Fountain Publishers, 1999), 121; Justus Mugaju, "On the Eve of the Rural Health Programme," in Rural Health Providers in South-West Uganda, ed. Mohammad Kisubi and Justus Mugaju (Kampala: Fountain Publishers, 1999), 125–26; Republic of Uganda, "Reproductive Health Division 5-Year Strategic Framework 2000–2004" (Kampala: Ministry of Health, July 2000), viii.

3. United Nations Development Program (UNDP), Human Development Report 2004 (New York: UNDP, 2004).

4. Republic of Uganda, "Some Salient Population and Development Indicators"; Uganda Bureau of Statistics (UBOS) and ORC Macros, Uganda Demographic and Health Survey 2000–2001, (Calverton, MD: UBOS and ORC Macro, 2001), 41.

5. Elena Prada, Florence Mirembe, Fatima H. Ahmed, Rose Nalwadda, and Charles Kiggundu, Abortion and Postabortion Care in Uganda: A Report from Health Care Professionals and Health Facilities, Occasional Report No. 17 (New York: Alan Guttmacher Institute, 2005), 5.

6. Lara Knudsen, "Limited Choices: A Look at Women's Access to Health Care in Uganda," Women's Studies Quarterly Nos. 3 and 4 (Winter 2004): 253–60.

7. Prada, et al., Abortion and Postabortion Care in Uganda, 5; Uganda Bureau of Statistics (UBOS) and ORC Macros, Uganda Demographic and Health Survey 2000–2001, 54.

8. Prada, et al., Abortion and Postabortion Care in Uganda, 5.

9. Jotham Jotham Musinguzi, head of Family Health Department, director of Population Secretariat, Ministry of Finance, Planning, and Economic Development. Interview March 27, 2002, Kampala, Uganda.

10. Lisa Ann Richey, "Uganda: HIV/AIDS and Reproductive Health," in Where Human Rights Begin: Essays on Health, Sexuality and Women, Ten Years after Vienna, Cairo and Beijing, ed. Wendy Chavkin and Ellen Chesler (New Brunswick, NJ: Rutgers University Press, 2005).

11. Uganda Bureau of Statistics (UBOS), 2002 Uganda Population and Housing Census (Kampala: UBOS, 2002), 12.

12. Florence A. O. Ebanyat, assistant commissioner, Reproductive Health, Ministry of Health. Interview March 18, 2002, Kampala, Uganda.

13. Miriam Sentongo, senior medical officer, project manager, Reproductive Health Division, Ministry of Health. Interview April 2, 2002, Kampala, Uganda.

14. Josephine Othieno, operations manager of Marie Stopes Uganda. Interview March 21, 2002, Kampala, Uganda; Stella Neema, research fellow, medical anthropologist, Makerere Institute of Social Research. Interview March 28, 2002, Kampala, Uganda; Priscila Monica Nswemu, midwife, Marie Stopes Uganda—Makerere Kavule. Interview March 6, 2002, Kampala, Uganda; Joy Kyazike Kyeyune, vice president, Association of Uganda Women Medical Doctors, project manager, Adolescent Friendly Reproductive Health Services Project. Interview April 3, 2002, Kampala, Uganda; Jane Atergire, vice sectretary, Uganda Private Midwives Association. Interview April 3, 2002, Kampala, Uganda.

15. Neema, interview; Atergire, interview.

16. Elly Mugumya, executive director, Family Planning Association of Uganda. Interview April 3, 2002, Kampala, Uganda.

17. Nswemu, interview.

18. Othieno, interview.

19. Ibid.; Uganda Bureau of Statistics (UBOS) and ORC Macros, Uganda

Demographic and Health Survey 2000–2001, 75.

20. Nswemu, interview.

21. Uganda Bureau of Statistics (UBOS), 2002 Uganda Population and Housing Census, 14.

22. Ibid., 13.

23. Musinguzi, interview.

24. Ebanyat, interview.

25. Alan Guttmacher Institute (AGI), "Adolescents in Uganda: Sexual and Reproductive Health," Issues in Brief, 2005 Series, No. 2, www.guttmacher.org/pubs/rib/2005/03/30/rib2–05.pdf (accessed July 21, 2005), 2.

26. Ibid.

27. Ibid., 1.

28. Ibid.

29. Michael A. Koenig, Iryna Zablotska, Tom Lutalo, Fred Nalugoda, Jennifer Wagman, and Ron Gray, "Coerced First Intercourse and Reproductive Health among Adolescent Women in Rakai, Uganda," International Family Planning Perspectives 30, no. 4 (December 2004): 156.

30. Mugaju, "On the Eve of the Rural Health Programme," 1–2.

31. Ibid., 3.

32. Owarwo M. Mugumya, "Capacity Building for Health," in Rural Health Providers in South-West Uganda, Mohammad Kisubi and Justus Mugaju (Kampala: Fountain Publishers, 1999), 63.

33. Gill Walt, Health Policy: An Introduction to Process and Power (Johannesburg: Witwatersrand University Press, 1994), 84.

34. Mohammad Kisubi, "The Impact of Decentralization on Rural Health Services," in Rural Health Providers in South-West Uganda, ed. Mohammad Kisubi and Justus Mugaju (Kampala: Fountain Publishers, 1999), 51.

35. Mugaju, "On the Eve of the Rural Health Programme," 5.

36. Mohammad Kisubi and Justus Mugaju, "Programme Design and Implementation 1985–1998: Progress and Challenges," in Rural Health Providers in South-West Uganda, ed. Mohammad Kisubi and Justus Mugaju (Kampala: Fountain Publishers, 1999), 35.

37. Republic of Uganda, "National Health Policy" (Kampala: Ministry of Health, September 1999).

38. Prada, et al., Abortion and Postabortion Care in Uganda, 5.

39. Uganda Bureau of Statistics (UBOS), 2002 Uganda Population and Housing Census, 4, 7.

40. Knudsen, "Limited Choices: A Look at Women's Access."

41. Mugaju, "District Rural Health Systems," 122–23.

42. Republic of Uganda, "Reproductive Health Division 5-Year," 22–23.

43. Mugumya, interview.

44. Stella Neema, "Women and Rural Health: The Gender Perspective," in Rural Health Providers in South-West Uganda, ed. Mohammad Kisubi and Justus Mugaju (Kampala: Fountain Publishers, 1999), 100.

45. Republic of Uganda, "National Adolescent Health Policy" (Entebbe: Ministry of Health, 2001), 7.

46. Ibid.

47. Kisubi, "The Impact of Decentralization," 57–59.

48. Republic of Uganda, "Some Salient Population and Development"; Marie Stopes International, "Uganda Profile," www.mariestopes.org.uk/uganda.html (accessed February 28, 2002).

49. Musinguzi, interview.

50. Atergire, interview.

51. Ibid.

52. Mugumya, interview.

53. Republic of Uganda, "Sexual and Reproductive Health Minimum Package for Uganda" (Kampala: Ministry of Health, Earnest Publishers, 1999), viii.

54. Anthony K. Mbonye, principal medical officer, Department of Community

Health, Ministry of Health. Email correspondence March 19, 2002.

55. Ebanyat, interview.

56. Knudsen, "Limited Choices: A Look at Women's Access."

57. Amandua Jacinto, "The Problem of Dual Employment of Health Workers in Uganda," Uganda Health Bulletin 7, no. 2 (April 2001): 5.

58. Knudsen, "Limited Choices: A Look at Women's Access."

59. AGI, "Adolescents in Uganda," 4.

60. Steve Berry, "HIV & AIDS in Uganda," July 2005, www.avert.org (accessed August 14, 2005).

61. Republic of Uganda, "Reproductive Health Division 5-Year," 3.

62. Neema, interview.

63. Ibid.

64. Ibid.

65. Neema, "Women and Rural Health," 96.

66. Kyeyune, interview.

67. Republic of Uganda, "Reproductive Health Division 5-Year," 51.

68. Republic of Uganda, "National Adolescent Health Policy," 7.

69. Ibid.

70. Neema, "Women and Rural Health," 102.

71. Nestor Owomuhangi, associate programme officer of RH Programme, UNFPA. Interview March 7, 2002, Kampala, Uganda.

72. Ebanyat, interview.

73. Kyeyune, interview.

74. Ibid., recounting the response of male reproductive health workers.

75. Ebanyat, interview; Kyeyune, interview; Owomuhangi, interview; Mugumya, interview.

76. Ebanyat, interview; Kyeyune, interview.

77. Ebanyat, interview.

78. Mugumya, interview.

79. Othieno, interview.

80. Musinguzi, interview.

81. Uganda Bureau of Statistics (UBOS), 2002 Uganda Population and Housing Census, 11.

82. Ibid.

83. Uganda Bureau of Statistics (UBOS) and ORC Macros, Uganda Demographic and Health Survey 2000–2001, 198; Centers for Disease Control, "Infant Deaths and Mortality," www.cdc.gov/nchs/fastats/infmort.htm (accessed August 3, 2005); Centers for Disease Control, "Morbidity and Mortality Weekly Report," www.cdc.gov/epo/mmwr/preview/mmwrhtml/00054602.htm (accessed November 14, 2002).

84. Uganda Bureau of Statistics (UBOS) and ORC Macros, Uganda Demographic and Health Survey 2000–2001, 198; Centers for Disease Control, "Infant Deaths and Mortality"; Centers for Disease Control, "Morbidity and Mortality Weekly Report."

85. Mugumya, interview.

86. Ebanyat, interview.

87. Edward K. Kirumira, "Developing a Population Policy for Uganda," in Developing Uganda, ed. Holger Bernt Hansen and Michael Twaddle (Kampala: Fountain Publishers, 1998), 186, 189.

88. United Nations Secretariat, Population Division, "Demographic Situation in High Fertility Countries," presented at Workshop on Prospects for Fertility Decline in High Fertility Countries, July 9–11, 2001, New York, New York.

89. United Nations Secretariat, Population Division, "Demographic Situation."

90. Mbonye, email correspondence.

91. Kirumira, "Developing a population policy," 192–93.

92. Uganda Bureau of Statistics (UBOS) and ORC Macros, Uganda Demographic and Health Survey 2000–2001, 54.

93. Musinguzi, interview.

94. AGI, "Adolescents in Uganda," 1.

95. Anita Hardon, Ann Mutua, Sandra Kabir, et al., Monitoring Family Planning and Reproductive Rights: A Manual for Empowerment (London: Zed Books, 1997), 32.

96. Mbonye, email correspondence; Knudsen, "Limited Choices: A Look at Women's Access."

97. Uganda Bureau of Statistics (UBOS) and ORC Macros, Uganda Demographic and Health Survey 2000–2001, 56.

98. Ibid.

99. Neema, interview.

100. Republic of Uganda, "Progress and Critical Needs in Population, Reproductive Health and Gender" (Kampala: Population Secretariat, Ministry of Planning and Economic Development) www.uganda.co.ug/population/report.htm (accessed February 21, 2002); Ebanyat, interview.

101. Mugumya, interview.

102. Ibid.

103. Nswemu, interview.

104. Ebanyat, interview.

105. Othieno, interview.

106. Neema, interview.

107. Owomuhangi, interview.

108. Ibid.

109. Mugumya, interview.

110. Ibid.

111. Kyeyune, interview; Ebanyat, interview; Owomuhangi, interview.

112. Uganda Bureau of Statistics (UBOS) and ORC Macros, Uganda Demographic and Health Survey 2000–2001, 67; Mugumya, interview.

113. AGI, "Adolescents in Uganda," 2; Othieno, interview; Nswemu, interview; Owomuhangi, interview; Ebanyat, interview; Musinguzi, interview; Mugumya, interview; Atergire, interview.

114. Mugumya, interview.

115. Republic of Uganda, "National Adolescent Health Policy," 9.

116. Othieno, interview.

117. Prada, et al., Abortion and Postabortion Care in Uganda, 6.

118. Ibid., 5; Owomuhangi, interview.

119. Owomuhangi, interview; Sentongo, interview.

120. Musinguzi, interview; Atergire, interview; Nswemu, interview; Mugumya, interview; Ebanyat, interview.

121. Ebanyat, interview.

122. Neema, interview; Sentongo, interview.

123. Sentongo, interview; Mugumya, interview; Owomuhangi, interview; Othieno, interview; Atergire, interview; Ebanyat, interview.

124. Atergire, interview.

125. Ebanyat, interview.

126. Musinguzi, interview.

127. Atergire, interview.

128. Kyeyune, interview; Neema, interview; Mbonye, email correspondence; Nswemu, interview; Sentongo, interview.

129. Kyeyune, interview.

130. Neema, interview.

131. Sentongo, interview.

132. Republic of Uganda, "Reproductive Health Division 5-Year," 20.

133. Mbonye, email correspondence.

134. Mugumya, interview.

135. Kyeyune, interview.

136. Ebanyat, interview.

137. Ibid.

138. Othieno, interview.

139. Nswemu, interview.

140. Prada, et al., Abortion and Postabortion Care in Uganda, 6.

141. Ibid., 7.

142. Atergire, interview.

143. Owomuhangi, interview.

144. Mbonye, email correspondence.

145. Ebanyat, interview.

146. Ibid.

147. Ibid.

148. Owomuhangi, interview; Neema, interview; Ebanyat, interview; Sentongo, interview; Kyeyune, interview.

149. Neema, interview.

150. Owomuhangi, interview.

151. Ebanyat, interview.

152. Kyeyune, interview.

153. Ibid.

154. Musinguzi, interview.

155. Prada, et al., Abortion and Postabortion Care in Uganda, 7.

156. Lisa Ann Richey and Stine Jessen Haakonsson, "Access to ARV Treatment: Aid, Trade, and Governance in Uganda," DIIS Working Paper 2004/19, Danish Institute for International Studies, 2004, 30.

157. AGI, "Adolescents in Uganda," 2.

158. Ebanyat, interview.

159. Ibid.

160. AGI, "Adolescents in Uganda," 2.

161. Berry, "HIV & AIDS in Uganda."

162. Richey, et al., "Access to ARV Treatment," 30.

163. AGI, "Adolescents in Uganda," 2.

164. Ibid., 3.

165. Ibid., 4.

166. Ebanyat, interview; Atergire, interview; Neema, interview.

167. AGI, "Adolescents in Uganda," 3.

168. Neema, interview.

169. AGI, "Adolescents in Uganda," 4.

170. Mugumya, interview.

171. Owomuhangi, interview; Mugumya, interview.

172. Owomuhangi, interview.

173. Ebanyat, interview; Musinguzi, interview.

174. Kirumira, "Developing a Population Policy," 185.

175. Ibid., 186.

176. Musinguzi, interview.

177. Republic of Uganda, "Progress and Critical Needs."

178. Republic of Uganda, "Annual Health Sector Performance Report Financial Year 2000–2001" (Kampala: Ministry of Health, September 2001), 24.

179. Republic of Uganda, "Health Sector Strategic Plan 2000/01–2004/05" (Kampala: Ministry of Health, August 2000), 24.

180. Republic of Uganda, "The State of Uganda Population Report 2001: Empowerment for Quality Life; Time for Action" (Kampala: Population Secretariat, Ministry of Finance and Economic Planning, 2001), 31.

181. Sentongo, interview.

182. Florence A. O. Ebanyat, "The Reproductive Health Programme in Uganda." (Kampala: Ministry of Health, 2001), 5, 8.

183. Ebanyat, interview; Mbonye, email correspondence.

184. Ebanyat, interview; Mbonye, email correspondence; Atergire, interview.

185. Musinguzi, interview.

186. Ibid.

187. Mohammad Kisubi, "Donor-funded Health Programmes: Prospects and Problems," in Rural Health Providers in South-West Uganda, ed. Mohammad Kisubi and Justus Mugaju (Kampala: Fountain Publishers, 1999), 141.

188. Kisubi, "Donor-funded Health Programmes," 141; Richey, et al., "Access to ARV Treatment," 30.

189. Owomuhangi, interview.

190. United Nations Population Fund (UNFPA), "Uganda Country Programme 2001 Annual Report to the Executive Director" (Kampala, Uganda: UNFPA, January 2002).

191. Ebanyat, interview.

192. Walt, Health Policy, 84–85.

193. Ebanyat, interview; Sentongo, interview.

194. Sentongo, interview.

195. Ebanyat, interview.

196. Kisubi, "Donor-funded Health Programmes," 147.

197. Owomuhangi, interview.

198. Richey, "Uganda: HIV/AIDS and Reproductive Health."

199. Kyeyune, interview.

200. Neema, interview.

201. Sentongo, interview.

3. Peru

1. Tammy Quintanilla Zapata, lawyer, Movimiento El Pozo. Interview November 10, 2003, Lima, Peru.

2. Alan Guttmacher Institute, "Abortion in Context: United States and Worldwide." Issues in Brief, Series 1 (New York: Alan Guttmacher Institute, 1999), 2.

3. Trixsi Vargas Vasquez, counseling coordinator, Apoyo a Programas de Poblacion (APROPO). Interview November 11, 2003, Lima, Peru.

4. Susana Chávez, director, Sexual Rights and Citizenship in Health Program, Centro de la Mujer Peruana Flora Tristán. Interview November 7, 2003, Lima, Peru.

5. Delicia Ferrando, Flora Tristán, and Pathfinder International, *El Aborto Clandestino en el Perú: Hechos y Cifras* (Lima: Pathfinder International, 2002), 11.

6. República del Perú, *Encuesta Demográfica y de Salud Familiar, 2000* (Lima: USAID, UNICEF, Measure/DHS+, and Macro International, 2001), 49.

7. Anna-Britt Coe, "From Anti-Natalist to Ultra-Conservative: Restricting Reproductive Choice in Peru" *Reproductive Health Matters*, 12, no. 24 (2004): 59–60.

8. Chávez, interview.

9. Cecilia Olea Mauleon, Centro de la Mujer Peruana Flora Tristán. Interview November 13, 2003, Lima, Peru.

10. Miguel Ramos, sociologist, Sexuality and Reproductive Health Unit, Universidad Nacional Cayetano Heredia. Interview November 13, 2003, Lima, Peru.

11. Rossina Guerrero, psychologist, Centro de la Mujer Peruana Flora Tristán. Interview October 31, 2003, Lima, Peru.

12. Chávez, interview.

13. Miguel Gutiérrez Ramos, medical director, Pathfinder International, president, Peruvian Society of Obstetrics and Gynecology. Interview November 12, 2003, Lima, Peru.

14. Guerrero, interview.

15. Centro de la Mujer Peruana Flora Tristán, "La salud de las mujeres rurales," Fact Sheet, 28 de Mayo Campana (Lima: Centro de la Mujer Peruana Flora Tristán, 2002).

16. Ramos, interview.

17. Chávez, interview.

18. Quintanilla, interview.

19. Chávez, interview.

20. Coe, "From Anti-Natalist to Ultra-Conservative," 57.

21. Daniel Gho Aspilcueta, CEO/president, Instituto Peruano de Paternidad Responsable (INPPARES). Interview November 12, 2003, Lima, Peru; Quintanilla, interview.

22. Quintanilla, interview.

23. Rocío Gutiérrez, Movimiento Manuela Ramos. Interview November 10, 2003, Lima, Peru.

24. República del Perú, Defensoría del Pueblo, *La Violencia Sexual: Un Problema de Seguridad Ciudadanía—Las Voces de las Víctimas* (Lima: Defensoría del Pueblo, 2000), 18–19.

25. Quintanilla, interview.

26. Ibid.

27. José Carlos Ugaz, lawyer, Benites, De Las Casas, Forno, Ugaz. Interview November 7, 2003, Lima, Peru.

28. Coe, "From Anti-Natalist to Ultra-Conservative," 59.

29. Ramos, interview.

30. Chávez, interview; Ramos, interview.

31. Chávez, interview.

32. Ramos, interview.

33. Ibid.

34. Centro de la Mujer Peruana Flora Tristán, *Informe: Derechos Sexuales y Derechos Reproductivos de las Mujeres* (Lima: Centro de la Mujer Peruana Flora Tristán, 2001), 27.

35. Chávez, interview.

36. Vargas, interview.

37. Chávez, interview.

38. Ugaz, interview.

39. Ibid.

40. Guerrero, interview.

41. Coe, "From Anti-Natalist to Ultra-Conservative," 65.

42. Chávez, interview.

43. Guerrero, interview.

44. Ibid.

45. Americo Mayorga Canales, medical director, Centro Universitario de Salud Pedro P. Díaz. Interview October 9, 2003, Arequipa, Peru.

46. Aspilcueta, interview.

47. Chávez, interview.

48. Mayorga, interview.

49. Ferrando, et al., *El Aborto Clandestino*, 25; República del Perú, *Encuesta Demográfica*, 1.

50. Quintanilla, interview.

51. M. Gutiérrez, interview.

52. Author's notes, November 13, 2003.

53. Olea, interview.

54. Ferrando, et al., *El Aborto Clandestino*, 22.

55. M. Gutiérrez, interview.

56. República del Perú, Ministerio de Salud, *Por la Vida y la Salud: Programa de Salud Reproductiva y Planificación Familiar 1996–2000* (Lima: Ministerio de Salud, 1996), 14.

57. M. Gutiérrez, interview.

58. Chávez, interview; Mayorga, interview; M. Gutiérrez, interview.

59. Chávez, interview.

60. Ramos, interview.

61. Ugaz, interview.

62. Ines Romero Bidegaray, *El Aborto Clandestino en el Perú: Una Aproximación desde los Derechos Humanos* (Lima: Centro de la Mujer Peruana Flora Tristán, 2002), 41.

63. M. Gutiérrez, interview.

64. Ibid.

65. Ramos, interview.

66. Ibid.

67. Ibid.

68. Olea, interview; Guerrero, interview.

69. Guerrero, interview.

70. Chávez, interview.

71. M. Gutiérrez, interview.

72. Aspilcueta, interview.

73. Author's notes, October 31, 2003.

74. Ibid.

75. Ugaz, interview.

76. Ibid.

77. Ibid.

78. Coe, "From Anti-Natalist to Ultra-Conservative," 62.

79. Ibid.

80. Olea, interview; Defensoría del Pueblo, *Anticoncepción Quirúrgica Voluntaria: Casos Investigados por la Defensoría del Pueblo* (Lima: Defensoría del Pueblo, 1998), 40, 46.

81. Guerrero, interview.

82. Coe, "From Anti-Natalist to Ultra-Conservative," 62.

83. Defensoría del Pueblo, *Anticoncepción Quirúrgica Voluntaria*, 33–34.

84. Defensoría del Pueblo, *La Aplicación de la Anticoncepción Quirúrgica y los Derechos Reproductivos II: Casos Investigados por la Defensoría del Pueblo* (Lima: Defensoría del Pueblo, 1999), 194.

85. Defensoría del Pueblo, *Anticoncepción Quirúrgica Voluntaria*, 35–37.

86. Ibid., 47–48. Emphasis added.

87. Guerrero, interview.

88. Coe, "From Anti-Natalist to Ultra-Conservative," 64.

89. Guerrero, interview.

90. BBC News, "Peruvian Sterilization Inquiry Reopens," news.bbc.co.uk/2/hi/Americas/3000454.stm (accessed June 18, 2003); Defensoría del Pueblo, *La Aplicación de la Anticoncepción Quirúrgica y los Derechos Reproductivos III* (Lima: Defensoría del Pueblo, 2002), 19.

91. Aspilcueta, interview.

92. Chávez, interview.

93. Ibid.

94. Mayorga, interview.

95. Coe, "From Anti-Natalist to Ultra-Conservative," 59.

96. Mayorga, interview.
97. Quintanilla, interview.
98. Ramos, interview.
99. M. Gutiérrez, interview.
100. Ramos, interview.
101. Ibid.
102. R. Gutiérrez, interview.
103. Quintanilla, interview.
104. R. Gutiérrez, interview.
105. Ibid.
106. Coe, "From Anti-Natalist to Ultra-Conservative," 62.
107. Ibid.
108. Ibid., 61, 62.
109. Ramos, interview.
110. R. Gutiérrez, interview.
111. Ramos, interview.
112. R. Gutiérrez, interview.
113. Quintanilla, interview.
114. M. Gutiérrez, interview.
115. Ramos, interview.
116. Aspilcueta, interview.
117. República del Perú, *Encuesta Demográfica*, 49.
118. Guerrero, interview.
119. R. Gutiérrez, interview.
120. Ibid.
121. Ibid.
122. Guerrero, interview.
123. R. Gutiérrez, interview.
124. Ramos, interview.

4. Denmark

1. Denmark StatisticBank, "Fertility Rates by Age, Region, and Time," www.statbank.dk/statbank5a/default.asp?w=1024 (accessed January 25, 2005).
2. Lisbeth B. Knudsen, "Recent Fertility Trends in Denmark—A Discussion of the Impact of Family Policy in a Period with Increasing Fertility," Danish Center for Demographic Research, SDU Odense University, Research Report 11, 1999, 3. (No relation to author)
3. Knudsen, "Recent Fertility Trends in Denmark," 15.

4. Lisbeth B. Knudsen, sociologist, Danish Center for Demographic Research, SDU Odense University. Interview June 4, 2002, Odense, Denmark.
5. Ibid.
6. Henry P. David, Janine M. Morgall, Mogens Osler, Niels K. Rasmussen, and Birgitte Jensen, "United States and Denmark: Different Approaches to Health Care and Family Planning," *Studies in Family Planning* 21, no. 1 (January-February 1990), 1.
7. Ibid.
8. Knudsen, interview.
9. Lisbeth B. Knudsen, "Induced Abortion in the Nordic countries," Danish Center for Demographic Research, SDU Odense University, Research Report 22, 2001, 1.
10. Nell Rasmussen and Danish Family Planning Association (DFPA), *Sexual and Reproductive Health and Rights for Youth: The Danish Experience* (Copenhagen: DFPA, 1996), 12.
11. David, et al., "United States and Denmark," 2.
12. Ibid., 4.
13. Knudsen, interview.
14. Helle Samuelsen, anthropologist, Institute of Public Health, Department of International Health, PANUM Institute. Interview June 10, 2002, Copenhagen, Denmark.
15. David, et al., "United States and Denmark," 13–14.
16. Ibid., 2.
17. Johan Seidenfaden, interim national program administrator, Danish Family Planning Association. Interview June 7, 2002, Copenhagen, Denmark; Charlotte Wilken-Jensen, medical director, DFPA contraceptive clinic, Frederiksberg Hospital OB/GYN clinic. Interview June 11, 2002, Copenhagen, Denmark.
18. David, et al., "United States and Denmark," 13–14.
19. Seidenfaden, interview.

20. Vibeke Rasch, Lisbeth B. Knudsen, and Tine Gammeltoft, *Nar der ikke er noget tredje valg: Social sarbarhed og valget af abort* [When There Is No Third Option: Social Vulnerability and the Choice of Induced Abortion] (Sundhedsstyrelsen, August 2004), 175.

21. Wilken-Jensen, Interview.

22. Denmark, Ministry of Health, "Health Care in Denmark." www.sum. dk/health/sider/print.htm (accessed May 5, 2002).

23. David, et al., "United States and Denmark," 5.

24. Ibid., 4.

25. Wilken-Jensen, interview.

26. United Nations Population Fund, *State of World Population 2003* (New York: UN, 2003), 72.

27. David, et al., "United States and Denmark," 12.

28. Wilken-Jensen, interview.

29. United Nations Population Division, Department of Economic and Social Affairs, *World Contraceptive Use*, 2004, www.un.org/esa/population/publications/contraceptive2003/WallChart_CP2003.pdf (accessed June 12, 2005); Rasch, et al., *When There Is No Third Option*, 177.

30. David, et al., "United States and Denmark," 6–7.

31. United Nations Population Division, *World Contraceptive Use.*

32. Wilken-Jensen, interview.

33. Knudsen, interview.

34. Ibid.

35. Wilken-Jensen, interview.

36. Sniff Nexoe, Ph.D. candidate, Institute of Public Health. Interview June 7, 2002, Copenhagen, Denmark.

37. Lau Esbensen, Ph.D. candidate, University of Copenhagen, Center for Women and Gender Studies. Interview June 6, 2002, Copenhagen, Denmark.

38. Ibid.

39. Ibid.

40. Ibid.

41. Ibid.; Nexoe, interview.

42. Nexoe, interview.

43. Ibid.

44. Ibid.; Knudsen, interview.

45. Nexoe, interview.

46. Esbensen, interview.

47. Ibid.

48. Rasmussen and Danish Family Planning Association, *Sexual and Reproductive Health and Rights,* 34, 36.

49. Knudsen, interview; Wilken-Jensen, interview.

50. Stanley K. Henshaw, Susheela Singh, and Taylor Haas, "Recent Trends in Abortion Rates Worldwide," *Family Planning Perspectives* 25, no. 1 (1999): 47; Knudsen, "Induced Abortion in the Nordic countries."

51. Wilken-Jensen, interview.

52. David, et al., "United States and Denmark," 8.

53. Wilken-Jensen, interview.

54. Knudsen, interview.

55. Rasmussen and Danish Family Planning Association, *Sexual and Reproductive Health and Rights,* 36.

56. Wilken-Jensen, interview.

57. Seidenfaden, interview.

58. Wilken-Jensen, interview.

59. Ibid.

60. Ibid.

61. Knudsen, interview; David, et al., "United States and Denmark," 8.

62. Knudsen, interview.

63. Kristeligt Folkeparti, www.krf. dk/hoejre.phtml?krf=1349 (accessed June 12, 2005).

64. Seidenfaden, interview.

65. Ibid.; Wilken-Jensen, interview.

66. Wilken-Jensen, interview.

67. Nexoe, interview; Seidenfaden, interview.

68. Samuelsen, interview.

69. Seidenfaden, interview.

70. Samuelsen, interview.

71. Knudsen, interview.

72. Wilken-Jensen, interview; Rasch, et al., *When There Is No Third Option*, 175.

73. Nexoe, interview.

74. Ibid.

75. Wilken-Jensen, interview.

76. Esbensen, interview.

77. Wilken-Jensen, interview.

78. Esbensen, interview.

79. Rasmussen and Danish Family Planning Association, *Sexual and Reproductive Health and Rights*, 39.

80. Esbensen, interview, citing A. M. Schmidt, P. L. Petersen, P. E. Helkjaer, et al., "Prenatal Diagnosis in the County of South Jutland: Review of 1,026 Amniocenteses," *Ugeskr Laeger* 148, no. 36 (September 1, 1986): 2289–91.

81. Esbensen, interview.

82. Knudsen, interview.

83. Wilken-Jensen, interview.

84. Esbensen, interview.

85. Ibid.

86. Denmark Statisticbank, *Population by Area, Marital Status, Age, Sex and Citizenship (1979–2005)*, www.statbank. dk/statbank5a/default.asp?w=1024 (accessed June 12, 2005).

87. Rasch, et al., *When There Is No Third Option*, 175.

88. Ibid., 54, 175.

89. A. Eskild, L. B. Helgadottir, F. Jerve, et al., "Provosert abort blant kvinner med fremmedkulturell bakgrunn i Oslo," [Induced Abortion among Women with Ethnic Background in Oslo] *Tidskrift for Norsk Laegeforening* 122, no. 14 (2002): 1355–57.

90. Seidenfaden, interview.

91. Ibid.

92. Ibid.; Rasch, et al., *When There Is No Third Option*, 175.

93. Seidenfaden, interview.

94. Ibid.

95. Ibid.

96. Ibid.

97. Samuelsen, interview.

5. United States

1. Dianne Jntl Forte and Karen Judd, "The South within the North: Reproductive Choice in Three U.S. Communities," in *Negotiating Reproductive Rights: Women's Perspectives Across Countries and Cultures*, ed. Rosalind P. Petchesky and Karen Judd (London: Zed Books, 1998), 263.

2. Ibid., 264.

3. Ibid., 264.

4. Government of the District of Columbia, Department of Health, *District of Columbia State Health Profile*, State Center for Health Statistics Administration, December 2003, 10–11.

5. Ibid., 41.

6. United States Government, U.S. Census Bureau, "Fertility of American Women, June 2000," October 2001, 1.

7. National Women's Law Center and Oregon Health and Science University, *Making the Grade on Women's Health: A National and State-by-State Report Card 2004* (Washington, DC: National Women's Law Center, 2004), 9.

8. Dorothy Roberts, *Killing the Black Body: Race, Reproduction, and the Meaning of Liberty* (New York: Vintage Books, 1997), 9. Emphasis in original.

9. Susan M. Reverby, "Cultural Memory and the Tuskegee Syphilis Study," *Hastings Center Report* 31, no. 5 (September-October 2001): 23.

10. Roberts, *Killing the Black Body*, 56.

11. Henry P. David, Janine M. Morgall, Mogens Osler, Niels K. Rasmussen, and Birgitte Jensen, "United States and Denmark: Different Approaches to Health Care and Family Planning," *Studies in Family Planning* 21, no. 1 (January-February 1990): 4.

12. Planned Parenthood Federation of America (PPFA), "Margaret Sanger," September 2004, www.ppfa.org/pp2/portal/files/portal/medicalinfo/birthcontrol/bio-margaret-sanger.xml (accessed August 11, 2005).

13. Ibid.

14. Ibid.

15. Ibid.

16. Angela Davis, quoted in Roberts, *Killing the Black Body*, 58.

17. Forte and Judd, "South within the North," 269.

18. Ibid.

19. Roberts, *Killing the Black Body*, 89.

20. Ibid., 69.

21. Ibid., 68.

22. Ibid., 67.

23. Ibid., 90.

24. Quoted in Ibid., 91.

25. Roberts, *Killing the Black Body*, 94; Jane Lawrence, "The Indian Health Service and the Sterilization of Native American Women," *American Indian Quarterly* 24, no. 3 (Summer 2000): 400, 408.

26. Lawrence, "Indian Health Service," 400.

27. Ibid., 401.

28. Ibid., 405.

29. Quoted in Roberts, *Killing the Black Body*, 95.

30. Lawrence, "Indian Health Service," 410.

31. Roberts, *Killing the Black Body*, 95.

32. Ibid.

33. Ibid., 95–96.

34. Ibid., 59

35. Ibid., 92.

36. Ibid., 119; Centers for Disease Control, "Births: Preliminary Data for 2000," www.cdc.gov/nchs/births.htm.

37. National Abortion Federation, *The Truth about Abortion*. 1996.

38. Ibid.

39. Ibid.

40. American College of Obstetricians and Gynecologists, *Birth Control: A Woman's Choice* (Washington, DC: ACOG, 2003), 75.

41. Henry J. Kaiser Family Foundation, *Fact Sheet: Sexually Transmitted Diseases in the United States*, February 2000.

42. David, et al., "United States and Denmark," 2, 3, 12–13.

43. Jane Ann White, co-owner, Downtown Women's Center. Interview January 16, 2000, Portland, Oregon.

44. David, et al., "United States and Denmark," 13.

45. Ibid.

46. National Latina Institute for Reproductive Health, "The Reproductive Health of Latinas in the US," Fact Sheet, March 2002, www.latinainstitute.org/pdf/ReproHealth/pdf (accessed July 20, 2005).

47. Roberts, *Killing the Black Body*, 118.

48. Patricia Donovan, "School-Based Sexuality Education: The Issues and Challenges," *Family Planning Perspectives* 30, no. 4 (July/August 1998): 188.

49. Devon Cloninger and Susan Pagliaro, "Sex Education: Curricula and Programs," Advocates for Youth, November 2002.

50. Ibid.

51. Ibid.

52. Advocates for Youth, "Myths and Facts about Sex Education," www.advocatesforyouth.org/rrr/mythsfacts.htm (accessed July 21, 2005).

53. Donovan, "School-Based Sexuality Education," 188.

54. Ibid.

55. Ibid.

56. Ibid., 190.

57. Ibid.

58. Terry Daley, abortion counselor, Downtown Women's Center. Interview March 7, 2000, Portland, Oregon.

59. Forte and Judd, "South within the North," 281.

60. Roberts, *Killing the Black Body*, 119.

61. David, et al., "United States and Denmark," 3.

62. National Women's Law Center, *Making the Grade on Women's Health*, 8; Marlene Gerber Fried and Sheila Clarke, "Expanding Abortion Access: The U.S.

Experience," in *Advocating for Abortion Access: Eleven Country Studies*, ed. Barbara Klugman and Debbie Budlender (Johannesburg, South Africa: Women's Health Project, 2001), 285.

63. Roberts, *Killing the Black Body*, 111.

64. Government of the District of Columbia, *District of Columbia State Health Profile*, 3, 4, 8.

65. Ann F. Osborne, PA-C, clinic director, Little Rock Family Planning Services. Interview May 23, 2003, Little Rock, Arkansas.

66. David, et al., "United States and Denmark," 6; US NGOs in Support of the Cairo Consensus, "Keeping America's Promises: U.S. Funding for Reproductive Health Care at Home and Abroad," Washington, DC, 1998, 5.

67. National Women's Law Center and Kaiser Family Foundation, *Women's Access to Care: A State-Level Analysis of Key Health Policies* (Menlo Park, CA: Kaiser Family Foundation, 2003), 2.

68. Ibid.

69. Roberts, *Killing the Black Body*, 184.

70. National Women's Law Center, *Women's Access to Care*, 4.

71. David, et al., "United States and Denmark," 5.

72. Rachel Atkins, vice president of Medical Services, Planned Parenthood of Northern New England. Phone interview May 18, 2004.

73. National Latina Institute for Reproductive Health, "The Reproductive Health of Latinas in the U.S."

74. United States Supreme Court, *Griswold v. Connecticut*, 381 U.S. 479, 1965.

75. United States Supreme Court, *Eisenstadt v. Baird*, 405 U.S. 438, 1972.

76. United Nations Development Program, *Human Development Report 2004* (New York: UNDP, 2004), 156.

77. David, et al., "United States and Denmark," 5.

78. AGI, *Contraceptive Use*.

79. Roberts, *Killing the Black Body*, 125.

80. University of Pittsburgh Medical Center, "Information for Patients: Norplant—Questions and Answers."

81. Roberts, *Killing the Black Body*, 105, 108.

82. Forte and Judd, "South within the North," 284.

83. Ibid.

84. Roberts, *Killing the Black Body*, 132.

85. Ibid., 109.

86. White, interview.

87. National Women's Law Center, *Women's Access to Care*, 78.

88. Ibid.

89. Ibid., 78–79.

90. David, et al., "United States and Denmark," 7.

91. Fried and Clarke, "Expanding Abortion Access," 287.

92. Ibid.

93. David, et al., "United States and Denmark," 7.

94. Fried and Clarke, "Expanding Abortion Access," 288.

95. Ibid.

96. Osborne, interview.

97. Daley, interview.

98. Osborne, interview.

99. Fried and Clarke, "Expanding Abortion Access," 288.

100. Ibid., 289.

101. Ibid., 292.

102. National Women's Law Center, *Women's Access to Care*, 81.

103. Roberts, *Killing the Black Body*, 231.

104. United States Supreme Court, *Harris v. McRae*, 448 U.S. 297, 1980.

105. United States Supreme Court, *Webster v. Reproductive Health Services*, 492 U.S. 490, 1989.

106. Forte and Judd, "South within the North," 267; Alan Guttmacher Institute (AGI), "Abortion in Context: United States and Worldwide," Issues in Brief, Series 1, 1999, 6.

107. National Abortion Federation, *Truth about Abortion*.

108. Ibid.

109. Fried and Clarke, "Expanding Abortion Access," 284.

110. National Abortion Federation, *Truth about Abortion*.

111. White, interview.

112. National Women's Law Center, *Women's Access to Care*, 59.

113. Ibid., 58.

114. National Abortion Federation, *Truth about Abortion*.

115. Ibid.

116. Forte and Judd, "South within the North," 268.

117. Roberts, *Killing the Black Body*, 101, 111.

118. Abbie Adams, abortion counselor, Abortion and Counseling Services. Interview May 26, 2003, Albuquerque, New Mexico.

119. Osborne, interview.

120. National Abortion Federation, *Truth about Abortion*.

121. Ibid.

122. All of the information in this paragraph is taken from Lara Knudsen, "Pregnant? Need Help? An Inside Account of Experiences at a Crisis Pregnancy Center," *Body Politic* 9, no. 5 (November/December 1999): 20–21.

123. United States Government, Department of Health and Human Services, "President Announces $43 Million in Grants from Compassion Capital Fund," August 3, 2004, www.hhs.gov/news/press/2004pres/20040803b.html (accessed July 18, 2005).

124. National Abortion Federation, *The Truth about Abortion*.

125. Osborne, interview.

126. Brittney Camp, counselor, Little Rock Family Planning Services. Interview May 23, 2003, Little Rock, Arkansas.

127. Atkins, interview.

128. Fried and Clarke, "Expanding Abortion Access," 284.

129. Planned Parenthood Federation of America (PPFA), "Teenagers, Abortion, and Government Intrusion Laws," 2004, www.plannedparenthood.org/pp2/portal/files/portal/medicalinfo/abortion/fact-teenagers-abortion-intrusion.xml (accessed July 21, 2005).

130. PPFA, "Teenagers, Abortion, and Government Intrusion Laws."

131. National Women's Law Center, *Women's Access to Care*, 76–77.

132. Ibid., 6.

133. Daley, interview.

134. Larry S. Rodick, president/CEO, Planned Parenthood of Alabama. Interview May 22, 2003, Birmingham, Alabama.

135. National Women's Law Center, *Women's Access to Care*, 6.

136. Ibid.

137. Julia Preston, "Appeals Court Voids Ban on 'Partial Birth' Abortions," *New York Times*, July 9, 2005, www.nytimes.com/2005/07/09/national/09abort.html (accessed July 19, 2005).

138. National Women's Law Center, *Women's Access to Care*, 72–73.

139. Daley, interview.

140. Adams, interview.

141. Fried and Clarke, "Expanding Abortion Access," 303.

142. The Abortion Access Project, "Fact Sheet: The Shortage of Abortion Providers," June 2003. www.abortionaccess.org/AAP/publica_resources/fact_sheets/shortage_provider.htm (accessed July 21, 2005).

143. National Abortion Federation, *Truth about Abortion*.

144. Ibid.; Forte and Judd, "South within the North," 268.

145. Abortion Access Project, "Fact Sheet: The Shortage of Abortion

Providers"; Fried and Clarke, "Expanding Abortion Access," 303.

146. Osborne, interview.

147. Adams, interview.

148. White, interview.

149. Fried and Clarke, "Expanding Abortion Access," 294.

150. Ibid.; Abortion Access Project, "Fact Sheet: The Shortage of Abortion Providers."

151. Abortion Access Project, "Fact Sheet: The Shortage of Abortion Providers."

152. Atkins, interview.

153. White, interview.

154. Osborne, interview.

155. Ibid.

156. Adams, interview.

157. Rodick, interview.

158. Lara Knudsen, "Justifying Murder? Front Row Seats to the Nuremberg Files Trial," *Body Politic* 9, no. 2 (March/April 1999): 3–5.

159. Ibid.

160. White, interview.

161. National Abortion Federation, *Truth about Abortion*; Fried and Clarke, "Expanding Abortion Access," 303.

162. Fried and Clarke, "Expanding Abortion Access," 304.

163. Rachel Benson Gold, "Hierarchy Crackdown Clouds Future of Sterilization, EC Provision at Catholic Hospitals," *Guttmacher Report* 5, no. 2 (May 2002), www.guttmacher.org/pubs/tgr/05/2/gr050211.html (accessed July 20, 2005).

164. Fried and Clarke, "Expanding Abortion Access," 303.

165. White, interview.

166. Abortion Access Project, "Fact Sheet: The Shortage of Abortion Providers."

167. Clinicians for Choice, "Professional Organizations Speak," 2004, www.prochoice.org/cfc/professional_organizations.html (accessed August 11, 2005).

168. Marlene B. Goldman, Jane S. Occhiuto, Laura E. Peterson, Jane G.

Zapka, and R. Heather Palmer, "Physician Assistants as Providers of Surgically Induced Abortion Services," *American Journal of Public Health* 94, no. 8 (August 2004): 1352–57.

169. Daley, interview.

170. Henry J. Kaiser Family Foundation, *Fact Sheet: Sexually Transmitted Diseases in the United States.*

171. State Family Planning Administrators, Office of Population Affairs, Department of Health and Human Services, *Healthy People 2010*, Center for Health Training, 2001, 25–5.

172. Ibid., 25–6; Government of the District of Columbia, *District of Columbia State Health Profile*, 24.

173. Henry J. Kaiser Family Foundation, *Fact Sheet: Sexually Transmitted Diseases in the United States.*

174. Government of the District of Columbia, *District of Columbia State Health Profile*, 27.

175. Ibid., 31; Institute of Medicine, *No Time to Lose: Getting More from HIV Prevention* (Washington, DC: IOM, 2000), 1.

176. Institute of Medicine, *No Time to Lose*, 2.

177. Devon A. Mihesuah, "A Few Cautions at the Millennium on the Merging of Feminist Studies with American Indian Women's Studies," *Signs* 25, no. 4 (Summer 2000): 1247; Yvette Roubideaux, Mel Zuckerman, and Enid Zuckerman, "A Review of the Quality of Health Care for American Indians and Alaska Natives," Commonwealth Fund, 2004, 13–14.

178. Velma McBride Murry and James J. Ponzetti Jr., "American Indian Female Adolescents' Sexual Behavior: A Test of the Life-Course Experience Theory," *Family and Consumer Sciences Research Journal* 26, no. 1 (September 1997): 75.

179. Ibid., 85–87.

180. Ibid., 79.

181. Adams, interview.

182. National Latina Institute for Reproductive Health, "Reproductive Health of Latinas in the U.S."

183. Ibid.

184. Ibid.

185. Government of the District of Columbia, *District of Columbia State Health Profile*, 36, 37.

186. Roberts, *Killing the Black Body*, 101, 111; Henry J. Kaiser Family Foundation, *Fact Sheet: Sexually Transmitted Diseases in the United States*.

187. Roberts, *Killing the Black Body*, 172–73.

188. Ibid., 163.

189. Ibid., 155.

190. Ibid., 175.

191. Ibid., 152–53, 161, 172, 177.

192. Ibid., 161, 189.

193. Ibid., 191.

194. Project Prevention, "How We Help the Children," www.projectprevention.org/program/index.html (accessed August 11, 2005).

195. Clare Murphy, "Selling Sterilisation to Addicts," BBC News Online, news.bbc.co.uk/2/hi/americas/3189763.stm (accessed September 2, 2003).

196. Murphy, "Selling Sterilisation to Addicts."

197. Judith M. Scully, "Cracking Open CRACK: Unethical Sterilization Movement Gains Momentum," *Different Takes* No. 2 (Spring 2000).

198. Murphy, "Selling Sterilisation to Addicts."

199. Scully, "Cracking Open CRACK."

200. Ibid.

201. Dorothy Roberts, professor of Law, Northwestern University. Phone Interview June 23, 2004.

202. US NGOs in Support of the Cairo Consensus, "Keeping America's Promises," 3.

203. Judith E. Jacobsen, "The United States," in *Promoting Reproductive Health: Investing in Health for Development*, ed. Shepard Forman and Romita Ghosh (Boulder: Lynne Rienner Publishers, 2000), 252.

204. Ibid., 254–55.

205. Ibid., 251.

206. Ibid., 260–61.

207. Ibid., 257.

208. US NGOs in Support of the Cairo Consensus, "Keeping America's Promises," 3.

209. Jacobsen, "United States," 255.

210. US NGOs in Support of the Cairo Consensus, "Keeping America's Promises," 3.

211. Jeffrey Sachs, "Weapons of Mass Salvation," *Economist*, October 24, 2002, www.economist.com/opinion/displayStory.cfm?story_id=1403544 (accessed July 20, 2005).

212. Jacobsen, "United States," 265, 273.

213. Forte and Judd, "South within the North," 266; Roberts, *Killing the Black Body*, 300.

214. Fried and Clarke, "Expanding Abortion Access," 295.

215. Roberts, interview.

216. Fried and Clarke, "Expanding Abortion Access," 295–96.

217. Ibid.

218. Roberts, *Killing the Black Body*, 99.

219. Ibid., 101.

220. Roberts, interview.

221. Fried and Clarke, "Expanding Abortion Access," 286; Roberts, interview.

222. Roberts, interview.

223. Forte and Judd, "South within the North," 266.

224. Ibid., 267.

225. Roberts, interview.

226. Jael Silliman, Marlene Gerber Fried, Loretta Ross, and Elena R. Gutierrez, *Undivided Rights: Women of Color Organize for Reproductive Justice* (Cambridge, MA: South End Press, 2004), 285.

227. Fried and Clarke, "Expanding Abortion Access," 284.

228. Ibid.

229. Ibid., 298.

230. Roberts, interview.

231. Ibid.

232. Ibid.

233. Atkins, interview.

234. Ibid.

235. Ibid.

236. Ibid.

237. White, interview.

238. Daley, interview.

239. Bruce Armstrong, "The Young Men's Clinic: Addressing Men's Reproductive Health and Responsibilities," *Perspectives on Sexual and Reproductive Health* 35, no. 5 (2003): 220.

240. Genevieve Sherrow, Tristan Ruby, Paula K. Braverman, Nathalie Bartle, Shawn Gibson, and Linda Hock-Long, "Man2Man: A Promising Approach to Addressing the Sexual and Reproductive Health Needs of Young Men," *Perspectives on Sexual and Reproductive Health* 35, no. 5 (2003): 215–16.

241. Roberts, interview.

6. Vietnam

1. Socialist Republic of Vietnam, National Committee for Population and Family Planning (NCPFP), *Vietnam Population Strategy 2001–2010* (Hanoi: NCPFP, 2001), 1.

2. Socialist Republic of Viet Nam, *Education in Viet Nam: Trends and Differentials* (Ha Noi: Statistical Publishing House, 1996), 1.

3. Socialist Republic of Vietnam, Committee for Population, Family and Children (CPFC), "Viet Nam 2002 Demographic and Health Survey: Major Findings," 2; UNFPA Viet Nam, "Situation at a Glance: Population and Reproductive Health in Vietnam," 1999.

4. Daniele Belanger, "Son Preference in a Rural Village in North Vietnam," *Studies in Family Planning* 33, no. 4 (2002): 321.

5. Annika Johansson, Nguyen Thu Nga, Tran Quang Huy, Doan Du Dat, and Kristina Holmgren, "Husbands' Involvement in Abortion in Vietnam," *Studies in Family Planning* 29, no. 4 (1998): 402.

6. Malin Fihnborg and Magnus Wulkan, *Population and Family Planning Policies in Vietnam: A Reproductive Rights Perspective*, Umea University Department of Law, Minor Field Study Report No. 21, 1999, 1; John Bryant, "Communism, Poverty, and Demographic Change in North Vietnam," *Population and Development Review* 24, no. 2 (June 1998): 236.

7. Socialist Republic of Vietnam, "Viet Nam 2002 Demographic and Health Survey," 2.

8. Ibid.

9. Nguyen Kim Cuc, standing vice-president, Viet Nam Family Planning Association (VINAFPA). Interview March 9, 2004, Hanoi, Vietnam.

10. Nguyen Thi Hoai Duc, director, Center for Reproductive and Family Health (RaFH). Interview March 11, 2004, Hanoi, Vietnam.

11. Daniel M. Goodkind, "Vietnam's One-or-Two-Child Policy in Action," *Population and Development Review* 21, no. 1 (March 1995): 89, 90.

12. Quach Thu Trang, program officer, Population and Development International (PDI). Interview March 10, 2004, Hanoi, Vietnam.

13. Goodkind, "Vietnam's One-or-Two-Child Policy," 99.

14. Ibid., 100.

15. Tine Gammeltoft, *Women's Bodies, Women's Worries: Health and Family Planning in a Vietnamese Rural Community* (Surrey, Great Britain: Curzon Press, 1999), 20, 59.

16. Vu Quy Nhan, director of research and capacity building, Population

Council. Interview March 16, 2004, Hanoi, Vietnam.

17. Nguyen Hoang Anh, "Women in Industry," in *Images of the Vietnamese Woman in the New Millennium,* ed. Le Thi Nham Tuyet, CGFED (Hanoi: Gioi Publishers, 2002), 134–35.

18. Nguyen Kim Cuc, interview.

19. Do Thi Thanh Nhan, senior expert, Department of Family and Social Affairs, Vietnam Women's Union. Interview March 15, 2004, Hanoi, Vietnam.

20. Tine Gammeltoft, medical anthropologist, Vietnamese Committee for Population, Family and Children. Interview March 26, 2004, Hanoi, Vietnam.

21. Goodkind, "Vietnam's One-or-Two-Child Policy in Action," 85; Gammeltoft, *Women's Bodies, Women's Worries,* 91.

22. Gammeltoft, interview.

23. Ibid.

24. Socialist Republic of Viet Nam, Committee for Population, Family and Children of Vietnam (CPFC), "Promulgation of the Population Ordinance" *Vietnam Population News* No. 26 (2003), 1.

25. Do Thi Thanh Nhan, interview.

26. Gammeltoft, interview.

27. Sita Michael Bormann, program coordinator, EU/UNFPA Reproductive Health Initiative for Youth in Asia (RHIYA). Interview March 24, 2004, Hanoi, Vietnam.

28. Quach Thu Trang, interview.

29. Vu Quy Nhan, interview.

30. Tine Gammeltoft, "Abortion Conventionalized, Abortion Ritualized: Defining Limits to Human Life in Contemporary Vietnam." Paper presented at AAS 2001, Chicago, 4.

31. Johansson, et al., "Husbands' Involvement," 401.

32. Leonard Swidler, "Confucianism for Modern Persons in Dialogue with Christianity and Modernity," *Journal of Ecumenical Studies* 40, nos. 1/2 (2003).

33. Bormann, interview.

34. Daniel M. Levitt, health and humanitarian program manager, United States Agency for International Development (USAID)—Vietnam. Interview March 24, 2004, Hanoi, Vietnam.

35. Quach Thu Trang, interview.

36. Swidler, "Confucianism for Modern Persons."

37. Nguyen Thi Hoai Duc, interview.

38. Le Thi Nham Tuyet, professor of Social Anthropology, director, Research Centre for Gender, Family and Environment in Development (CGFED). Interview March 23, 2004, Hanoi, Vietnam.

39. Nina R. McCoy, public health specialist, Family Health International. Interview March 23, 2004, Hanoi, Vietnam.

40. Socialist Republic of Viet Nam, Committee for Population, Family, and Children (CPFC); and Population Reference Bureau, *Adolescents and Youth in Viet Nam* (Hanoi: Center for Population Studies and Information, 2003), 37–38.

41. McCoy, interview.

42. Khuat Thu Hong, "Study on Sexuality in Vietnam: The Known and Unknown Issues," Population Council, South & East Asia Regional Working Paper No. 11. Hanoi, 1998, 28.

43. Do Thi Thanh Nhan, interview; McCoy, interview.

44. Le Thi Nham Tuyet, interview.

45. Ibid.

46. McCoy, interview.

47. Population Council, *Annual Report 2001: South and East Asia,* 2001, 28.

48. Ibid.

49. Bormann, interview.

50. Vu Quy Nhan, interview.

51. Ibid.

52. Ibid.

53. Ibid.

54. Nguyen Kim Cuc, interview; Le Thi Nham Tuyet, interview.

55. Lisa J. Messersmith, program officer, The Ford Foundation. Interview

March 15, 2004, Hanoi, Vietnam; Levitt, Interview.

56. McCoy, interview.

57. Gammeltoft, interview.

58. Le Thi Nham Tuyet, interview.

59. Nguyen Thi Bich Hang, country representative, Marie Stopes International. Interview March 16, 2004, Hanoi, Vietnam.

60. United Nations Country Team— Viet Nam, *IDT/MDG Progress—Viet Nam* (Hanoi: Office of the United Nations Resident Coordinator, July 2001), 15.

61. Nguyen Thi Bich Hang, interview.

62. World Health Organization, "Health and Ethnic Minorities in Viet Nam," Technical Series No. 1, June 2003, 15.

63. Gammeltoft, *Women's Bodies, Women's Worries*, 20.

64. Nguyen Kim Cuc, interview.

65. Do Trong Hieu, "Reproductive Health Care in Rural Areas," *Population Family Planning News* No. 6 (1998): 7.

66. World Health Organization, "Health and Ethnic Minorities in Viet Nam," 2–4.

67. Messersmith, interview.

68. World Health Organization, "Health and Ethnic Minorities in Viet Nam," 9–10.

69. Ibid., 1, 6.

70. Nguyen Hoang Anh, "Women and Health Care," in *Images of the Vietnamese Woman in the New Millennium*, ed. Le Thi Nham Tuyet, CGFED (Hanoi: Gioi Publishers, 2002), 121.

71. Quach Thu Trang, interview.

72. World Health Organization, "Health and Ethnic Minorities in Viet Nam," 21.

73. Gammeltoft, *Women's Bodies, Women's Worries*, 23.

74. World Health Organization, "Health and Ethnic Minorities in Viet Nam," 21.

75. Levitt, interview.

76. Nguyen Thi Bich Hang, interview.

77. Nguyen Van Phai, et al., "Fertility and family planning in Vietnam," 7; Socialist Republic of Vietnam, "Viet Nam 2002 Demographic and Health Survey," 2.

78. Bryant, "Communism, Poverty, and Demographic Change," 255.

79. Ibid.

80. Vu Quy Nhan, interview; Messersmith, interview.

81. Le Thi Nham Tuyet, Pham Xuan Tieu, and Hoang Ba Thinh, "Country Study of Vietnam," In *Some Studies on Reproductive Health in Vietnam Post-Cairo*, ed. Le Thi Nham Tuyet and Hoang Ba Thinh, CGFED (Hanoi: National Political Publishing House, 1999), 18.

82. Gammeltoft, interview.

83. Nguyen Van Phai, John Knodel, Mai Van Cam, and Hoang Xuyen, "Fertility and Family Planning in Vietnam: Experience from the 1994 Inter-censal Demographic Survey," *Studies in Family Planning* 27, no. 1 (1996): 6; Socialist Republic of Vietnam, "Viet Nam 2002 Demographic and Health Survey," 2.

84. Nguyen Kim Cuc, interview.

85. Vu Quy Nhan, Le Thi Phuong Mai, Nguyen Trong Hau, et al., *A Situation Analysis of Public Sector Reproductive Health Services in Seven Provinces of Vietnam* (Hanoi: Population Council, August 2000), v.

86. Bormann, interview.

87. Messersmith, interview.

88. Gammeltoft, *Women's Bodies, Women's Worries*, 20.

89. Quach Thu Trang, interview.

90. Do Thi Thanh Nhan, interview.

91. Gammeltoft, interview.

92. Ibid.

93. Nguyen Kim Cuc, interview; Nguyen Thi Bich Hang, interview.

94. Quach Thu Trang, interview.

95. Bormann, interview.

96. Nguyen Thi Hoai Duc, interview.

97. UNDP, UNFPA, WHO, and World Bank, "Abortion in Viet Nam: An Asssessment of Policy, Programme, and Research Issues,"whqlibdoc.who.int/ hq/1999/WHO_RHR_HRP_ITT_99.2.pdf (accessed March 17, 2004), (Geneva:

WHO, 1999), 1–2.

98. Nguyen Thi Hoai Duc, interview.

99. Daniel Goodkind, "Abortion in Vietnam: Measurements, Puzzles, and Concerns," *Studies in Family Planning* 25, no. 6 (1994): 342; Alan Guttmacher Institute, *Sharing Responsibility: Women, Society, and Abortion Worldwide* (New York: Alan Guttmacher Institute, 1999), 27.

100. Bela Ganatra, Marc Bygdeman, Phan Bich Thuy, Nguyen Duc Vinh, and Vu Manh Loi, "Introducing Medical Abortion into Service Delivery in Vietnam: Report of an Assessment Conducted by the Ministry of Health, Ipas, and WHO" (Hanoi: Ford Foundation, MOH, WHO, March 2003), 9.

101. Mike Chinoy, "Vietnam's Abortion Rate Rises as 'Baby Boomers' Come of Age," CNN, February 6, 1999, www.cnn.com/WORLD/asiapcf/9902/06/vietnam.abortion/index.html (accessed February 24, 2004).

102. Johansson, et al., "Husbands' Involvement," 401–2.

103. UNDP, et al., "Abortion in Viet Nam: An Assessment of Policy," 10.

104. Le Thi Nham Tuyet, interview.

105. Nguyen Kim Cuc, interview; Nguyen Thi Hoai Duc, interview.

106. Vu Quy Nhan, interview.

107. Ibid.

108. Gammeltoft, *Women's Bodies, Women's Worries*, 97.

109. Annika Johansson, *Dreams and Dilemmas: Women and Family Planning in Rural Vietnam* (Stockholm: Karolinska Institutet, 1998), 49.

110. Do Thi Thanh Nhan, interview.

111. Messersmith, interview.

112. Goodkind, "Abortion in Vietnam," 345.

113. Vu Quy Nhan, et al., *A Situation Analysis*, v.

114. Annika Johansson, Le Thi Nham Tuyet, Nguyen The Lap, and Kajsa Sundstrom, "Abortion in Context: Women's Experience in Two Villages in Thai Binh Province, Vietnam," *International Family Planning Perspectives* 22, no. 3 (1996): 106.

115. Messersmith, interview.

116. Vu Quy Nhan, interview.

117. Gammeltoft, interview.

118. Gammeltoft, *Women's Bodies, Women's Worries*, 89–90.

119. Gammeltoft, interview.

120. Ibid.

121. Goodkind, "Abortion in Vietnam," 344; Gammeltoft, "Abortion Conventionalized, Abortion Ritualized," 22.

122. UNDP, et al., "Abortion in Viet Nam: An Assessment of Policy," 12.

123. Ganatra, et al., "Introducing Medical Abortion," 12.

124. Nguyen Thi Hoai Duc, interview; Vu Quy Nhan, interview.

125. Messersmith, interview.

126. Jonathan Haughton and Dominique Haughton, "Son Preference in Vietnam," *Studies in Family Planning* 26, no. 6 (1995), 325.

127. Nguyen Thi Bich Hang, interview; Nguyen Thi Hoai Duc, interview.

128. Pham Thi Hue, "Marriage and Fertility in Recent Studies," *Family and Women Studies*, Center for Family and Women Studies of Vietnam, No. 1 (2002): 42.

129. Belanger, "Son Preference," 328–29.

130. Le Thi Nham Tuyet, "Closing Remarks," in *Images of the Vietnamese Woman in the New Millennium*, ed. Le Thi Nham Tuyet, CGFED (Hanoi: Gioi Publishers, 2002), 262–63.

131. Ibid.

132. Belanger, "Son Preference," 325–26.

133. Pham Thi Hue, "Marriage and Fertility," 40.

134. Daniel Goodkind, "Rising Gender Inequality in Vietnam since Reunification," *Pacific Affairs* 68, no. 3 (1995): 349–50.

135. Gammeltoft, interview; Vu Quy Nhan, interview.

136. Vu Quy Nhan, interview.
137. Ibid.
138. Belanger, "Son Preference," 332–33; Johansson, *Dreams and Dilemmas*, 58–59.
139. Nguyen Thi Hoai Duc, interview.
140. Gammeltoft, interview.
141. Thomas T. Kane, Jennifer Middleton, and Kathy Shapiro, *Strategic Appraisal of the Reproductive Health Program of Vietnam*, Reproductive Health Program, December 2000, 52; Community of Concerned Partners, "HIV/AIDS: A Social and Economic Challenge for Viet Nam," CG Meeting, December 2003, Hanoi, 2.
142. Levitt, interview; McCoy, interview.
143. Levitt, interview.
144. Bormann, interview.
145. Nina McCoy, Thomas T. Kane, and Rosanne Rushing, *HIV/AIDS Prevention and Care in Viet Nam: Lessons Learned from the FHI/Impact Project, 1996–2003* (Hanoi: Family Health International Viet Nam, 2004), 51.
146. McCoy, interview; Bormann, interview.
147. Levitt, interview.
148. Gammeltoft, interview.
149. Levitt, interview.
150. Nguyen Minh Luan, "Vietnamese Women and the Environment," in *Images of the Vietnamese Woman in the New Millennium*, ed. Le Thi Nham Tuyet, CGFED (Hanoi: Gioi Publishers, 2002), 220.
151. Socialist Republic of Vietnam, "Viet Nam 2002 Demographic and Health Survey," 2.
152. Do Thi Thanh Nhan, interview; Nguyen Thi Bich Hang, interview; Quach Thu Trang, interview.
153. Quach Thu Trang, interview.
154. McCoy, interview.
155. Ibid.
156. Ibid.
157. Gammeltoft, interview.
158. McCoy, interview.
159. Nguyen Kim Cuc, interview; McCoy, interview; Nguyen Thi Bich Hang, interview; Vu Quy Nhan, interview.
160. Le Thi Nham Tuyet, interview.
161. Vu Quy Nhan, et al, *A Situation Analysis*, 27.
162. Socialist Republic of Viet Nam, National Committee for Population and Family Planning (NCPFP), "Population Control Results Promising," *Population-Family Planning News* No. 8 (1998): 2.
163. Socialist Republic of Vietnam, *Vietnam Population Strategy 2001–2010*, 27.
164. Gammeltoft, interview.
165. Le Thi Nham Tuyet, interview.
166. Gammeltoft, interview.
167. McCoy, interview.
168. Levitt, interview.
169. Messersmith, interview.
170. Levitt, interview.
171. David Sokal, Do Trong Hieu, Debra H. Weiner, Dao Quang Vinh, Trinh Huu Vach, and Robert Hanenberg, "Long-term Follow-up after Quinacrine Sterilization in Vietnam: Part 1—Interim Efficacy Analysis," *Fertility and Sterility* 74 (2000): 1084–85.
172. Levitt, interview.
173. Bormann, interview.
174. Nguyen Thi Hoai Duc, interview.
175. Nguyen Kim Cuc, interview.
176. Messersmith, interview.
177. Gammeltoft, interview.
178. Levitt, interview.
179. Messersmith, interview.
180. Goodkind, "Vietnam's One-or-Two-Child Policy in Action," 86.
181. Goodkind, "Rising Gender Inequality," 343.
182. Johansson, *Dreams and Dilemmas*, 21; Sophie Quinn-Judge, "Women in the Early Vietnamese Communist Movement: Sex, Lies, and Liberation," *South East Asia Research* 9, no. 3 (2001): 247.
183. Quinn-Judge, "Women in the Early Vietnamese," 21.

184. Le Thi Nham Tuyet and Hoang Ba Thinh, "Indicators of Action on Women's Health and Rights after Beijing," in *Some Studies on Reproductive Health in Vietnam—Post-Cairo*, ed. Le Thi Nham Tuyet and Hoang Ba Thinh, CGFED (Hanoi: National Political Publishing House, 1999), 59, 61; Center for American Women and Politics, "Women Serving in the 109th Congress, 2005–2007," www.cawp.rutgers.edu/Facts/Officeholders/cong-current.html (accessed July 5, 2005).

185. Messersmith, interview; Nguyen Thi Hoai Duc, interview.

186. Nguyen Thi Hoai Duc, interview; Do Thi Thanh Nhan, interview.

187. Nguyen Thi Bich Hang, interview.

188. Goodkind, "Rising Gender Inequality," 350–51; Vu Quy Nhan, interview.

189. Nguyen Kim Thuy, "Rural Women in Vietnam," in *Images of the Vietnamese Woman in the New Millennium*, ed. Le Thi Nham Tuyet, CGFED (Hanoi: Gioi Publishers, 2002), 36.

190. Gammeltoft, interview.

191. Quach Thu Trang, interview.

192. Vu Quy Nhan, et al., *A Situation Analysis*, vi.

193. Bormann, interview.

194. Gammeltoft, interview.

195. Levitt, interview.

196. Gammeltoft, interview.

197. Bormann, interview.

198. Nguyen Kim Cuc, interview.

7. Jordan

1. Hashemite Kingdom of Jordan, Department of Statistics (DOS), and ORC Macro, *Jordan Population and Family Health Survey 2002* (Calverton, MD: ORC Macro, 2003), 2.

2. Hashemite Kingdom of Jordan, et al., *Jordan Population and Family Health Survey 2002*, 1.

3. United Nations Development Fund for Women (UNIFEM), Arab State Regional Office, "Paving the Road towards Empowerment: Egypt, Jordan, Lebanon, Palestine, Syria, the United Arab Emirates and Yemen," (Amman: UNIFEM, 2002), 2.

4. UNIFEM, "Paving the Road," 4, 7.

5. J. Schoemaker, M. N. Sarayrah, A. Yassa, and S. Farah, *2001 Men's Involvement in Reproductive Health Survey: Impact Assessment of a National Communication Campaign* (Baltimore, MD: Johns Hopkins Bloomberg School of Public Health Center for Communication Programs, 2002), 1.

6. Hashemite Kingdom of Jordan, National Committee for Women (JNCW), "Jordanian Women: Mapping the Journey on the Road to Equality" (Amman: JNCW, 2002), 6.

7. Schoemaker, et al., *2001 Men's Involvement*, 24; Hashemite Kingdom of Jordan, et al., *Jordan Population and Family Health Survey 2002*, 20.

8. Schoemaker, et al., *2001 Men's Involvement*, 5; Hashemite Kingdom of Jordan, et al., *Jordan Population and Family Health Survey 2002*, 19.

9. Mehtab S. Karim, "Reproductive Behavior in Muslim Countries," DHS Working Papers No. 23 (Calverton, MD: Macro International, UNFPA, 1997), 3, 9; Hashemite Kingdom of Jordan, et al., *Jordan Population and Family Health Survey 2002*, 36.

10. Karim, "Reproductive Behavior," 3, 9; Hashemite Kingdom of Jordan, et al., *Jordan Population and Family Health Survey 2002*, 45.

11. Hashemite Kingdom of Jordan, et al., *Jordan Population and Family Health Survey 2002*, 84.

12. Lina Qardan, deputy resident advisor, Johns Hopkins University School of Hygiene and Public Health, Center for Communication Programs. Interview March 30, 2004, Amman, Jordan.

13. Ayman Abdel-Mohsen, deputy project director, reproductive health advisor, Primary Health Care Initiatives (PHCI). Interview April 4, 2004, Amman, Jordan.

14. Issa Al-Masarweh, associate professor, College of Social Sciences (University of Jordan). Interview April 6, 2004, Amman, Jordan.

15. Basma Khraisat, country director, IMPACT Project, Family Health International. Interview April 20, 2004, Amman, Jordan.

16. Hashemite Kingdom of Jordan, National Population Commission, General Secretariat (NPC/GS), "National Reproductive Health and Life Planning Communication Strategy for Jordanian Youth 2000–2005" (Amman: Population Publication Series, no date), 4.

17. Hashemite Kingdom of Jordan, et al., *Jordan Population and Family Health Survey 2002*, 44; National Abortion Federation, *The Truth about Abortion*, 1996.

18. Malhas, personal communication, July 26, 2005.

19. Seifeldin Abbaro, country representative, UNFPA. Interview April 8, 2004, Amman, Jordan.

20. Abbaro, interview.

21. Qardan, interview; Abbaro, interview.

22. Qardan, interview; Nouf Al-Omari, nurse, medical program director, Commerical Market Strategies. Interview March 31, 2004, Amman, Jordan.

23. Asma Bishara, program officer, Johns Hopkins University School of Hygiene and Public Health, Center for Communication Programs. Interview March 30, 2004, Amman, Jordan.

24. Abbaro, interview; Kholoud Abu Zaid, former senior program coordinator, Save the Children. Interview April 7, 2004, Amman, Jordan.

25. Hashemite Kingdom of Jordan, National Population Commission, General Secretariat (NPC/GS), "Highlights on the Jordanian Youth: Reproductive Health, Life Planning, Education and Employment" (Amman, Jordan: Population Publication Series, April 2001), 15.

26. Abbaro, interview.

27. Ibid.

28. Bernhart, personal communication, July 17, 2005.

29. Abbaro, interview.

30. Al-Omari, interview; Leila Hamarneh, director of projects, Arab Women Organization of Jordan. Interview April 14, 2004, Amman, Jordan.

31. Al-Omari, interview.

32. Qardan, interview; Bernhart, personal communication, July 17, 2005.

33. Zeinab Abu Al-Sha'ar, director of medical services, Jordanian Association for Family Planning and Protection (JAFPP). Interview April 4, 2004, Amman, Jordan; Bishara, Interview; Basem Abu Ra'ad, executive director, Jordanian Association for Family Planning and Protection (JAFPP). Interview April 4, 2004, Amman, Jordan.

34. Bishara, interview.

35. Ibid.

36. Ibid.

37. Nouf Al-Omari and Michael Bernhart, "Client Preference regarding Provider for IUD Insertion," Commercial Market Strategies, November 2002, 1.

38. Al-Omari, interview.

39. Abdel-Mohsen, interview.

40. Al-Omari, interview.

41. Abbaro, interview.

42. United Nations Population Fund (UNFPA), "Towards Family Planning Policy in Jordan," Working Paper No. 9, May 1994, 12, 13.

43. Qteit, personal communication, August 5, 2005.

44. Abbaro, interview; Qardan, interview.

45. Abbaro, interview.

46. Zuhair J. Al-Zu'bi, chief, Field Health Programme, United Nations Relief and Works Agency (UNRWA)—Jordan. Interview April 25, 2004, Amman, Jordan.

47. Hamarneh, interview.

48. Ibid.

49. UNFPA, "Towards Family Planning Policy in Jordan," 5.

50. Ibid., 7.

51. Nisreen Haddadin Bitar, former program manager, EngenderHealth. Interview April 26, 2004, Amman, Jordan.

52. Al-Zu'bi, interview.

53. Bitar, interview.

54. Bernhart, personal communication, July 17, 2005.

55. Abdel-Mohsen, interview.

56. Hashemite Kingdom of Jordan, et al., *Jordan Population and Family Health Survey 2002*, 47.

57. Ibid., 16.

58. Schoemaker, et al., *2001 Men's Involvement*, 31; Salwa Bitar Qteit, senior project management specialist, Office of Population and Family Health, United States Agency for International Development (USAID). Interview April 15, 2004, Amman, Jordan.

59. EngenderHealth, "Trends in Female Sterilization in Jordan, 1998–2000" (Amman: EngenderHealth, May 2002), 1.

60. Abu Ra'ad, interview; Suneeta Sharma and Issa Almasarweh, "Family Planning Market Segmentation in Jordan: An Analysis of the Family Planning Market in Jordan to Develop an Effective and Evidence-based Strategic Plan for Attaining Contraceptive Security," POLICY Project, Draft Report, March 2004, 1, 4.

61. Michael Bernhart, resident advisor—Jordan, Commercial Market Strategies. Interview March 31, 2004, Amman, Jordan.

62. Bitar, interview.

63. Hashemite Kingdom of Jordan, "National Reproductive Health and Life Planning Communication Strategy," 5.

64. Nisreen Bitar, Rasha Dabash, Salah Mawajdeh, Manal Shahrouri, and Ramez Habash, "Attitudes towards Tubal Ligation among Users, Potential Users,

and Husbands in Jordan" (Amman: EngenderHealth, October 2003), 1.

65. EngenderHealth, "Jordanian Providers' Knowledge, Attitudes and Practices Regarding Female Sterilization and Long-Acting Hormonal Methods" (Amman: EngenderHealth, May 2002), 7.

66. Nadine Khoury and Michael Bernhart, "Perceptions of Contraceptives: A Projective Study," Commercial Market Strategies, November 2000, 7; Bitar, interview.

67. Schoemaker, et al., *2001 Men's Involvement*, 17, 46.

68. Khraisat, interview; Hashemite Kingdom of Jordan, et al., *Jordan Population and Family Health Survey 2002*, 47.

69. Bishara, interview; Bernhart, interview.

70. Bernhart, interview.

71. Ibid.

72. Ibid.

73. Schoemaker, et al., *2001 Men's Involvement*, 20–21.

74. Nisreen Bitar, Janet Muzlan Turan, Saleh Mawajdeh, and Manal Shahrouri, "Client Perceptions of Norplant and Depo Provera at JAFPP Clinics" (Amman: EngenderHealth, May 2002), 6.

75. Bitar, et al., "Client Perceptions," 8.

76. Bernhart, interview; Al-Omari, interview; Michael Bernhart, Tara Muayad, Abdul Rahman, and Nesreen Salim Khraisha, "Reasons for Non-adoption of Modern Methods: An In-depth Field Study," Commercial Market Strategies, November 2003, 2; Qardan, interview.

77. Qardan, interview; Bitar, interview.

78. Qardan, interview.

79. Hashemite Kingdom of Jordan, et al., *Jordan Population and Family Health Survey 2002*, 58.

80. Bernhart, interview.

81. Ibid.

82. Dana Khan N. Malhas, national programme officer, United Nations Development Fund for Women (UNIFEM),

Arab States Regional Office. Interview April 25, 2004, Amman, Jordan.

83. Bishara, interview; Hamarneh, interview.

84. Hamarneh, interview.

85. Khraisat, interview.

86. Qardan, interview.

87. Bernhart, interview; Abdul Rahim Ma'ayta, coordinator, program officer, Higher Population Council General Secretariat. Interview April 5, 2004, Amman, Jordan; Hashemite Kingdom of Jordan, et al., *Jordan Population and Family Health Survey 2002*, 42.

88. Karim, "Reproductive Behavior," 29.

89. Ma'ayta, interview.

90. Qardan, interview.

91. Ibid.

92. Bishara, interview; Al-Masarweh, interview.

93. Bernhart, interview.

94. UNFPA, "Towards Family Planning Policy in Jordan," 4.

95. Hashemite Kingdom of Jordan, et al., *Jordan Population and Family Health Survey 2002*, 68.

96. Bishara, interview.

97. AbuZaid, interview.

98. Qardan, interview.

99. Ibid.; Schoemaker, et al., *2001 Men's Involvement*, 35.

100. Michel Farsoun, Nadine Khoury, and Carol Underwood, "In Their Own Words: A Qualitative Study of Family Planning in Jordan," IEC Field Report No. 6 (Baltimore, MD: Johns Hopkins Center for Communication Programs, 1996), ix.

101. Abu Al-Sha'ar, interview; Al-Omari, interview; Khoury and Bernhart, "Perceptions of Contraceptives," 15.

102. Al-Omari, interview.

103. Mousa Shteiwi and Michael Bernhart, "The Contraception Adoption Process," Commercial Market Strategies, August 2000.

104. Al-Zu'bi, interview.

105. Hamarneh, interview; Issa S. Al-Masarweh, "Adolescent and Youth Reproductive Health in Jordan: Status, Issues, Policies, and Programs," POLICY Project, January 2003, 11.

106. Hashemite Kingdom of Jordan, et al., *Jordan Population and Family Health Survey 2002*, 7.

107. Al-Masarweh, personal communication, July 19, 2005 (citing unpublished data from *Population and Family Health Survey 2002*).

108. Michael Bernhart, Rania Abu Baker, and Ghada Abu Ali, "Sources of Doctors' Knowledge of Contraceptives," Commercial Market Strategies, November 2001, 1; Hashemite Kingdom of Jordan, et al., *Jordan Population and Family Health Survey 2002*, 42.

109. Al-Zu'bi, interview.

110. Bitar, interview.

111. Qteit, interview.

112. Qardan, interview; Bishara, interview; Bitar, interview.

113. Bitar, interview.

114. Al-Omari, interview.

115. Hamarneh, interview.

116. Abbaro, interview.

117. Bernhart, interview.

118. Al-Zu'bi, interview.

119. Aida Seif El Dawla, Amal Abdel Hadi, and Nadia Abdel Wahab, "Women's Wit over Men's: Trade-offs and Strategic Accommodations in Egyptian Women's Reproductive Lives," in *Negotiating Reproductive Rights: Women's Perspectives Across Countries and Cultures*, ed. Rosalind P. Petchesky and Karen Judd (London: Zed Books, 1998), 75.

120. Bernhart, interview.

121. Qteit, interview.

122. Al-Omari, interview.

123. Hamarneh, interview.

124. Lamis Nasser, Bashir Belbeisi, and Diana Atiyat, "Violence against Women in Jordan: Demographic Characteristics of Victims and Perpetrators" (Amman: UNIFEM, WHO, 1998), 8; UNIFEM—

Arab State Regional Office, "Evaluating the Status of Jordanian Women in Light of the Beijing Platform for Action" (Amman: UNIFEM, 2003), 34; Bernhart, personal communication, July 17, 2005.

125. Nasser, et al., "Violence against Women in Jordan," 8; Queen Noor, *Leap of Faith: Memoirs of an Unexpected Life* (New York: Miramax Books, 2003), 388.

126. Noor, *Leap of Faith*, 388.

127. Rana Ahmen Husseini, "Current Challenges facing the Arab Women's Movements," *Al-Raida* 20, no. 100 (Winter 2003): 36; Hashemite Kingdom of Jordan, "Jordanian Women: Mapping the Journey," 20.

128. Al-Masarweh, interview.

129. Ibid.; Salwa Nasser, executive director, Jordan Forum for Business and Professional Women. Interview April 15, 2004, Amman, Jordan.

130. AbuZaid, interview; Nasser, interview; Hamarneh, interview; Abbaro, interview; Khraisat, interview.

131. Hamarneh, interview.

132. Abbaro, interview.

133. Al-Masarweh, "Adolescent and Youth Reproductive Health in Jordan," 6.

134. Nasser, et al., "Violence against Women in Jordan," 27.

135. Bernhart, personal communication, July 17, 2005.

136. Khraisat, interview.

137. Nasser, interview.

138. Ibid.

139. Khraisat, interview.

140. Bernhart, interview.

141. Nasser, et al., "Violence against Women in Jordan," 14; Bernhart, interview.

142. Abu Ra'ad, interview.

143. Ibid.

144. Abbaro, interview.

145. Qardan, interview.

146. Hashemite Kingdom of Jordan, National Population Commission, General Secretariat (NPC/GS), Johns Hopkins University Population Communication Services, "Family Planning Knowledge, Attitudes and Public Advocacy: Findings from the 1997 Survey of Muslim Religious Leaders in Jordan" (Baltimore, MD: Johns Hopkins School of Public Health, 1998), 14.

147. Abu Al-Sha'ar, interview; Ma'ayta, interview.

148. Khraisat, interview.

149. Ibid.

150. A. Asa'ad, B. Khraisat, C. Soliman, R. Qutob, and M. Al Kahteeb, "Prevalence of Reproductive Tract Infection (RTI)/Sexually Transmitted Infection (STI) in Symptomatic Women in Urban Jordan," presented at Fifteenth International AIDS Conference, Bangkok, Thailand, July 11–16, 2004.

151. Khraisat, interview.

152. Ibid.

153. Schoemaker, et al., *2001 Men's Involvement*, 52.

154. Ma'ayta, interview; Al-Masarweh, "Adolescent and Youth Reproductive Health," 9.

155. Khraisat, interview.

156. Nasser, interview.

157. Hashemite Kingdom of Jordan, et al., *Jordan Population and Family Health Survey 2002*, 143, 146.

158. Ibid., 14.

159. Malhas, personal communication, July 26, 2005.

160. Malhas, interview.

161. Khraisat, interview.

162. UNAIDS, "AIDS News," (in Arabic) November 1, 2003, 14; Malhas, interview; Khraisat, interview.

163. Al-Zu'bi, interview.

164. Khraisat, interview.

165. Ibid.

166. Ibid.

167. Abdel-Mohsen, interview; Bernhart, interview.

168. Abu Ra'ad, interview.

169. Al-Zu'bi, interview.

170. Bernhart, personal communication, July 17, 2005.

171. Al-Masarweh, interview.

172. Bitar, interview.
173. Malhas, interview.
174. Bitar, interview.
175. Al-Masarweh, interview; Bishara, interview; Qteit, interview.
176. Sharma, Almasarweh, "Family Planning Market Segmentation," 27.
177. Bitar, interview.
178. Qteit, interview; USAID brochure.
179. Bitar, interview.
180. Ibid.
181. Ibid.
182. Al-Masarweh, interview.
183. Abbaro, interview.
184. Al-Masarweh, interview.
185. Qardan, interview.
186. Al-Masarweh, interview.
187. Qardan, interview.
188. Representative of Jordan, United Nations, "Programme of Action of the International Conference on Population and Development," www.unfpa.org/icpd/icpd_poa.htm#pt2ch1 (accessed July 12, 2005) (Cairo, Egypt: United Nations, 1994).
189. Abdel-Mohsen, interview.
190. Qardan, interview; Hashemite Kingdom of Jordan, National Committee for Women (JNCW), Introductory brochure.
191. Bernhart, interview.
192. Al-Masarweh, "Adolescent and Youth Reproductive Health," 17.
193. Sharma, Almasarweh, "Family Planning Market Segmentation," 5.
194. Hashemite Kingdom of Jordan, National Population Commission, General Secretariat (NPC/GS), "National Population Strategy Reproductive Health Action Plan, Stage 1: 2003–2007" (Amman: National Population Commission, April 2003), 1.
195. Ibid., 5, 9.
196. Ibid., 10.
197. Ibid., 50–51.
198. Hashemite Kingdom of Jordan, National Committee for Women (JNCW), "The National Strategy for Women in Jordan" (Amman: JNCW, September 1993), 2.

199. All the history in this paragraph is taken from Sherry R. Lowrance, "After Beijing: Political Liberalization and the Women's Movement in Jordan," *Middle Eastern Studies*, July 1998, 5–9.
200. Bernhart, interview.
201. Malhas, interview.
202. Ibid.
203. Ibid.
204. Lowrance, "After Beijing," 3.
205. Malhas, interview.
206. Bitar, interview.
207. AbuZaid, interview.
208. Ibid.
209. Ibid.
210. Malhas, interview.
211. Ibid.
212. Ibid.
213. Fatima Mernissi, *The Veil and the Male Elite: A Feminist Interpretation of Women's Rights in Islam,* trans. Mary Jo Lakeland (Cambridge, MA: Perseus Books, 1991), 118, 138–39.
214. Malhas, interview.
215. Hamarneh, interview.
216. Qteit, interview.
217. Hamarneh, interview.
218. Ibid.
219. Ibid.
220. Bitar, interview.
221. Bishara, interview.
222. UNFPA, "Towards Family Planning Policy in Jordan," 4.
223. Nasser, et al., "Violence against Women in Jordan," 6.
224. Bishara, interview.
225. Nasser, interview.
226. Ibid.
227. UNIFEM, "Evaluating the Status of Jordanian Women," 27.
228. AbuZaid, interview.
229. Ibid.
230. UNIFEM, "Evaluating the Status of Jordanian Women," 22.
231. Qardan, interview.
232. Ibid.
233. Nasser, interview.

234. Hashemite Kingdom of Jordan, "Highlights on the Jordanian Youth," 6; Hashemite Kingdom of Jordan, "Jordanian Women: Mapping the Journey," 15.

235. Nasser, interview.

236. AbuZaid, interview.

237. Qardan, interview.

238. Hamarneh, interview.

239. Anonymous, "The Gender-Sensitive Fact-File: Profiles of the Arab League Countries—Jordan," Al- Raida 20, no. 100 (Winter 2003): 106–7.

240. Hashemite Kingdom of Jordan, "Jordanian Women: Mapping the Journey," 20.

241. Nasser, et al., "Violence against Women in Jordan," 7.

242. Ibid., 8.

243. Anonymous, "Gender-Sensitive Fact-File," 106–7.

244. Hashemite Kingdom of Jordan, National Committee for Women (JNCW), "Jordanian Women: Major Socio-economic Indicators" (no date).

245. Anonymous, "Gender-Sensitive Fact-File," 106–7.

246. UNIFEM, "Paving the Road towards Empowerment," 43.

247. Hashemite Kingdom of Jordan, "Jordanian Women: Major Socio-economic Indicators."

248. Nasser, et al., "Violence against Women in Jordan," 5.

Conclusion

Special thanks to the Feminist Press for permission to reprint parts of Lara Knudsen, "Limited Choices: A Look at Women's Access to Health Care in Uganda," *Women's Studies Quarterly* Nos. 3 and 4 (Winter 2004): 253–60.

1. Rosalind P. Petchesky, "Cross-country Comparisons and Political Visions," in *Negotiating Reproductive Rights: Perspectives across Countries and Cultures,* ed. Rosalind P. Petchesky and Karen Judd (London: Zed Books, 1998), 300.

2. Jael Silliman, Marlene Gerber Fried, Loretta Ross, and Elena R. Gutierrez, *Undivided Rights: Women of Color Organize for Reproductive Justice* (Cambridge, MA: South End Press, 2004), 287.

3. Petchesky, "Cross-country Comparisons," 313.

4. Dorothy Roberts, *Killing the Black Body: Race, Reproduction, and the Meaning of Liberty* (New York: Vintage Books, 1997), 95.

5. Roberts, *Killing the Black Body,* 138.

6. Zuhair J. Al-Zu'bi, chief, Field Health Programme, United Nations Relief and Works Agency (UNRWA)—Jordan. Interview April 25, 2004, Amman, Jordan.

7. Rosalind P. Petchesky, "Introduction," in *Negotiating Reproductive Rights: Women's Perspectives across Countries and Cultures,* ed. Rosalind P. Petchesky and Karen Judd (London: Zed Books, 1998), 7.

8. Roberts, *Killing the Black Body,* 6.

9. Trixsi Vargas Vasquez, coordinadora de consejeria, Apoyo a Programas de Poblacion (APROPO). Interview November 11, 2003, Lima, Peru.

10. Elisabeth Ahman and Iqbal Shah, "Unsafe Abortion: Worldwide Estimates for 2000," *Reproductive Health Matters* 10, no. 19 (May 2002): 13.

11. Alan Guttmacher Institute, *Sharing Responsibility: Women, Society, and Abortion Worldwide* (New York: Alan Guttmacher Institute, 1999), 32.

12. Alan Guttmacher Institute, "Abortion in Context: United States and Worldwide," Issues in Brief, Series 1 (New York: Alan Guttmacher Institute, 1999), 1.

13. Miguel Gutiérrez Ramos, obstetrician/gynecologist, medical director of Pathfinder International, president-elect of la Sociedad Peruana de Obstetricia y Ginecología. Interview November 12, 2003, Lima, Peru.

14. Rossina Guerrero, psychologist, Programa de Derechos Sexuales y Ciudadanía en Salud, Centro de la Mujer Peruana Flora Tristán. Interview October 31, 2003, Lima, Peru.

15. Vargas, interview.

16. Nestor Owomuhangi, associate programme officer of RH Programme, UNFPA. Interview March 7, 2002, Kampala, Uganda.

17. Salwa Bitar Qteit, senior project management specialist, Office of Population and Family Health, United States Agency for International Development (USAID). Interview April 15, 2004, Amman, Jordan.

18. Daniel Gho Aspilcueta, obstetrician/gynecologist, CEO/president, Instituto Peruano de Paternidad Responsable (INPPARES). Interview November 12, 2003, Lima, Peru.

19. Tersia Cruywagen, owner, Reproductive Choices. Interview May 19, 2000, Johannesburg, South Africa.

20. Janet Cole, obstetrician/gynecologist, former head of Termination of Pregnancy Services, Gynaecological Oncology Unit, Groote Schuur Hospital. Interview April 18, 2000, Cape Town, South Africa.

21. Tammy Quintanilla Zapata, lawyer, Movimiento El Pozo. Interview November 10, 2003, Lima, Peru.

22. Joy Kyazike Kyeyune, vice president, Association of Uganda Women Medical Doctors, project manager, Adolescent Friendly Reproductive Health Services Project. Interview April 3, 2002, Kampala, Uganda.

Bibliographies

Introduction

Ahman, Elisabeth, and Iqbal Shah. "Unsafe Abortion: Worldwide Estimates for 2000." *Reproductive Health Matters* 10, no. 19 (May 2002): 13–17.

Alan Guttmacher Institute. "Abortion in Context: United States and Worldwide." Issues in Brief, Series 1. New York: Alan Guttmacher Institute, 1999.

Alan Guttmacher Institute. *Sharing Responsibility: Women, Society, and Abortion Worldwide.* New York: Alan Guttmacher Institute, 1999.

Ashford, Lori S. "New Population Policies: Advancing Women's Health and Rights." *Population Bulletin* 56, no. 1 (March 2001). www.prb.org (accessed March 16, 2002).

Basu, Alaka M. "The New International Population Movement: A Framework for a Constructive Critique." *Health Transition Review* 7, suppl. 4 (1997): 7–31. www.nceph. anu.edu.au/htc/html/htrV7.htm (accessed March 9, 2002).

Bhatia, Rajani. "Ten Years after Cairo: The Resurgence of Coercive Population Control in India." *DifferenTakes* no. 31 (Spring 2005).

Caldwell, John C. "Reaching a Stationary Global Population: What We Have Learnt, and What We Must Do." *Health Transition Review* 7, suppl. 4 (1997): 37–42. www.nceph. anu.edu.au/htc/html/htrV7.htm (accessed March 9, 2002).

Casterline, John B., and Steven W. Sinding. "Unmet Need for Family Planning in Developing Countries and Implications for Population Policy." Population Council, 2000. www.popcouncil.org/pdfs/wp/135.pdf (accessed March 16, 2002).

Center for Reproductive Rights. *Breaking the Silence: The Global Gag Rule's Impact on Unsafe Abortion.* New York: Center for Reproductive Rights, 2003.

Corner House, The. "A Decade after Cairo: Women's Health in a Free Market Economy." Briefing 31, The Corner House, June 2004.

Dorn, Harold F. "World Population Growth." In *The Population Dilemma*, ed. Philip M. Hauser, 7–28. American Assembly, Columbia University. Englewood Cliffs, NJ: Prentice Hall, 1963.

Dreze, J., and M. Murthi. "Womens' Education is the Most Important Factor Explaining Fertility Differences in India." Programme for the Study of Economic Organisation and Public Policy, 2000. www.eldis.org/static/DOC7804.htm (accessed April 7, 2003).

Ehrlich, Paul. *The Population Bomb.* New York: Ballantine Books, 1968.

Garcia-Moreno, Claudia, and Amparo Claro. "Challenges from the Women's Health Movement: Women's Rights versus Population Control." www.hsph.harvard.edu/rt21/globalism/CLARO.html (accessed March 3, 2002).

Grimes, Seamus. "Controlling Third World Population Growth: A Major Theme of the UN Population Conference in Cairo." www.hsph.harvard.edu/rt21/globalism/Grimes.html (acessed March 3, 2002).

Hardon, Anita, Ann Mutua, Sandra Kabir, and Elly Engelkes. *Monitoring Family Planning and Reproductive Rights: A Manual for Empowerment.* London: Zed Books, 1997.

Hartmann, Betsy. *Reproductive Rights and Wrongs: The Global Politics of Population Control and Contraceptive Choice.* New York: Harper & Row, 1987. Also available at www.hsph.harvard.edu/rt21/globalism/HARTMANNc1.html (accessed March 3, 2002).

Haslegrave, Marianne. "Implementing the ICPD Program of Action: What a Difference a Decade Makes." *Reproductive Health Matters* 12, no. 23 (2004): 12–19.

Jacobsen, Judith E. "The United States." In *Promoting Reproductive Health: Investing in Health for Development,* ed. Shepard Forman and Romita Ghosh, 251–77. Boulder, CO: Lynne Rienner Publishers, 2000.

Lorimer, Frank. "Issues of Population Policy." In *The Population Dilemma,* ed. Philip M. Hauser, 143–78. American Assembly, Columbia University. Englewood Cliffs, NJ: Prentice Hall, 1963.

Lyons, Maryinez, Evasius K. Bauni, Peter Riwa, Stella Neema, Elanor Preston-Whyte, and William Muhuwava. "Family Planning and Sexual Behaviour in the Era of STI and HIV/AIDS: Review of the Literature." World Health Organization, Department of Reproductive Health and Research. Geneva, Switzerland, February 2001. (Unpublished report.)

Malthus, Thomas. *On Population.* London: unknown press, 1798; reprint, New York: Random House, 1960.

Mollmann, Marianne, and Susana Chávez. *La regla de la mordaza y la acción política en la lucha por la despenalización del aborto.* Lima: Centro de la Mujer Peruana Flora Tristán, 2003.

Morsy, Soheir A. "Deadly Reproduction among Egyptian Women: Maternal Mortality and the Medicalization of Population Control." In *Conceiving the New World Order,* ed. Faye D. Ginsburg and Rayna Rapp, 162–76. Berkeley and Los Angeles: University of California Press, 1995.

Petchesky, Rosalind P. "Introduction." In *Negotiating Reproductive Rights: Women's Perspectives Across Countries and Cultures,* ed. Rosalind P. Petchesky and Karen Judd, 1–30. London: Zed Books, 1998.

Richey, Lisa. "Does Economic Policy Conflict with Population Policy? A Case Study of Reproductive Health in Tanzania." Working paper, Centre for Development Research. Copenhagen, Denmark, 2001.

Richey, Lisa. "Is Overpopulation Still the Problem? Global Discourse and Reproductive Health Challenges in the Time of HIV/AIDS." Working paper, Centre for Development Research. Copenhagen, Denmark, 2002.

Roberts, Dorothy. *Killing the Black Body: Race, Reproduction, and the Meaning of Liberty.* New York: Vintage Books, 1997.

Sai, Fred T. "The ICPD Program of Action: Pious Hope or a Workable Guide?" *Health Transition Review* 7, suppl. 4 (1997): 1–5. www.nceph.anu.edu.au/htc/html/htrV7.htm (accessed March 9, 2002).

Sanders, David, and Richard Carver. *The Struggle for Health: Medicine and the Politics of Underdevelopment.* Hong Kong: MacMillan Education, 1985.

United Nations. "Program of Action of the International Conference on Population and Development." http://www.un.org/popin/icpd/conference/offeng/poa.html (accessed April 7, 2003). Cairo, Egypt: United Nations, 1994.

United Nations Secretariat, Population Division. "Demographic Situation in High Fertility Countries." Presented at "Workshop on Prospects for Fertility Decline in High Fertility Countries." July 9–11, 2001. New York, New York.

United States Government, Office of President George W. Bush. "Memorandum of March 28, 2001: Restoring the Mexico City Policy." *Federal Register* 66, no. 61 (2001).

US NGOs in Support of the Cairo Consensus. "Keeping America's Promises: US Funding for Reproductive Health Care at Home and Abroad." Washington, DC, 1998.

Watkins, Susan Cotts, and Dennis Hodgson. "Feminists and Neo-Malthusians: Past and Present Alliances." *Population and Development Review* 23, no. 3 (September 1997): 469–523.

Werner, David. *Where There Is No Doctor: A Village Health Care Handbook.* Second ed. London: Macmillan Press, 1993.

World Bank. "Population and Development: Implications for the World Bank." 1994. www.worldbank.org/html/extdr/hnp/population/pop_dev.htm (accessed March 17, 2002).

World Health Organization, Department of Reproductive Health and Research. "Improving Reproductive Health—A Global Imperative." Biennial Report, 2002–2003. Geneva: WHO, 2004.

South Africa

Adamo, Marie. Deputy Director of Reproductive Health for the Provincial Administration, Western Cape. Department of Health and Social Services. Personal communication, June 15, 2005.

Baleta, Adele. "Concern Voiced over 'Dry Sex' Practices in South Africa." *Lancet,* October 17, 1998, 1292.

Bennett, Trude. "Reproductive Health in South Africa." *Public Health Reports* 114, no. 1 (January 1999): 88.

Berry, Steve. "HIV & AIDS in South Africa." July 2005. www.avert.org/aidssouthafrica.htm (accessed August 15, 2005).

Burman, Sandra, and Patricia Van der Spuy. "The Illegitimate and the Illegal in a South African City: The Effects of Apartheid on Births out of Wedlock." *Journal of Social History* 29, no. 3 (Spring 1996): 613–35.

Center for Reproductive Law and Policy, International Federation of Women Lawyers— Kenya Chapter. *Women of the World: Laws and Policies Affecting Their Reproductive Lives (Anglophone Africa).* New York: Center for Reproductive Law and Policy, 1997.

Cole, Janet. Obstetrician/gynecologist, former Head of Termination of Pregnancy Services. Gynaecological Oncology Unit, Groote Schuur Hospital. Interview April 18, 2000. Cape Town, South Africa.

Cruywagen, Tersia. Owner, Reproductive Choices. Interview May 19, 2000. Johannesburg, South Africa.

Dickson, Kim Eva, Rachel K. Jewkes, Heather Brown, Jonathan Levin, Helen Rees, and Luyanda Mavuya. "Abortion Service Provision in South Africa Three Years after Liberalization of the Law." *Studies in Family Planning* 34, no. 4 (Dec. 2003): 277–84.

Dickson-Tetteh, Kim. Clinical Director. Reproductive Health Research Unit, Department of Obstetrics and Gynaecology, Chris Baragwanath Hospital. Interview May 24, 2000. Soweto, South Africa.

Dickson-Tetteh, Kim, and Deborah L. Billings. "Abortion Care Services Provided by Registered Midwives in South Africa." *International Family Planning Perspectives* 28, no. 3 (2002): 144–50.

Dickson-Tetteh, Kim, and Helen Rees. "Efforts to Reduce Abortion-Related Mortality in South Africa." In *Safe Motherhood Initiatives: Critical Issues*, ed. Marge Berer and T. K. Ravindran, 190–97. Oxford: Blackwell Science, 1999.

Ewan, Mandy. Clinic worker/administrator. Marie Stopes Clinic. Interview April 19, 2000. Cape Town, South Africa.

Garenne, Michel, Stephen Tollman, and Kathleen Kahn. "Premarital Fertility in Rural South Africa: A Challenge to Existing Population Policy." *Studies in Family Planning* 31, no. 1 (March 2000): 47.

Goosen V., and B. Klugman, eds. *The South African Women's Health Book*. Women's Health Project. Cape Town: Oxford University Press, 1996.

Haslegrave, Marianne. "Implementing the ICPD Program of Action: What a Difference a Decade Makes." *Reproductive Health Matters* 12, no. 23 (2004): 12–19.

Jewkes, Rachel, Heather Brown, Kim Dickson-Tetteh, Jonathan Levin, and Helen Rees. "Prevalence of Morbidity Associated with Abortion before and after Legalisation in South Africa." *British Medical Journal* 324, no. 7348 (May 25, 2002): 1252–53.

Klugman, Barbara. Program Officer in Sexuality and Reproductive Health. Ford Foundation. Personal communication April 25, 2005.

Klugman, Barbara. "Responding to Demands, Initiating Policy: The Story of the South African Women's Health Project." In *African Women's Health*, ed. Meredith Turshen, 193–215. Trenton: Africa World Press, 2000.

Klugman, Barbara, Marion Stevens, and Alex van den Heever. "South Africa." In *Promoting Reproductive Health: Investing in Health for Development*, ed. Shepard Forman and Remita Ghosh, 147–81. Boulder, CO: Lynne Rienner Publishers, 2000.

Klugman, Barbara, Marion Stevens, Alex van den Heever, and Meryl Federl. *From Words to Action: Sexual and Reproductive Rights, Health Policies and Programming in South Africa, 1994–1998*. Johannesburg: Women's Health Project, 1998.

Kuumba, Monica Bahati. "Perpetuating Neo-colonialism through Population Control: South Africa and the United States." *Africa Today*. 40, no. 3 (Summer 1993): 79–85.

LoveLife. "Young people flock to trendy loveLife clinics." June 19, 2002. www.lovelife.org.za/corporate/media_room/article.php?uid=124 (accessed August 11, 2005).

Magardie, Khadija. "Abortion in South Africa." *LOLA press*, July–October 2002, 32–35.

Manjezi, Ntuthu. Project Manager for Community-Based Reproductive Health Services. Planned Parenthood Association of South Africa—Western Cape. Interview April 17, 2000. Cape Town, South Africa.

Mitchell, E. M. H., K. A. Trueman, M. C. Gabriel, A. Fine, and N. Manentsa. "Accelerating the Pace of Progress in South Africa: An Evaluation of the Impact of Values Clarification Workshops on Termination of Pregnancy Access in Limpopo Province." Johannesburg, South Africa: Ipas, 2004.

Mogale, Claudia. Head Nurse, Family Planning Clinic. Johannesburg Hospital. Interview May 22, 2000. Johannesburg, South Africa.

Mokoena, Gloria. Nurse-Midwife, Head Nurse. Hillcare Women's Clinic. Interview May 16, 2000. Johannesburg, South Africa.

Moss, Margaret. Head of Contraceptive and Sexual Health Services. Department of Obstetrics and Gynecology, Groote Schuur Hospital. Interview April 17, 2000. Cape Town, South Africa.

Ngubane, Phindile. "Stigma of Abortion Leaves Facilities Unused." *Star*, April 20, 2000.

Ntuli, Antoinette, Solani Khosa, and David McCoy. *The Equity Gauge*. Durban: Health Systems Trust, 1999.

Phillips, Barnaby. "Ministry Attacks Mbeki Aids Stance." BBC News. September 21, 2001. news.bbc.co.uk/1/hi/world/africa/1556715.stm (accessed August 15, 2005).

Ramphora, Rachel. Head Nurse, Termination of Pregnancy Services. Johannesburg Hospital. Interview May 22, 2000. Johannesburg, South Africa.

Republic of South Africa. *Constitution of the Republic of South Africa, 1996*. Act 108 of 1996.

Republic of South Africa, Department of Health and Social Services. "Western Cape Cumulative Monthly TOP Statistics Sheet." Collected by Marie Adamo, Deputy Director of Reproductive Health for the Provincial Administration Western Cape. 2000.

Republic of South Africa, Department of Health. "HIV/AIDS/STD Strategic Plan for South Africa, 2000–2005." Pretoria: Department of Health, 2000.

Republic of South Africa, Department of Health. *South Africa Demographic and Health Survey 1998: Full Report*. Johannesburg: Department of Health, 1998.

Republic of South Africa, National Committee on Confidential Enquiries into Maternal Deaths (NCCEMD). "Shortfall in Provision of Abortion Services has Serious Consequences." 1998.

Republic of South Africa, President's Office. *Choice on Termination of Pregnancy Act, 1996*. No. 1891. November 22, 1996.

Republic of South Africa, Statistics South Africa. "Census 2001." www.statssa.gov.za/census01/html/default.asp (accessed January 15, 2005).

Republic of South Africa, Statistics South Africa. "Earning and Spending in South Africa: Selected Findings and Comparisons from the Income and Expenditure Surveys of October 1995 and October 2000." Pretoria: Statistics South Africa, 2002.

Republic of South Africa. *Sterilization Act 44 of 1998*.

Sapa. "Contraceptive Jab Gets a Clean Bill of Health." *Star*, April 20, 2000.

Senne, Motsomi. Nurse-Midwife and Chief Executive Officer. Planned Parenthood Association of South Africa. Interview May 19, 2000. Johannesburg, South Africa.

Sonko, Rita, David McCoy, Eva Gosa, Christoph Hamelmann, Nzapfurundi Chabikuli, Anne Moys, Arthi Ramkissoon, and Jabu Hlazo. "Sexually Transmitted Infections: An Overview of Issues on STI Management and Control in South Africa." Durban: Health Systems Trust, March 2003.

Taitz, Laurice. "Medics Refuse to Perform Abortions." *Sunday Times*, June 4, 2000.

Tint, Khin San. Senior Researcher. Department of Community Health, University of Witwatersrand. Interview May 24, 2000. Johannesburg, South Africa.

UNAIDS. *2004 Report on the Global AIDS Epidemic*. Geneva: UNAIDS, June 2004.

Varga, Christine A. "How Gender Roles Influence Sexual and Reproductive Health among South African Adolescents." *Studies in Family Planning* 34, no. 3 (September 2003): 160–72.

————. "Pregnancy Termination among South African Adolescents." *Studies in Family Planning* 33, no. 4 (December 2002): 283–98.

Varkey, Sanjani Jane, and Sharon Fonn. "Termination of Pregnancy." In *South African Health Review: 1999*, Health Systems Trust, 357–68. Durban: Health Systems Trust, 1999.

Varkey, Sanjani Jane, Sharon Fonn, and Mpefe Ketlhapile. "The Role of Advocacy in Implementing the South African Abortion Law." *Reproductive Health Matters* 8 (November 2000): 103–11.

Women's Legal Centre. "South Africa: Reflection on 10 Years after Cairo." 2004. www.wlce.co.za/advocacy/article1.php (accessed June 15, 2005).

Uganda

Akite, Lydia, ed. "Adolescent Sexual Reproductive Health in Uganda Schools." Kampala: Straight Talk Foundation, 2001.

Alan Guttmacher Institute. "Adolescents in Uganda: Sexual and Reproductive Health." *Issues in Brief.* 2005 Series, no. 2. www.guttmacher.org/pubs/rib/2005/03/30/rib2–05.pdf (accessed July 21, 2005).

Ashford, Lori S. "New Population Policies: Advancing Women's Health and Rights." *Population Bulletin* 56, no. 1 (March 2001). www.prb.org (accessed March 16, 2002).

Atergire, Jane, Vice Secretary, Uganda Private Midwives Association. Interview April 3, 2002. Kampala, Uganda.

Berry, Steve. "HIV and AIDS in Uganda." July 2005. www.avert.org/aidsuganda.htm (accessed August 14, 2005).

Centers for Disease Control. "Infant Deaths and Mortality." www.cdc.gov/nchs/fastats/infmort.htm (accessed August 3, 2005).

Centers for Disease Control. "Morbidity and Mortality Weekly Report." www.cdc.gov/epo/mmwr/preview/mmwrhtml/00054602.htm (accessed November 14, 2002).

Ebanyat, Florence A. O. (MD). Assistant Commissioner, Reproductive Health, Ministry of Health. Interview March 18, 2002. Kampala, Uganda.

Ebanyat, Florence A. O. "The Reproductive Health Programme in Uganda." Kampala: Ministry of Health. 2001.

Gupta, Neeru, Charles Katende, and Ruth Bessinger. "Associations of Mass Media Exposure with Family Planning Attitudes and Practices in Uganda." *Studies in Family Planning* 34, no. 1 (March 2003): 19–31.

Hardon, Anita, Ann Mutua, Sandra Kabir, and Elly Engelkes. *Monitoring Family Planning and Reproductive Rights: A Manual for Empowerment.* London: Zed Books, 1997.

Hultberg, Bobby. "Community Involvement in Health." In *Rural Health Providers in South-West Uganda*, ed. Mohammad Kisubi and Justus Mugaju, 78–95. Kampala: Fountain Publishers, 1999.

Jacinto, Amandua. "The Problem of Dual Employment of Health Workers in Uganda." *Uganda Health Bulletin* 7, no. 2 (April 2001): 5–7.

Kirumira, Edward K. "Developing a Population Policy for Uganda." In *Developing Uganda*, ed. Holger Bernt Hansen and Michael Twaddle, 185–93. Kampala: Fountain Publishers, 1998.

Kisubi, Mohammad. "Donor-funded Health Programmes: Prospects and Problems." In *Rural Health Providers in South-West Uganda*, ed. Mohammad Kisubi and Justus Mugaju, 141–60. Kampala: Fountain Publishers, 1999.

———. "The Impact of Decentralization on Rural Health Services." In *Rural Health Providers in South-West Uganda*, ed. Mohammad Kisubi and Justus Mugaju, 35–62. Kampala: Fountain Publishers, 1999.

———. "The Way Forward." In *Rural Health Providers in South-West Uganda*, ed. Mohammad Kisubi and Justus Mugaju, 161–65. Kampala: Fountain Publishers, 1999.

Kisubi, Mohammad, and Justus Mugaju. "Programme Design and Implementation 1985–1998: Progress and Challenges." In *Rural Health Providers in South-West Uganda*, ed. Mohammad Kisubi and Justus Mugaju, 16–34. Kampala: Fountain Publishers, 1999.

Knudsen, Lara. "Limited Choices: A Look at Women's Access to Health Care in Uganda." *Women's Studies Quarterly* Nos. 3 and 4 (Winter 2004): 253–60.

Koenig, Michael A., Iryna Zablotska, Tom Lutalo, Fred Nalugoda, Jennifer Wagman, and Ron Gray. "Coerced First Intercourse and Reproductive Health among Adolescent Women in Rakai, Uganda." *International Family Planning Perspectives* 30, no. 4 (December 2004): 156–63.

Kyeyune, Joy Kyazike. Vice President, Association of Uganda Women Medical Doctors. Project Manager, Adolescent Friendly Reproductive Health Services Project. Interview April 3, 2002. Kampala, Uganda.

Leah, Okoth. "AIDS Kills More than Malaria." *Monitor,* October 5, 2001, 7.

Lloyd, Cynthia B. "Negotiating Reproductive Outcomes in Uganda (book review)." *Population and Development Review* 24, no. 1 (March 1998): 171–72.

Marie Stopes International. "Uganda Profile." www.mariestopes.org.uk/uganda.html (accessed February 28, 2002).

Mbonye, Anthony K. (MD). Principal Medical Officer, Department of Community Health, Ministry of Health. Email correspondence March 19, 2002.

Mirembe, Florence, Freddie Ssengooba, and Rosalind Lubanga. "Cairo in Action: Uganda Profile." Draft. July 1998.

Mugaju, Justus. "On the Eve of the Rural Health Programme." In *Rural Health Providers in South-West Uganda*, ed. Mohammad Kisubi and Justus Mugaju, 1–15. Kampala: Fountain Publishers, 1999.

Mugaju, Justus. "District Rural Health Systems: Case Studies of Bushenyi, Kisoro, and Sembabule." In *Rural Health Providers in South-West Uganda*, ed. Mohammad Kisubi and Justus Mugaju, 119–40. Kampala: Fountain Publishers, 1999.

Mugumya, Elly. Social Worker and Executive Director, Family Planning Association of Uganda. Interview April 3, 2002. Kampala, Uganda.

Mugumya, Owarwo M. "Capacity Building for Health." In *Rural Health Providers in South-West Uganda*, ed. Mohammad Kisubi and Justus Mugaju, 63–77. Kampala: Fountain Publishers, 1999.

Musinguzi, Jotham (MD/MPH). Head of Family Health Department and Director of Population Secretariat, Ministry of Finance, Planning, and Economic Development. Interview March 27, 2002. Kampala, Uganda.

Musisi, Elizabeth. Nurse-Midwife, Nursing Officer In-Charge, Mulago Hospital Family Planning Clinic. Interview March 28, 2002. Kampala, Uganda.

Neema, Stella (Ph.D.). Research Fellow, Medical Anthropologist, Makerere Institute of Social Research. Interview March 28, 2002. Kampala, Uganda.

Neema, Stella. "Women and Rural Health: The Gender Perspective." In *Rural Health Providers in South-West Uganda*, ed. Mohammad Kisubi and Justus Mugaju, 96–118. Kampala: Fountain Publishers, 1999.

nSalasatta, Dan. "Bear Children by Choice, not Chance." *New Vision*, October 10, 2001, 30.

Nswemu, Priscila Monica. Registered Nurse-Midwife. Marie Stopes Uganda—Makerere Kavule. Interview March 6, 2002. Kampala, Uganda.

Ntozi, James P. M. High Fertility in Rural Uganda: The Role of Socioeconomic and Biological Factors. Kampala: Fountain Publishers, 1995.

Othieno, Josephine, Nurse, Operations Manager of Marie Stopes Uganda. Interview March 21, 2002. Kampala, Uganda.

Owomuhangi, Nestor, Associate Programme Officer of RH Programme, UNFPA. Interview March 7, 2002. Kampala, Uganda.

Prada, Elena, Florence Mirembe, Fatima H. Ahmed, Rose Nalwadda, and Charles Kiggundu. Abortion and Postabortion Care in Uganda: A Report from Health Care Professionals and Health Facilities. Occasional Report, no. 17. New York: Alan Guttmacher Institute, 2005.

Republic of Uganda. "Annual Health Sector Performance Report Financial Year 2000–2001." Kampala: Ministry of Health, September 2001.

———. "Health Sector Strategic Plan 2000/01–2004/05. Kampala: Ministry of Health, August 2000.

———. "National Adolescent Health Policy." Entebbe: Ministry of Health, 2001.

———. "National Health Policy." Kampala: Ministry of Health, September 1999.

———. "National Population Policy: For Sustainable Development." Kampala: Population Secretariat, Ministry of Finance and Economic Planning, January 1995.

———. "Population and Development Situation." Kampala: Population Secretariat, Ministry of Planning and Economic Development. www.uganda.co.ug/population/report. htm (accessed February 21, 2002).

———. "Population Levels, Trends and Characteristics." Kampala: Population Secretariat, Ministry of Planning and Economic Development. www.uganda.co.ug/population/report.htm (accessed February 21, 2002).

———. "Progress and Critical Needs in Population, Reproductive Health and Gender." Kampala: Population Secretariat, Ministry of Planning and Economic Development. www.uganda.co.ug/population/report.htm (accessed February 21, 2002).

———. "Reproductive Health Division 5-Year Strategic Framework 2000–2004." Kampala: Ministry of Health, July 2000.

———. "Sexual and Reproductive Health Minimum Package for Uganda." Kampala: Ministry of Health, Earnest Publishers, 1999.

———. "Some Salient Population and Development Indicators for Uganda." Population Secretariat, Ministry of Planning and Economic Development. Based on 1991 census.

———. "The State of Uganda Population Report 2001: Empowerment for Quality Life; Time for Action." Kampala: Population Secretariat, Ministry of Finance and Economic Planning. 2001.

———. "Uganda Health Profile." Uganda Health Bulletin 7, no. 1 (January 2001): 74–76. Kampala: Ministry of Health, Policy Analysis Unit.

Richey, Lisa Ann. "Uganda: HIV/AIDS and Reproductive Health." In Where Human Rights Begin: Essays on Health, Sexuality and Women, Ten Years after Vienna, Cairo and Beijing, ed. Wendy Chavkin and Ellen Chesler. New Brunswick, NJ: Rutgers University Press, 2005.

Richey, Lisa Ann, and Stine Jessen Haakonsson. "Access to ARV Treatment: Aid, Trade, and Governance in Uganda." DIIS Working Paper 2004/19. Danish Institute for International Studies, 2004.

Sentongo, Miriam (MD). Senior Medical Officer and Project Manager, Reproductive Health Division, Ministry of Health. Interview April 2, 2002. Kampala, Uganda.

Strudsholm, Jesper. "Uganda: AIDS Pressure Creates a New Openness." In Women's Voices, Women's Choices—on Reproductive Health, ed. Linda Nordahl Jakobsen and Nell Rasmussen, 41–48. Copenhagen: Danish Family Planning Association, 1998.

Tamale, Sylvia. When Hens Begin to Crow: Gender and Parliamentary Politics in Uganda. Kampala: Fountain Publishers, 1999.

Uganda Bureau of Statistics (UBOS). 2002 Uganda Population and Housing Census. Kampala: UBOS, 2002.

Uganda Bureau of Statistics (UBOS) and ORC Macros. Uganda Demographic and Health Survey 1995. Calverton, MD: UBOS and ORC Macro, 1995.

———. Uganda Demographic and Health Survey 2000–2001. Calverton, MD: UBOS and ORC Macro, 2001.

United Nations Population Fund (UNFPA). "Uganda Country Programme 2001 Annual Report to the Executive Director." Kampala, Uganda. January 2002.

United Nations Secretariat, Population Division. "Demographic Situation in High Fertility Countries." Presented at "Workshop on Prospects for Fertility Decline in High Fertility Countries." July 9–11, 2001. New York, New York.

Walt, Gill. Health Policy: An Introduction to Process and Power. Johannesburg: Witwatersrand University Press, 1994.

Peru

Almeyda Castro, Luis. "Atención del aborto en adolescentes." In Adolescencia y Salud Reproductiva, by República del Perú, Ministerio de Salud, 105–7. Lima: Ministerio de Salud, 2000.

Andreas, Carol. When Women Rebel: The Rise of Popular Feminism in Peru. Westport, Connecticut: Lawrence Hill, 1985.

BBC News. "Peruvian Sterlization Inquiry Reopens." news.bbc.co.uk/2/hi/americas/3000454.stm (accessed June 18, 2003).

Bosch, Xavier. "Former Peruvian Government Censured over Sterilizations." British Medical Journal 325, no. 7358 (August 3, 2002): 236.

Castro Martin, Teresa, and Fatima Juárez. "Women's Education and Fertility in Latin America: Exploring the Significance of Education for Women's Lives." DHS Working Paper, no. 10. Calverton, MD: Macro International, 1994.

Centro de la Mujer Peruana Flora Tristán. Informe: Derechos Sexuales y Derechos Reproductivos de las Mujeres. Lima: Centro de la Mujer Peruana Flora Tristán, 2001.

———. "La Salud de las Mujeres Rurales." Fact Sheet, 28 de mayo Campaign. Lima: Centro de la Mujer Peruana Flora Tristán, 2002.

———. Sexualidad y Derechos Ciudadanos. Lima: Centro de la Mujer Peruana Flora Tristán, 2001.

Centro de la Mujer Peruana Flora Tristán, DEMUS (Estudio para la Defensa de los Derechos de la Mujer). *Mortalidad Materna y Aborto Inseguro: Enfrentando la Realidad.* "Pronunciamiento." Roundtable, October 14, 1999, Lima.

Chávez, Susana. Director. Programa de Derechos Sexuales y Ciudadanía en Salud, Centro de la Mujer Peruana Flora Tristán. Interview November 7, 2003. Lima, Peru.

Coe, Anna-Britt. "From Anti-Natalist to Ultra-Conservative: Restricting Reproductive Choice in Peru." *Reproductive Health Matters* 12, no.24 (2004): 56–69.

Faundes, Anibal. "Asistencia a la mujer víctima de violencia sexual." In *Taller "Violencia de Género" para Perú y la Region Andina*, by Sociedad Peruana de Obstetricia y Ginecología, 27–34. Lima: Sociedad Peruana de Obstetricia y Ginecología, 2003.

Ferrando, Delicia. "Frecuencia del aborto en el Perú." In *Manual del Curso Nacional Aborto y Salud Reproductiva*, by República del Perú, Instituto Materno Perinatal (MINSA), 7–21. Lima: Ministerio de Salud, 1997.

Ferrando, Delicia, Centro de la Mujer Peruana Flora Tristán, and Pathfinder International. *El Aborto Clandestino en el Perú: Hechos y Cifras.* Lima: Centro de la Mujer Peruana Flora Tristán, Pathfinder International, 2002.

Ferrando, Delicia, and Pathfinder International. *Programa de Atención Integral del Aborto Incompleto en el Perú.* Lima: DFID, Ministerio de Salud (MINSA), Pathfinder International, 2001.

Gho Aspilcueta, Daniel. Obstetrician/Gynecologist, CEO/President, Instituto Peruano de Paternidad Responsable (INPPARES). Interview November 12, 2003. Lima, Peru.

Grupo Impulsor Nacional Mujeres por Igualdad Real. *Mujeres y Ciudadanía en el Perú.* Lima: Grupo Impulsor Nacional Mujeres por Igualdad Real, 1998.

Guerrero, Rossina. Psychologist. Programa de Derechos Sexuales y Ciudadanía en Salud, Centro de la Mujer Peruana Flora Tristán. Interview October 31, 2003. Lima, Peru.

Guezmes, Ana. "Estado actual de la violencia de género en el Perú." In *Taller "Violencia de Género" para Perú y la Region Andina*, by Sociedad Peruana de Obstetricia y Ginecología, 17–22. Lima: Sociedad Peruana de Obstetricia y Ginecología, 2003.

Guezmes, Ana, Nancy Palomino, and Miguel Ramos. *Violencia Sexual y Física contra las Mujeres en el Perú.* Lima: World Health Organization, Centro de la Mujer Peruana Flora Tristán, Universidad Peruana Cayetano Heredia, 2002.

Gutiérrez, Miguel. "Frente al aborto, nuestra responsabilidad es creer conciencia social informada." In *Mortalidad Materna y Aborto Inseguro: Enfrentando la Realidad*, by Centro de la Mujer Peruana Flora Tristán, DEMUS (Estudio para la Defensa de los Derechos de la Mujer), 11–30. Roundtable, October 14, 1999, Lima.

Gutiérrez Ramos, Miguel. Obstetrician/Gynecologist, Medical Director of Pathfinder International, and President-Elect of la Sociedad Peruana de Obstetricia y Ginecología. Interview November 12, 2003. Lima, Peru.

Gutiérrez, Miguel, and Delicia Ferrando. "Incidencia del aborto y sus efectos sobre la fecundidad." Draft. CEPAL-CELADE UN Series Seminar and Conferences, forthcoming.

Gutiérrez, Rocío. Movimiento Manuela Ramos. Interview November 10, 2003. Lima, Peru.

Marckwardt, Albert M., and Luis H. Ochoa. *Population and Health Data for Latin America.* Columbia, MD: Macro International, USAID, Pan-American Health Organization, 1993.

Mayorga Canales, Americo. Obstetrician/Gynecologist, Medical Director. Centro Universitario de Salud Pedro P. Díaz. Interview October 9, 2003. Arequipa, Peru.

Mensch, Barbara, Mary Arends-Kuenning, and Anrudh Jain. "The Impact of Quality of Family Planning Services on Contraceptive Use in Peru." *Studies in Family Planning* 27, no. 2 (March-April 1996): 59–75.

Miloslavich Tupac, Diana. "Las mujeres en los gobiernos locales y regionales: Garantía para la sostenibilidad de la arquitectura institucional de género." In *La Mitad del Poder: Instancias y Mecanismos para el Adelanto de la Mujer*, ed. Diana Miloslavich Tupac. Lima: Centro de la Mujer Peruana Flora Tristán, 2002.

Mollmann, Marianne, and Susana Chávez. *La Regla de la Mordaza y la Acción Política en la Lucha por la Despenalización del Aborto*. Lima: Centro de la Mujer Peruana Flora Tristán, 2003.

Mostajo, Desiree. "Consecuencias ginecológicas y obstétricas de la violencia." In *Taller 'Violencia de Género' para Perú y la Region Andina*, by Sociedad Peruana de Obstetricia y Ginecología, 23–26. Lima: Sociedad Peruana de Obstetricia y Ginecología, 2003.

Nugent, Guillermo. "Prólogo." In *Estado Laico: A la Sombra de la Iglesia*, by Centro de la Mujer Peruana Flora Tristán, 9–12. Lima: Centro de la Mujer Peruana Flora Tristán, 2003.

Olea Mauleon, Cecilia. Programa de Derechos Sexuales y Ciudadanía en Salud, Centro de la Mujer Peruana Flora Tristán. Interview November 13, 2003. Lima, Peru.

Palomino, Nancy, Miguel Ramos, Rocío Valverde, and Ernesto Vasquez. *Entre el Placer y la Obligación: Derechos Sexuales y Derechos Reproductivos de Mujeres y Varones de Huamanga y Lima*. Lima: Universidad Nacional Cayetano Heredia, Population Concern, 2003.

Quintanilla Zapata, Tammy. Lawyer, Movimiento El Pozo. Interview November 10, 2003. Lima, Peru.

Quintanilla Zapata, Tammy Lorena. "Información sobre el aborto en el Perú: Estudio comparativo de la regulación juridical del aborto en América Latina y el Caribe." CLADEM. Lima, August 1997, www.cladem.org/espanol/nacionales/peru/aborto_peru. asp (accessed November 2, 2003).

Ramos, Miguel. Sociologist. Unidad de Sexualidad y Salud Reproductiva, Universidad Nacional Cayetano Heredia. Interview November 10, 2003. Lima, Peru.

República del Perú. *Encuesta Demográfica y de Salud Familiar, 2000*. Calverton, Maryland: Macro International, USAID, UNICEF, Measure/DHS+, 2001.

República del Perú, Defensoría del Pueblo (Rocío Villanueva Flores). *Anticoncepción Quirúrgica Voluntaria: Casos Investigados por la Defensoría del Pueblo*. Lima: Defensoría del Pueblo, 1998.

————. *La Aplicación de la Anticoncepción Quirúrgica y los Derechos Reproductivos II: Casos Investigados por la Defensoría del Pueblo*. Lima: Defensoría del Pueblo, 1999.

————. *La Aplicación de la Anticoncepción Quirúrgica y los Derechos Reproductivos III*. Lima: Defensoría del Pueblo, 2002.

República del Perú, Defensoría del Pueblo. *Resolución Defensorial N°03-DP-2000*. Lima: Defensoría del Pueblo, 2000.

————. *La Violencia Sexual: Un Problema de Seguridad Ciudadana—Las Voces de las Víctimas*. Second edition. Lima: Defensoría del Pueblo, 2000.

República del Perú, Ministerio de Salud, Instituto Materno Perinatal. *Adolescencia y Salud Reproductiva*. Lima: Ministerio de Salud, 1997.

República del Perú, Ministerio de Salud, Dirección General de Salud de las Personas, Dirección Ejecutiva de Gestión Sanitaria. "Gestantes adolescente atendida/gestantes esperadas 2000–2002." Lima: Ministerio de Salud, 2002.

República del Perú, Ministerio de Salud. *Por la Vida y la Salud: Programa de Salud Reproductiva y Planificación Familiar 1996–2000.* Lima: Ministerio de Salud, 1996.

República del Perú, Ministerio de Salud, Programa Nacional de Planificación Familiar. "Producción de aervicios (parejas protegidas)." Lima: Ministerio de Salud, 2002.

República del Perú, PROMUDEH (now MIMDES). "Situación de la mujer Afroperuana: Obstáculos que vulneran, limitan y/o impiden el ejercicio de sus derechos." Lima: PROMUDEH, 2001.

Romero Bidegaray, Ines. *El Aborto Clandestino en el Perú: Una Aproximación desde los Derechos Humanos.* Lima: Centro de la Mujer Peruana Flora Tristán, 2002.

Sociedad Peruana de Obstetricia y Ginecología. *Seminario Internacional: Responsabilidad de las Sociedades de Obstetricia y Ginecología Frente al Manejo del Aborto para Reducir la Mortalidad Materna.* Lima: Sociedad Peruana de Obstetricia y Ginecología, 1998.

Tam, Luis. "Rural-to-Urban Migration in Bolivia and Peru: Association with Child Mortality, Breastfeeding Cessation, Maternal Care, and Contraception." Working Paper, no. 8. Calverton, MD: Demographic and Health Surveys, Macro International, 1994.

Ugaz, José Carlos. Lawyer. Benites, De Las Casas, Forno, y Ugaz. Interview November 7, 2003. Lima, Peru.

Ugaz, José. "Los aportes del derecho penal y la despenalización del aborto." In *Mortalidad Materna y Aborto Inseguro: Enfrentando la Realidad*, by Centro de la Mujer Peruana Flora Tristán, DEMUS (Estudio para la Defensa de los Derechos de la Mujer), 31–43. Roundtable, October 14, 1999, Lima.

Vargas Vasquez, Trixsi. Coordinadora de Consejeria, Apoyo a Programas de Poblacion (APROPO). Interview November 11, 2003. Lima, Peru.

Yamin, Alicia Ely. *Castillos de Arena en el Camino Hacia la Modernidad: Una Perspectiva desde los Derechos Humanos sobre el Proceso de Reforma del Sector Salud en el Perú (1990–2000) y sus Implicancias en la Muerte Materna.* Lima: Centro de la Mujer Peruana Flora Tristán, 2003.

Yupanqui, Samuel B. Abad. "Libertad religiosa y estado democráticos a propósito del debate constitucional." In *Estado Laico: A la Sombra de la Iglesia*, by Centro de la Mujer Peruana Flora Tristán, 61–76. Lima: Centro de la Mujer Peruana Flora Tristán, 2003.

Denmark

Anonymous. "Abortion Figures Tumble." *Copenhagen Post*, December 1, 2001. cphpost. periskop.dk/default.asp?id=12761 (accessed May 23, 2002).

Anonymous. "Abortion Laws to Be Tightened." *Copenhagen Post*, January 28, 1999. cphpost.periskop.dk/default.asp?id=7000 (accessed May 23, 2002).

Anonymous. "Abortion Pill Gets the Go Ahead." *Copenhagen Post*, September 7, 1998. cphpost.periskop.dk/default.asp?id=2948 (accessed May 23, 2002).

Anonymous. "Hospitals Proclaim Abortion Pill a Success." *Copenhagen Post*, January 10, 1998. cphpost.periskop.dk/default.asp?id=6451 (accessed May 23, 2002).

Anonymous. "Police to Remove Pro-Life Memorial." *Copenhagen Post*, January 28, 1999. cphpost.periskop.dk/default.asp?id=7001 (accessed May 23, 2002).

Anonymous. "Safe Sex Is Not a Teenage Priority, Survey Says." *Copenhagen Post*, June 21, 1999. cphpost.periskop.dk/default.asp?id=11277 (accessed May 23, 2002).

Anonymous. "Sex education—the Danish method." *Copenhagen Post*. 212.130.58.21.91/default.asp?id=11579 (accessed November 15, 2000).

Anonymous. "Teenage Abortions High in Capital." *Copenhagen Post*, August 20, 1998. cphpost.periskop.dk/default.asp?id=3257 (accessed May 23, 2002).

Anonymous. "Twenty-Five Years of Legalised Abortion." *Copenhagen Post*, January 10, 1998. cphpost.periskop.dk/default.asp?id=6449 (accessed May 23, 2002).

Correa, Sonia. *Population and Reproductive Rights: Feminist Perspectives from the South*. London: Zed Books, 1994.

David, Henry P, Janine M. Morgall, Mogens Osler, Niels K. Rasmussen, and Birgitte Jensen. "United States and Denmark: Different Approaches to Health Care and Family Planning." *Studies in Family Planning* 21, no. 1 (January-February 1990): 1–19.

Denmark, Ministry of the Interior and Health. *The Danish Healthcare Sector in Figures 2001/2002*. Ministry of the Interior and Health, May 2002.

Denmark, Ministry of Health. "Health Care in Denmark." www.sum.dk/health/sider/print.htm (accessed May 5, 2002).

———. "Health Conditions." www.um.dk/english/danmark/danmarksbog/kap3/3–7.asp (accessed May 5, 2002).

Denmark. "Denmark Law No.350 of 13 June 1973 on the Interruption of Pregnancy." cyber.law.harvard.edu/population/abortion/Denmark.abo.htm (accessed May 5, 2002).

Denmark StatisticBank, "Fertility Rates by Age, Region, and Time." www.statbank.dk/statbank5a/default.asp?w=1024 (accessed January 25, 2005).

———. "Population by Area, Marital Status, Age, Sex and Citizenship (1979–2005)." www.statbank.dk/statbank5a/default.asp?w=1024 (accessed June 12, 2005).

Esbensen, Lau Sander. Ph.D. student. University of Copenhagen, Center for Women and Gender Studies. Interview June 6, 2002. Copenhagen, Denmark.

Eskild, A., L. B. Helgadottir, F. Jerve, E. Qvigstad, S. Stray-Pedersen, and A. Loset. "Provosert abort blant kvinner med fremmedkulturell bakgrunn i Oslo." [Induced Abortion among Women with Ethnic Background in Oslo]. *Tidskrift for Norsk Laegeforening* 122, no. 14 (2002): 1355–57.

Foreningen Sex og Samfund (the Danish Family Planning Association). Annual Reports 2000, 2001.

———. *Sexual and Reproductive Health and Rights for Youth: The Danish Experience*. 1996.

———. *Ung 99—En Seksuel Profil: En Beskrivelse, Rapport 1*. Frederiksberg, 1999.

Henshaw, Stanley K., Susheela Singh, and Taylor Haas. "Recent Trends in Abortion Rates Worldwide." *Family Planning Perspectives* 25, no. 1 (1999): 44–48.

International Planned Parenthood Federation. "Denmark Country Profile." ippfnet.ippf.org/pub/IPPF_Regions/IPPF_CountryProfile.asp?ISOCode=DK (accessed May 5, 2002).

Knudsen, Lisbeth B. Sociologist, Associate Research Professor. Demografisk Forskningcenter, Syddansk Universitet (Danish Center for Demographic Research—SDU Odense University). (Since January 1, 2003, Associate Professor at Aalborg University.) Interview June 4, 2002. Odense, Denmark.

———. "Induced Abortion and Family Formation in Europe." In *Family Life and Family Policies in Europe: Problems and Issues in Comparative Perspective*, ed. F-x Kaufmann et al. Vol. 2. Oxford: Clarendon Press, 2002.

———. "Induced Abortions in Denmark." *Acta Obstetricia et Gynecologica Scandinavica* 76, supp. 164 (1997): 54–59.

———. "Induced Abortion in the Nordic Countries." Danish Center for Demographic Research—SDU Odense University. Research Report 22, 2001.

———. "Recent Fertility Trends in Denmark—A Discussion of the Impact of Family Policy in a Period with Increasing Fertility." Danish Center for Demographic Research—SDU Odense University. Research Report 11, 1999.

———. "Social Differentials in the Fertility Pattern—How Strong is the Influence of Control on the Fertility Development in Denmark?" In *Ongoing Research at the Danish Center for Demographic Research—a Report from a Meeting in the Danish Demographic Society*. Danish Center for Demographic Research—SDU Odense University. Research Report 13, 2000.

Knudsen, Lisbeth B., and Mike Murphy. "Registers as Data Source in Studies of Reproductive Behavior." Danish Center for Demographic Research—SDU Odense University. Research Report 12, 1999.

Knudsen, Lisbeth B., and Hanne Wielandt. "Legally Induced Abortion—Experiences from Denmark." Danish Center for Demographic Research—SDU Odense University. Research Report 18, 2000.

Kristeligt Folkeparti. www.krf.dk/hoejre.phtml?krf=1349 (accessed June 12, 2005).

Nexoe, Sniff. Ph.D. student. Institute of Public Health. Interview June 7, 2002. Copenhagen, Denmark.

Rasch, Vibeke, Lisbeth B. Knudsen, and Tine Gammeltoft. *Nar der ikke er noget tredje valg: Social sarbarhed og valget af abort.* [When There Is No Third Option: Social Vulnerability and the Choice of Induced Abortion.] Sundhedsstyrelsen, August 2004.

Rasch, Vibeke, Lisbeth B. Knudsen, and Hanne Wielandt, "Pregnancy Planning and Acceptance among Danish Pregnant Women." *Acta Obstetricia et Gynecologica Scandinavica* 80 (2001): 1030–35.

Rasmussen, Nell, and Danish Family Planning Association. *Sexual and Reproductive Health and Rights for Youth: The Danish Experience.* n.d.

Samuelsen, Helle. Anthropologist, Associate Professor. Institute of Public Health, Department of International Health, University of Copenhagen. Interview June 10, 2002. Copenhagen, Denmark.

Schmidt, A. M., P. L. Petersen, P. E. Helkjaer, J. Kjeldsen, C. Lampe, and B. N. Pedersen. "Prenatal Diagnosis in the County of South Jutland: Review of 1,026 Amniocenteses." *Ugeskr Laeger* 148, no. 36 (September 1986): 2289–91.

Seidenfaden, Johan. Interim National Program Administrator, Foreningen Sex og Samfund (Danish Family Planning Association). Interview June 7, 2002. Copenhagen, Denmark.

Sexual and Reproductive Health Assocations from Denmark, Sweden, Norway, Finland, and Iceland. "The Nordic Resolution on Adolescent Sexual Health and Rights." Helsinki, October 1998.

United Nations Population Division, Department of Economic and Social Affairs. *World Contraceptive Use, 2004.* www.un.org/esa/population/publications/contraceptive2003/WallChart_CP2003.pdf (accessed June 12, 2005).

United Nations Population Fund. *State of World Population 2003.* New York: UN, 2003.

Vallgarda, Signild, Allan Krasnik, and Karsten Vrangbaek. *Health Care Systems in Transition: Denmark.* Copenhagen: European Observatory on Health Care Systems, 2001.

Wielandt, Hanne, and Lisbeth B. Knudsen. "Birth Control: Some Experiences from Denmark." *Contraception* 55 (1997): 301–6.

———. "Sexual Activity and Pregnancies among Adolescents in Denmark—Trends during the Eighties." *Nordisk Sexologi* 15 (1997): 75–88.

Wilken-Jensen, Charlotte. OB/GYN, Medical consultant, Head of DFPA's Contraceptive Clinic. Interview June 11, 2002. Frederiksberg, Denmark.

World Health Organization—Regional Office for Europe. *Denmark: Highlights on Women's Health.* World Health Organization, 2000.

United States

Abma, J., A. Chandra, W. Mosher, L. Peterson, and L. Piccinino. "Fertility, Family Planning, and Women's Health: New Data from the 1995 National Survey of Family Growth." National Center for Health Statistics. *Vital Health Statistics* 23, no. 19. Hyattsville, MD: National Center for Health Statistics, 1997.

Abma, J. C., G. M. Martinez, W. D. Mosher, and B. S. Dawson. "Teenagers in the United States: Sexual Activity, Contraceptive Use, and Childbearing, 2002." National Center for Health Statistics. *Vital Health Statistics* 23, no. 24 (2004).

Abortion Access Project. "Fact Sheet: The Shortage of Abortion Providers." June 2003. www.abortionaccess.org/AAP/publica_resources/fact_sheets/shortage_provider.htm (accessed July 21, 2005).

Adams, Abbie. Abortion Counselor. Abortion and Counseling Services. Interview May 26, 2003. Albuquerque, New Mexico.

Advocates for Youth, "Myths and Facts about Sex Education." www.advocatesforyouth. org/rrr/mythsfacts.htm (accessed July 21, 2005).

Alan Guttmacher Institute. "Abortion in Context: United States and Worldwide." Issues in Brief, Series 1, 1999.

———. *Contraceptive Use.* New York: Alan Guttmacher Institute, 2002. www.agi-usa. org/pubs/fb_contr_use.html (accessed July 19, 2005).

———. *Family Planning Annual Report: 2004 Summary.* New York: Alan Guttmacher Institute, 2005.

———. *Sharing Responsibility: Women, Society, and Abortion Worldwide.* New York: Alan Guttmacher Institute, 1999.

American College of Obstetricians and Gynecologists, *Birth Control: A Woman's Choice.* Washington, DC: ACOG, 2003.

Armstrong, Bruce. "The Young Men's Clinic: Addressing Men's Reproductive Health and Responsibilities." *Perspectives on Sexual and Reproductive Health* 35, no. 5 (2003): 220–25.

Atkins, Rachel. Vice President of Medical Services. Planned Parenthood of Northern New England. Phone interview May 18, 2004.

Camp, Brittney. Counselor. Little Rock Family Planning Services. Interview May 23, 2003. Little Rock, Arkansas.

Centers for Disease Control. "Births: Preliminary Data for 2000." National Center for Health Statistics. www.cdc.gov/nchs/births.htm

Center for Reproductive Law and Policy. *The World's Abortion Laws 2000.* Poster.

Clinicians for Choice, "Professional Organizations Speak." 2004. www.prochoice.org/cfc/ professional_organizations.html (accessed August 11, 2005).

Cloninger, Devon, and Susan Pagliaro. "Sex Education: Curricula and Programs." Advocates for Youth, November 2002.

Daley, Terry. Abortion Counselor. Downtown Women's Center. Interview March 7, 2000. Portland, Oregon.

David, Henry P, Janine M. Morgall, Mogens Osler, Niels K. Rasmussen, and Birgitte Jensen. "United States and Denmark: Different Approaches to Health Care and Family Planning." *Studies in Family Planning* 21, no. 1 (January-February 1990): 1–19.

Donovan, Patricia. "School-Based Sexuality Education: The Issues and Challenges." *Family Planning Perspectives* 30, no. 4 (July/August 1998).

Dorn, Harold F. "World Population Growth." In *The Population Dilemma*, ed. American Assembly, Columbia University, 7–28. Englewood Cliffs, NJ: Prentice Hall, 1963.

Ehrlich, Paul. *The Population Bomb*. New York: Ballantine Books, 1968.

Forte, Dianne Jntl, and Karen Judd. "The South within the North: Reproductive Choice in Three U.S. Communities." In *Negotiating Reproductive Rights: Women's Perspectives Across Countries and Cultures*, ed. Rosalind P. Petchesky and Karen Judd, 256–94. London: Zed Books, 1998.

Fried, Marlene Gerber, and Sheila Clarke. "Expanding Abortion Access: The U.S. Experience." In *Advocating for Abortion Access: Eleven Country Studies*, ed. Barbara Klugman and Debbie Budlender, 283–313. Johannesburg, South Africa: Women's Health Project, 2001.

Gold, Rachel Benson. "Hierarchy Crackdown Clouds Future of Sterilization, EC Provision at Catholic Hospitals." *Guttmacher Report* 5, no. 2 (May 2002). www.guttmacher.org/pubs/tgr/05/2/gr050211.html (accessed July 20, 2005).

Goldman, Marlene B., Jane S. Occhiuto, Laura E. Peterson, Jane G. Zapka, and R. Heather Palmer. "Physician Assistants as Providers of Surgically Induced Abortion Services." *American Journal of Public Health* 94, no. 8 (August 2004): 1352–57.

Government of the District of Columbia, Department of Health. *District of Columbia State Health Profile*. December 2003. State Center for Health Statistics Administration.

Haslegrave, Marianne. "Implementing the ICPD Program of Action: What a Difference a Decade Makes." *Reproductive Health Matters* 12, no. 23 (2004): 12–19.

Henry J. Kaiser Family Foundation. *Fact Sheet: Sexually Transmitted Diseases in the United States*. February 2000.

———. *Fact Sheet: Women and HIV/AIDS*. May 2001.

Institute of Medicine. *No Time to Lose: Getting More from HIV Prevention*. Washington, DC: Institute of Medicine, 2000.

Jacobsen, Judith E. "The United States." In *Promoting Reproductive Health: Investing in Health for Development*, ed. Shepard Forman and Romita Ghosh, 251–77. Boulder, CO: Lynne Rienner Publishers, 2000.

Jones, James H. "The Tuskegee Legacy: AIDS and the Black Community." *Hastings Center Report* 22, no. 6 (November-December 1992): 38–40.

Knudsen, Lara. "Justifying Murder? Front Row Seats to the Nuremberg Files Trial." *Body Politic* 9, no. 2 (March/April 1999): 3–5.

———. "Pregnant? Need Help? An Inside Account of Experiences at a Crisis Pregnancy Center." *Body Politic* 9, no. 5 (November/December 1999): 20–21.

Lawrence, Jane. "The Indian Health Service and the Sterilization of Native American Women." *American Indian Quarterly* 24, no. 3 (Summer 2000): 400–19.

Lorimer, Frank. "Issues of Population Policy." In *The Population Dilemma*, ed. American Assembly, Columbia University, 143–78. Englewood Cliffs, NJ: Prentice Hall, 1963.

Malthus, Thomas Robert. *On Population*. New York: Random House, 1960. First published in London, 1798.

Mihesuah, Devon A. "A Few Cautions at the Millennium on the Merging of Feminist Studies with American Indian Women's Studies." *Signs* 25, no. 4 (Summer 2000): 1247.

———. "Commonality of Difference: American Indian Women and History." *American Indian Quarterly* 20, no. 1 (Winter 1996): 15–27.

Mosher, William D., Gladys M. Martinez, Anjani Chandra, Joyce C. Abma, and Stephanie J. Wilson. "Use of Contraception and Use of Family Planning Services in the United States, 1982–2002." *Advance Data from Vital and Health Statistics*, no. 350. Hyattsville, MD: National Center for Health Statistics, 2004.

Murphy, Clare. "Selling Sterilisation to Addicts." BBC News Online. news.bbc.co.uk/2/hi/americas/3189763.stm (accessed September 2, 2003).

Murry, Velma McBride, and James J. Ponzetti Jr. "American Indian Female Adolescents' Sexual Behavior: A Test of the Life-Course Experience Theory." *Family and Consumer Sciences Research Journal* 26, no. 1 (September 1997): 75–95.

National Abortion Federation. *The Truth about Abortion*. 1996.

National Latina Institute for Reproductive Health. "The Reproductive Health of Latinas in the US." Fact Sheet. March 2002. www.latinainstitute.org/pdf/ReproHealth/pdf (accessed July 20, 2005).

National Women's Law Center, and Kaiser Family Foundation. *Women's Access to Care: A State-Level Analysis of Key Health Policies*. Menlo Park, CA: Kaiser Family Foundation, 2003.

National Women's Law Center, Oregon Health and Science University. *Making the Grade on Women's Health: A National and State-by-State Report Card 2004*. Washington, DC: National Women's Law Center, 2004.

Notestein, Frank W., Dudley Kirk, and Sheldon Segal. "The Problem of Population Control." In *The Population Dilemma*, by American Assembly, Columbia University, 125–42. Englewood Cliffs, NJ: Prentice Hall, 1963.

Osborne, Ann F., PA-C, Clinic Director. Little Rock Family Planning Services. Interview May 23, 2003. Little Rock, Arkansas.

Planned Parenthood Federation of America. "Margaret Sanger." September 2004. www.ppfa.org/pp2/portal/files/portal/medicalinfo/birthcontrol/bio-margaret-sanger.xml (accessed August 11, 2005).

———. "Teenagers, Abortion, and Government Intrusion Laws." 2004. www.plannedparenthood.org/pp2/portal/files/portal/medicalinfo/abortion/fact-teenagers-abortion-intrusion.xml (accessed July 21, 2005).

Pollitt, Katha. "Anti-Choice, Anti-Child." *Nation*, November 15, 1999, 10.

Preston, Julia. "Appeals Court Voids Ban on 'Partial Birth' Abortions." *New York Times*. July 9, 2005. www.nytimes.com/2005/07/09/national/09abort.html (accessed July 19, 2005).

Project Prevention, "How We Help the Children." www.projectprevention.org/program/index.html (accessed August 11, 2005).

Reverby, Susan M. "Cultural Memory and the Tuskegee Syphilis Study." *Hastings Center Report* 31, no. 5 (September–October 2001): 22–29.

Roberts, Dorothy. Professor of Law. Northwestern University. Phone Interview June 23, 2004.

———. *Killing the Black Body: Race, Reproduction, and the Meaning of Liberty*. New York: Vintage Books, 1997.

———. "Reconstructing the Patient: Starting with Women of Color." In *Feminism and Bioethics: Beyond Reproduction*, ed. Susan M. Wolf, 116–43. New York: Oxford University Press, 1996.

Rodick, Larry S. President/CEO. Planned Parenthood of Alabama. Interview May 22, 2003. Birmingham, Alabama.

———. President/CEO. Planned Parenthood of Alabama. Email correspondence December 16, 2003.

Roubideaux, Yvette, Mel Zuckerman, and Enid Zuckerman. "A Review of the Quality of Health Care for American Indians and Alaska Natives." Commonwealth Fund, 2004.

Sachs, Jeffrey. "Weapons of Mass Salvation." *Economist*, October 24, 2002. www.economist.com/opinion/displayStory.cfm?story_id=1403544 (accessed July 20, 2005).

Scully, Judith M. "Cracking Open CRACK: Unethical Sterilization Movement Gains Momentum." *Different Takes*, no. 2 (Spring 2000).

Sherrow, Genevieve, Tristan Ruby, Paula K. Braverman, Nathalie Bartle, Shawn Gibson, and Linda Hock-Long, "Man2Man: A Promising Approach to Addressing the Sexual and Reproductive Health Needs of Young Men." *Perspectives on Sexual and Reproductive Health* 35, no. 5 (2003): 215–19.

Silliman, Jael, Marlene Gerber Fried, Loretta Ross, and Elena R. Gutierrez. *Undivided Rights: Women of Color Organize for Reproductive Justice.* Cambridge, MA: South End Press, 2004.

State Family Planning Administrators, Office of Population Affairs, Department of Health and Human Services. *Healthy People 2010.* Center for Health Training, 2001.

Taeuber, Irene B. "Population Growth in Underdeveloped Areas." In *The Population Dilemma*, by American Assembly, Columbia University, 29–45. Englewood Cliffs, NJ: Prentice Hall, 1963.

United Nations Development Program. *Human Development Report 2004.* New York: UNDP, 2004.

United States Government, Department of Health and Human Services. "President Announces $43 Million in Grants from Compassion Capital Fund." August 3, 2004. www.hhs.gov/news/press/2004pres/20040803b.html (accessed July 18, 2005).

United States Government, U.S. Census Bureau. "Fertility of American Women, June 2000." October 2001.

United States Supreme Court. *Eisenstadt v. Baird*, 405 U.S. 438, 1972.

———. *Griswold v. Connecticut*, 381 U.S. 479, 1965.

———. *Harris v. McRae*, 448 U.S. 297, 1980.

———. *Webster vs. Reproductive Health Services*, 492 U.S. 490, 1989.

University of Pittsburgh Medical Center. "Information for Patients: Norplant—Questions and Answers." 2003. www.patienteducation.upmc.com/Pdf/Norplant.pdf (accessed July 19, 2005).

US NGOs in Support of the Cairo Consensus. "Keeping America's Promises: US Funding for Reproductive Health Care at Home and Abroad." Washington, DC, 1998.

Ventura, S. J., J. C. Abma, W. D. Mosher, and S. Henshaw. "Estimated Pregnancy Rates for the United States, 1990–2000: An Update." National Center for Health Statistics. *National Vital Statistics Reports* 52, no. 23 (2004).

Ventura, S. J., W. D. Mosher, S. C. Curtin, J. C. Abma, and S. Henshaw. "Trends in Pregnancies and Pregnancy Rates by Outcome: Estimates for the United States, 1976–1996." National Center for Health Statistics. *Vital Health Statistics* 21, no. 56 (2000).

White, Jane Ann. Nurse, co-owner. Downtown Women's Center. Interview January 16, 2000. Portland, Oregon.

Vietnam

(All Vietnamese names are listed by their first name, then second, third [surname is first name].)

Alan Guttmacher Institute. *Sharing Responsibility: Women, Society, and Abortion Worldwide.* New York: Alan Guttmacher Institute, 1999.

Anonymous. "Quinacrine Sterilization Method Found Effective among Women in Vietnam." *International Family Planning Perspectives* 19 (1993): 157–58.

Belanger, Daniele. "Son Preference in a Rural Village in North Vietnam." *Studies in Family Planning* 33, no. 4 (December 2002): 321–34.

Bormann, Sita Michael. Program Coordinator, RHIYA (EU/UNFPA Reproductive Health Initiative for Youth in Asia). Interview March 24, 2004. Hanoi, Vietnam.

Bryant, John. "Communism, Poverty, and Demographic Change in North Vietnam." *Population and Development Review* 24, no. 2 (June 1998): 235–69.

Center for American Women and Politics. "Women Serving in the 109th Congress, 2005–2007." www.cawp.rutgers.edu/Facts/Officeholders/cong-current.html (accessed July 5, 2005).

Center for Reproductive and Family Health. "Some Opinions on the Situation of Access to Health Care Service for the Poor." *Suc Khoe Sinh San* (Hanoi), December 2003, 5–6.

Chinoy, Mike. "Vietnam's Abortion Rate Rises as 'Baby Boomers' Come of Age." CNN. February 6, 1999. www.cnn.com/WORLD/asiapcf/9902/06/vietnam.abortion/index.html (accessed February 24, 2004).

Community of Concerned Parnters. "HIV/AIDS: A Social and Economic Challenge for Viet Nam." CG Meeting, December 2–3, 2003, Hanoi.

Community of Concerned Partners. *Key Issues in Viet Nam's Fight against HIV/AIDS.* UNDP. No date.

Dang Nguyen Anh. "Current Issues of Population and Human Resources for Development in Vietnam." *Family and Women Studies* (Center for Family and Women Studies of Vietnam) No. 1 (2002): 54–62.

Do Thi Thanh Nhan. Senior Expert, Department of Family and Social Affairs, Vietnam Women's Union. Interview March 15, 2004. Hanoi, Vietnam.

Do Trong Hieu. "Reproductive Health Care in Rural Areas." *Population-Family Planning News* No. 6 (January–March 1998): 7.

Feuerstein, Marie-Therese. "Family Planning in Vietnam." *Lancet* 342, no. 8865 (July 24, 1993): 188–89.

Fihnborg, Malin, and Magnus Wulkan. *Population and Family Planning Policies in Vietnam: A Reproductive Rights Perspective.* Umea University Department of Law, Minor Field Study Report No. 21. 1999.

Gammeltoft, Tine. Medical Anthropologist, Vietnamese Committee for Population, Family and Children. Interview March 26, 2004. Hanoi, Vietnam.

———. "Abortion Conventionalized, Abortion Ritualized: Defining Limits to Human Life in Contemporary Vietnam." Paper presented at AAS 2001, Chicago (unpublished).

———. "Vietnam: A Will to Create Changes." In *Women's Voices, Women's Choices—on Reproductive Health,* ed. Linda Nordahl Jakobsen and Nell Rasmussen, 80–90. Copenhagen: Danish Family Planning Association, 1998.

———. *Women's Bodies, Women's Worries: Health and Family Planning in a Vietnamese Rural Community.* Surrey, UK: Curzon Press, 1999.

Ganatra, Bela, Marc Bygdeman, Phan Bich Thuy, Nguyen Duc Vinh, and Vu Manh Loi. "Introducing Medical Abortion into Service Delivery in Vietnam: Report of an Assessment Conducted by the Ministry of Health, Ipas, and WHO." Hanoi: Ford Foundation, MOH, WHO, March 2003.

Goodkind, Daniel. "Abortion in Vietnam: Measurements, Puzzles, and Concerns." *Studies in Family Planning* 25, no. 6 (November–December 1994): 342–52.

———. "Rising Gender Inequality in Vietnam since Reunification." *Pacific Affairs* 68, no. 3 (Fall 1995): 342–59.

———. "Vietnam's One-or-Two-Child Policy in Action." *Population and Development Review* 21, no. 1 (March 1995): 85–111.

H. T. Hoa, N. V. Toan, A. Johansson, V. T. Hoa, B. Hojer, and L. A. Persson. "Child Spacing and Two Child Policy in Rural Vietnam: Cross Sectional Survey." *British Medical Journal* 313, no. 7065 (November 2, 1996): 1113–16.

Haughton, Jonathan, and Dominique Haughton. "Son Preference in Vietnam." *Studies in Family Planning* 26, no. 6 (November–December 1995): 325–37.

Hoang Ba Thinh. "Gender and Justice." In *Images of the Vietnamese Woman in the New Millennium,* ed. Le Thi Nham Tuyet, CGFED, 224–44. Hanoi: Gioi Publishers, 2002.

———. "Gender Viewpoint and Population Policy." In *Some Studies on Reproductive Health in Vietnam—Post-Cairo,* ed. Le Thi Nham Tuyet and Hoang Ba Thinh, CGFED, 155–76. Hanoi: National Political Publishing House, 1999.

———. "Marriage." In *Images of the Vietnamese Woman in the New Millennium,* ed. Le Thi Nham Tuyet, CGFED, 170–79. Hanoi: Gioi Publishers, 2002.

———. "Problem on Girl Adolescents." In *Images of the Vietnamese Woman in the New Millennium,* ed. Le Thi Nham Tuyet, CGFED, 180–91. Hanoi: Gioi Publishers, 2002.

———. "Relationship between Family Members." In *Images of the Vietnamese Woman in the New Millennium,* ed. Le Thi Nham Tuyet, CGFED, 139–56. Hanoi: Gioi Publishers, 2002.

———. "Reproduction and Family Happiness." In *Some Studies on Reproductive Health in Vietnam—Post-Cairo,* ed. Le Thi Nham Tuyet and Hoang Ba Thinh, CGFED, 185–92. Hanoi: National Political Publishing House, 1999.

———. *Sexual Exploitation of Children.* Hanoi: Gioi Publishers, 1999.

———. "Some Solutions Aiming at Preventing HIV/AIDS in Vietnam from the Gender Viewpoint." In *Some Studies on Reproductive Health in Vietnam—Post-Cairo,* ed. Le Thi Nham Tuyet and Hoang Ba Thinh, CGFED, 284–303. Hanoi: National Political Publishing House, 1999.

Johansson, Annika. *Dreams and Dilemmas: Women and Family Planning in Rural Vietnam.* Stockholm: Karolinska Institutet, 1998.

Johansson, Annika, Hoang Thi Hoa, Nguyen The Lap, Vinod Diwan, and Bo Eriksson. "Population Policies and Reproductive Patterns in Vietnam." *Lancet* no. 9014 (June 1, 1996): 1529–32.

Johansson, Annika, Le Thi Nham Tuyet, Nguyen The Lap, and Kajsa Sundstrom. "Abortion in Context: Women's Experience in Two Villages in Thai Binh Province, Vietnam." *International Family Planning Perspectives* 22, no. 3 (September 1996): 103–7.

Johansson, Annika, Nguyen Thu Nga, Tran Quang Huy, Doan Du Dat, and Kristina Holmgren. "Husbands' Involvement in Abortion in Vietnam." *Studies in Family Planning*
29, no. 4 (December 1998): 400–13.

Kane, Thomas T., Jennifer Middleton, and Kathy Shapiro. *Strategic Appraisal of the Reproductive Health Program of Vietnam.* Reproductive Health Program, December 2000.

Khuat Thu Hong. "Study on Sexuality in Vietnam: The Known and Unknown Issues."
Population Council, South and East Asia Regional Working Paper No. 11. Hanoi,
1998.

Le Thi Nham Tuyet. Professor of Social Anthropology, Director, Research Centre for Gender, Family and Environment in Development (CGFED). Interview March 23, 2004.
Hanoi, Vietnam.

————. "Closing Remarks." In *Images of the Vietnamese Woman in the New Millennium*,
ed. Le Thi Nham Tuyet, CGFED, 262–65. Hanoi: Gioi Publishers, 2002.

————. "Introduction: The Vietnamese Woman Today—Who Is She?" In *Images of the
Vietnamese Woman in the New Millennium*, ed. Le Thi Nham Tuyet, CGFED, 1–8.
Hanoi: Gioi Publishers, 2002.

Le Thi Nham Tuyet, and Hoang Ba Thinh. "Indicators of Action on Women's Health and
Rights after Beijing." In *Some Studies on Reproductive Health in Vietnam—Post-Cairo*,
ed. Le Thi Nham Tuyet and Hoang Ba Thinh, CGFED, 40–154. Hanoi: National Political Publishing House, 1999.

Le Thi Nham Tuyet, Pham Xuan Tieu, and Hoang Ba Thinh. "Country Study of Vietnam."
In *Some Studies on Reproductive Health in Vietnam—Post-Cairo*, ed. Le Thi Nham
Tuyet and Hoang Ba Thinh, CGFED, 9–39. Hanoi: National Political Publishing
House, 1999.

Levitt, Daniel M. Health and Humanitarian Program Manager, USAID Vietnam. Interview
March 24, 2004. Hanoi, Vietnam.

McCoy, Nina R. Public Health Specialist, Family Health International. Interview March
23, 2004. Hanoi, Vietnam.

McCoy, Nina, Thomas T. Kane, and Rosanne Rushing. *HIV/AIDS Prevention and Care in
Viet Nam: Lessons Learned from the FHI/Impact Project, 1996–2003.* Hanoi: Family
Health International Viet Nam, 2004.

Messersmith, Lisa J. Ph.D., MPH. Program Officer, Ford Foundation. Interview March 15,
2004. Hanoi, Vietnam.

Nguyen Hoang Anh. "Women and Health Care." In *Images of the Vietnamese Woman in
the New Millennium*, ed. Le Thi Nham Tuyet, CGFED, 115–28. Hanoi: Gioi Publishers, 2002.

Nguyen Hoang Anh. "Women in Industry." In *Images of the Vietnamese Woman in the New
Millennium*, ed. Le Thi Nham Tuyet, CGFED, 129–38. Hanoi: Gioi Publishers, 2002.

Nguyen Kim Cuc. Standing Vice-President, Viet Nam Family Planning Association (VIN-
AFPA). Interview March 9, 2004. Hanoi, Vietnam.

Nguyen Kim Thuy. "Rural Women in Vietnam." In *Images of the Vietnamese Woman in
the New Millennium*, ed. Le Thi Nham Tuyet, CGFED, 33–45. Hanoi: Gioi Publishers,
2002.

Nguyen Minh Luan. "Vietnamese Women and the Environment." In *Images of the Vietnamese Woman in the New Millennium*, ed. Le Thi Nham Tuyet, CGFED, 216–23.
Hanoi: Gioi Publishers, 2002.

Nguyen The Lap, Le Thi Nham Tuyet, and Annika Johansson. "Factors Affecting the Acceptance of Male and Female Sterilisation in Thaibinh Province." In *Some Studies on*

Reproductive Health in Vietnam—Post-Cairo, ed. Le Thi Nham Tuyet and Hoang Ba Thinh, CGFED, 259–83. Hanoi: National Political Publishing House, 1999.

———. "The Socio-psychological Factors of Women Giving Birth to 3rd Child upward in a Province of Red River Delta, North Vietnam." In *Some Studies on Reproductive Health in Vietnam—Post-Cairo,* ed. Le Thi Nham Tuyet and Hoang Ba Thinh, CGFED, 304–18. Hanoi: National Political Publishing House, 1999.

Nguyen The Lap, Le Thi Nham Tuyet, Annika Johansson, and Nguyen Thi Thu Huyen. "The Socio-psychological Factors Relating to Late Abortion." In *Some Studies on Reproductive Health in Vietnam—Post-Cairo,* ed. Le Thi Nham Tuyet and Hoang Ba Thinh, CGFED, 319–33. Hanoi: National Political Publishing House, 1999.

Nguyen Thi Bich Hang. Country Representative, Marie Stopes International. Interview March 16, 2004. Hanoi, Vietnam.

Nguyen Thi Hoai Duc. Director, Center for Reproductive and Family Health (RaFH). Interview March 11, 2004. Hanoi, Vietnam.

Nguyen Thi Thom, and Ann Larson. "DMPA Use Needs Better Side-Effect Management." *Population-Family Planning News* (NCPFP) No. 4 (Jan-June 1997): 5.

Nguyen Thu Nga. "Abortion Patterns and Women's Decision-Making in Abortion." Master's in Public Health thesis. Karolinska Institutet, Stockholm, 2000.

Nguyen Van Phai, Johan Knodel, Mai Van Cam, and Hoang Xuyen. "Fertility and Family Planning in Vietnam: Evidence from the 1994 Inter-censal Demographic Survey." *Studies in Family Planning* 27, no. 1 (January–February 1996): 1–16.

Pham Thi Hue. "Marriage and Fertility in Recent Studies." *Family and Women Studies* (Center for Family and Women Studies of Vietnam) No. 1 (2002): 38–44.

Population Council. *A Situation Analysis of Public Sector Reproductive Health Services in Seven Provinces of Vietnam.* Hanoi: Population Council, August 2000.

———. *Annual Report, 2001: South and East Asia.*

Quach Thu Trang. Program Officer, Population and Development International (PDI). Interview March 10, 2004. Hanoi, Vietnam.

Quinn-Judge, Sophie. "Women in the Early Vietnamese Communist Movement: Sex, Lies, and Liberation." *South East Asia Research* 9, no. 3 (2001): 245–69.

Socialist Republic of Viet Nam, Committee for Population, Family, and Children of Vietnam (CPFC). "Promulgation of the Population Ordinance." *Vietnam Population News* No. 26 (January-March 2003): 1.

———. "Results of the 2002 Population Change and Family Planning Survey." *Vietnam Population News* No. 26 (January-March 2003): 4–6.

———. "Situation of HIV/AIDS in Vietnam." *Vietnam Population News* No. 26 (January–March 2003): 6.

———. "Viet Nam 2002 Demographic and Health Survey: Major Findings." *Vietnam Population News* No. 28 (July–September 2003): 1–4.

Socialist Republic of Viet Nam, Committee for Population, Family, and Children of Vietnam (CPFC), Population Reference Bureau (PRB). *Adolescents and Youth in Viet Nam.* Hanoi: Center for Population Studies and Information, 2003.

Socialist Republic of Viet Nam, General Statistics Office. *1999 Population and Housing Census; Census Monograph on Marriage, Fertility and Mortality in Viet Nam: Levels, Trends and Differentials.* Hanoi: Statistical Publishing House, 2001.

Socialist Republic of Viet Nam, National Committee for Population and Family Planning (NCPFP). "Population Control Results Promising." *Population-Family Planning News* No. 8 (July–September 1998): 2.

————. "Strict Punishments Applied to Sexual Infringements on Children in Vietnam." *Family and Children Magazine*, January 2003, 12–13.

————. *Vietnam Population Strategy 2001–2010*. Hanoi: NCPFP, 2001.

Socialist Republic of Viet Nam, National Committee for Population and Family Planning, Centre for Population Studies and Information. *Selected Data of Some Censuses and General Survey Servicing Population-Family Planning Activities*. Hanoi: Ethnic Culture Publishing House, 1998.

Socialist Republic of Viet Nam. *Birth Spacing and Child Mortality in Viet Nam*. Ha Noi: Statistical Publishing House, 1996.

————. *Education in Viet Nam: Trends and Differentials*. Ha Noi: Statistical Publishing House, 1996.

Sokal, David, Do Trong Hieu, Debra H. Weiner, Dao Quang Vinh, Trinh Huu Vach, and Robert Hanenberg. "Long-term Follow-up after Quinacrine Sterilization in Vietnam. Part 1: Interim Efficacy Analysis." *Fertility and Sterility* 74 (2000): 1084–91.

Swidler, Leonard. "Confucianism for Modern Persons in Dialogue with Christianity and Modernity." *Journal of Ecumenical Studies* 40 (2003): 12–25.

Tran Thi Phuong Mai. Minister/Chairwoman, Committee for Population, Family, and Children. Deputy Director, Department of Reproductive Health, Ministry of Health. Interview March 10, 2004. Hanoi, Vietnam.

United Nations. *2000 Annual Report of the UN Resident Coordinator in Viet Nam*. Ha Noi: UN, 2000.

United Nations Country Team—Viet Nam. *IDT/MDG Progress—Viet Nam*. Hanoi: Office of the United Nations Resident Coordinator, July 2001.

UNAIDS, WHO. *AIDS Epidemic Update—December 2003*. Geneva: Joint UN Program on HIV/AIDS (UNAIDS), December 2003.

UNDP, UNFPA, WHO, and World Bank. "Abortion in Viet Nam: An Assessment of Policy, Programme, and Research Issues." Geneva: WHO, 1999. whqulibdoc.who.int/hq/1999/WHO_RHR_HRP_ITT_99.2.pdf (accessed March 17, 2004).

UNFPA Viet Nam. "Situation at a Glance: Population and Reproductive Health in Vietnam." No date.

Victor, Birgit Westphal, Do Thi Phuong, Tran Hung Minh, Hoan Tu Anh, Bui Thi Thanh Mai, Nguyen Thu Huong, and Nguyen Thi Kim Thanh. *Village Volunteers and Women's Reproductive Health*. Hanoi: Danish Red Cross, Viet Nam Red Cross, 1999.

Vu Hong Phong. "Expectations of Both Sexes Looking for Their Partners." In *Images of the Vietnamese Woman in the New Millennium*, ed. Le Thi Nham Tuyet, CGFED, 253–61. Hanoi: Gioi Publishers, 2002.

Vu Ngoc Bao, Philip Guest, Julie Pulerwitz, Le Thuy Lan Thao, Duong Xuan Dinh, Tran Thi Kim Xuyen, and Ann Levin. "Expanding Workplace HIV/AIDS Prevention Activities for a Highly Mobile Population: Construction Workers in Ho Chi Minh City." Horizons Program, Population Council. 2003.

Vu Quy Nhan. M.D., Ph.D. Director of Research and Capacity Building, Population Council. Interview March 16, 2004. Hanoi, Vietnam.

Vu Quy Nhan, Le Thi Phuong Mai, Nguyen Trong Hau, Robert A. Miller, Thomas T. Kane, John Stoeckel, Lynellyn D. Long, Bui Thi Thu Ha, Chu Phuc Thi, and Nguyen Thi Thom. *A Situation Analysis of Public Sector Reproductive Health Services in Seven Provinces of Vietnam*. Hanoi: Population Council, August 2000.

World Bank. "Vietnam Development Report: Poverty." November 26, 2003. www.worldbank.org.vn/news/press37_01.htm (accessed January 29, 2004).

World Health Organization. "Health and Ethnic Minorities in Viet Nam." Technical Series No. 1. WHO, June 2003.

Jordan

Abbaro, Seifeldin. Country Representative, UNFPA. Interview April 8, 2004. Amman, Jordan.

Abdel-Mohsen, Ayman. Deputy Project Director, Reproductive Health Advisor, Primary Health Care Initiatives (PHCI). Interview April 4, 2004. Amman, Jordan.

Abu Al-Sha'ar, Zeinab. Director of Medical Services, Jordanian Association for Family Planning and Protection (JAFPP). Interview April 4, 2004. Amman, Jordan.

Abu Ra'ad, Basem. Executive Director, Jordanian Association for Family Planning and Protection (JAFPP). Interview April 4, 2004. Amman, Jordan.

Abu Zaid, Kholoud. Former Senior Program Coordinator, Save the Children. Interview April 7, 2004. Amman, Jordan.

Al-Masarweh, Issa. Associate Professor, College of Social Sciences, University of Jordan. Interview April 6, 2004. Amman, Jordan.

Al-Masarweh, Issa S. "Adolescent and Youth Reproductive Health in Jordan: Status, Issues, Policies, and Programs." POLICY Project, January 2003.

Al-Omari, Nouf. Nurse, Medical Program Director, Commercial Market Strategies. Interview March 31, 2004. Amman, Jordan.

Al-Omari, Nouf, and Michael Bernhart. "Client Preference Regarding Provider for IUD Insertion." Unpublished ms. Commercial Market Strategies, November 2002.

Al-Zu'bi, Zuhair J. Chief, Field Health Programme, United Nations Relief and Works Agency (UNRWA)—Jordan. Interview April 25, 2004. Amman, Jordan.

Anonymous. "The Gender-Sensitive Fact-File: Profiles of the Arab League Countries—Jordan." *Al-Raida* 20, no. 100 (Winter 2003): 106–7.

Arab Women Organization. "Arab Women Organization: Making a Difference through Empowerment." Brochure, No date.

Asa'ad, A., B. Khraisat, C. Soliman, R. Qutob, and M. Al Kahteeb. "Prevalence of Reproductive Tract Infection (RTI)/Sexually Transmitted Infection (STI) in Symptomatic Women in Urban Jordan." Presented at Fifteenth International AIDS Conference, Bangkok, Thailand, July 11–16, 2004.

Bernhart, Michael. Resident Advisor—Jordan, Commercial Market Strategies. Interview March 31, 2004. Amman, Jordan.

Bernhart, Michael, Tara Muayad, Abdul Rahman, and Nesreen Salim Khraisha. "Reasons for Non-adoption of Modern Methods: An In-depth Field Study." Unpublished ms. Commercial Market Strategies, November 2003.

Bernhart, Michael, Rania Abu Baker, and Ghada Abu Ali. "Sources of Doctors' Knowledge of Contraceptives." Unpublished ms. Commercial Market Strategies, November 2001.

Bishara, Asma. Program Officer, Johns Hopkins University School of Hygiene and Public Health, Center for Communication Programs. Interview March 30, 2004. Amman, Jordan.

Bitar, Nisreen Haddadin. Former Program Manager, EngenderHealth. Interview April 26, 2004. Amman, Jordan.

Bitar, Nisreen, Janet Muzlan Turan, Saleh Mawajdeh, and Manal Shahrouri. "Client Perceptions of Norplant and Depo Provera at JAFPP Clinics." Amman: EngenderHealth, May 2002.

Bitar, Nisreen, Rasha Dabash, Salah Mawajdeh, Manal Shahrouri, and Ramez Habash. "Attitudes towards Tubal Ligation among Users, Potential Users, and Husbands in Jordan." Amman: EngenderHealth, October 2003.

El-Sarayrah, Mohamed Najib, Ali Oqla Njadat, Hatim Alawneh, Mohammad Jihad Al-Shraida, and Amjad Badr Al-Quadhi. "Population and Reproductive Health Issues in the Jordanian Daily Press: A Longitudinal Content Analysis 1994–1997–2000." Jordanian National Committee for Women (JNCW), Johns Hopkins University Center for Communication Programs, 2002.

Elsadda, Hoda. "Remaking Women: Feminism and Modernity in the Middle East." *Middle East Journal* 55, no. 1 (Winter 2001): 162.

EngenderHealth. "Jordanian Providers' Knowledge, Attitudes, and Practices Regarding Female Sterilization and Long-Acting Hormonal Methods." Amman: EngenderHealth, May 2002.

EngenderHealth. "Trends in Female Sterilization in Jordan, 1998–2000." Amman: EngenderHealth, May 2002.

Fargues, Philippe. "Population Dilemmas in the Middle East: Essays in Political Demography and Economy." *Population and Development Review* 25, no. 1 (March 1999): 177(4).

Farsoun, Michel, Nadine Khoury, and Carol Underwood. "In Their Own Words: A Qualitative Study of Family Planning in Jordan." IEC Field Report No. 6. Baltimore, MD: Johns Hopkins Center for Communication Programs, 1996.

Hamarneh, Leila. Director of Projects, Arab Women Organization of Jordan. Interview April 14, 2004. Amman, Jordan.

Hashemite Kingdom of Jordan, Department of Statistics (DOS), and Macro International Inc. (MI). *Jordan Population and Family Health Survey 1997*. Calverton, MD: Department of Statistics and Macro International, 1998.

Hashemite Kingdom of Jordan, Department of Statistics (DOS), and ORC Macro. *Jordan Population and Family Health Survey 2002*. Calverton, MD: ORC Macro, 2003.

Hashemite Kingdom of Jordan, Ministry of Health (MOH), Department of Statistics (DOS), Primary Health Care Initiatives (PHCI), Abt Associates, and United States Agency for International Development (USAID). *Jordan Healthcare Utilization and Expenditure Survey 2000*. Amman: Ministry of Health, 2000.

Hashemite Kingdom of Jordan, National Committee for Women (JNCW). Introductory brochure. No date.

———. "Jordanian Women: Major Socio-economic Indicators." No date.

———. "Jordanian Women: Mapping the Journey on the Road to Equality." Amman: JNCW, 2002.

———. "The National Strategy for Women in Jordan." Amman: JNCW, September 1993.

Hashemite Kingdom of Jordan, National Population Commission, General Secretariat (NPC/GS). "Highlights on the Jordanian Youth: Reproductive Health, Life Planning, Education and Employment." Amman, Jordan: Population Publication Series, April 2001.

———. "National Population Strategy Reproductive Health Action Plan, Stage 1: 2003–2007." Amman, Jordan: National Population Commission, April 2003.

─────. "National Reproductive Health and Life Planning Communication Strategy for Jordanian Youth 2000–2005." Amman, Jordan: Population Publication Series, no date.

Hashemite Kingdom of Jordan, National Population Commission, General Secretariat (NPC/GS), and Johns Hopkins University Population Communication Services. "Family Planning Knowledge, Attitudes, and Public Advocacy: Findings from the 1997 Survey of Muslim Religious Leaders in Jordan." Baltimore, MD: Johns Hopkins School of Public Health, 1998.

Hashim, Iman. "Reconciling Islam and Feminism." *Gender and Development* 7, no. 1 (March 1999): 7–14.

Husseini, Rana Ahmen. "Current Challenges Facing the Arab Women's Movements." *Al-Raida* 20, no. 100 (Winter 2003): 69–72.

Ilkkaracan, Pinar. "Women, Sexuality, and Social Change in the Middle East and the Maghreb." *Social Research* 69, no. 3 (Fall 2002): 753–79.

Karim, Mehtab S. "Reproductive Behavior in Muslim Countries." DHS Working Papers No. 23. Macro International Inc. and United Nations Population Fund. Calverton, MD: MI and UNFPA, October 1997.

Khoury, Nadine, and Michael Bernhart. "Perceptions of Contraceptives: A Projective Study." Unpublished ms. Commercial Market Strategies, November 2000.

Khraisat, Basma. Country Director, IMPACT Project, Family Health International. Interview April 20, 2004. Amman, Jordan.

Laloge, Michel. Social Sector for EC/Yemen, European Union—Delegation of the Commission to Jordan. Interview April 13, 2004. Amman, Jordan.

Lowrance, Sherry R. "After Beijing: Political Liberalization and the Women's Movement in Jordan." *Middle Eastern Studies* 34, no.3 (July 1998): 83.

Ma'ayta, Abdul Rahim. Coordinator, Program Officer, Higher Population Council General Secretariat. Interview April 5, 2004. Amman, Jordan.

Majid, Anouar. "The Politics of Feminism in Islam." *Signs* 23, no. 2 (Winter 1998): 321–61.

Malhas, Dana Khan N. National Programme Officer, United Nations Development Fund for Women (UNIFEM), Arab States Regional Office. (With Shatha Mahmoud, Project Coordinator, Migrant Women Workers Project.) Interview April 25, 2004. Amman, Jordan.

Mayer, Ann Elizabeth. "Comment on Majid's 'The Politics of Feminism in Islam.' " *Signs* 23, no. 2 (Winter 1998): 369–77.

Mernissi, Fatima. *The Veil and the Male Elite: A Feminist Interpretation of Women's Rights in Islam.* Trans. Mary Jo Lakeland. Cambridge, MA: Perseus Books, 1991.

Moghadam, Valentine M. "Islamic Feminism and Its Discontents: Toward a Resolution of the Debate." *Signs* 27, no. 4 (Summer 2002): 1135–72.

Nasser, Lamis, Bashir Belbeisi, and Diana Atiyat. "Violence against Women in Jordan: Demographic Characteristics of Victims and Perpetrators." Amman: UNIFEM, WHO, 1998.

Nasser Salwa. Executive Director, Jordan Forum for Business and Professional Women. Interview April 15, 2004. Amman, Jordan.

National Abortion Federation. *The Truth about Abortion.* 1996.

Qardan, Lina. Deputy Resident Advisor, Johns Hopkins University School of Hygiene and Public Health, Center for Communication Programs. Interview March 30, 2004. Amman, Jordan.

Qteit, Salwa Bitar. Senior Project Management Specialist, Office of Population and Family Health, United States Agency for International Development (USAID). Interview April 15, 2004. Amman, Jordan.

Queen Noor. *Leap of Faith: Memoirs of an Unexpected Life.* New York: Miramax Books, 2003.

Schoemaker, J., M. N. Sarayrah, A. Yassa, and S. Farah. *2001 Men's Involvement in Reproductive Health Survey: Impact assessment of a national communication campaign.* Baltimore, MD: Johns Hopkins Bloomberg School of Public Health Center for Communication Programs, 2002.

Seif El Dawla, Aida, Amal Abdel Hadi, and Nadia Abdel Wahab. "Women's Wit over Men's: Trade-offs and Strategic Accommodations in Egyptian Women's Reproductive Lives." In *Negotiating Reproductive Rights: Women's Perspectives Across Countries and Cultures,* ed. Rosalind P. Petchesky and Karen Judd, 69–107. London: Zed Books, 1998.

Sharma, Suneeta, and Issa Almasarweh. "Family Planning Market Segmentation in Jordan: An Analysis of the Family Planning Market in Jordan to Develop an Effective and Evidence-based Strategic Plan for Attaining Contraceptive Security." POLICY Project, Draft Report, March 2004.

Shteiwi, Mousa, and Michael Bernhart. "The Contraception Adoption Process." Unpublished ms. Commercial Market Strategies, August 2000.

Tabbarah, Riad. "Family, Gender, and Population in the Middle East: Policies in Context." (book review) *Population and Development Review* 23, no. 3 (Sept 1997): 666–68.

United Nations. "Programme of Action of the International Conference on Population and Development." www.unfpa.org/icpd/icpd_poa.htm#pt2ch1 (accessed April 7, 2003). Cairo, Egypt: United Nations, 1994.

United Nations Development Fund for Women (UNIFEM), Arab State Regional Office. "Evaluating the Status of Jordanian Women in Light of the Beijing Platform of Action." Amman: UNIFEM, 2003.

———. "Paving the Road towards Empowerment: Egypt, Jordan, Lebanon, Palestine, Syria, the United Arab Emirates and Yemen." Amman: UNIFEM, 2002.

———. "Violence against Women Campaign." Amman: UNIFEM, 1999.

UNAIDS. "AIDS News." (in Arabic) November 1, 2003.

United Nations Population Fund (UNFPA). "Towards Family Planning Policy in Jordan." Working Paper No. 9. May 1994.

United Nations Relief and Works Agency (UNRWA). "Fact Sheet on Health Programme in Jordan." Unpublished, no date.

Zurayk, Huda. "The Meaning of Reproductive Health for Developing Countries: The Case of the Middle East." *Gender and Development* 9, no. 2 (July 2001): 22–27.

Conclusion

Ahman, Elisabeth, and Iqbal Shah. "Unsafe Abortion: Worldwide Estimates for 2000." *Reproductive Health Matters* 10, no. 19 (May 2002): 13–17.

Al-Zu'bi, Zuhair J. Chief, Field Health Programme, United Nations Relief and Works Agency (UNRWA)—Jordan. Interview April 25, 2004. Amman, Jordan.

Alan Guttmacher Institute. "Abortion in Context: United States and Worldwide." Issues in Brief, Series 1. New York: Alan Guttmacher Institute, 1999.

Alan Guttmacher Institute. *Sharing Responsibility: Women, Society, and Abortion Worldwide.* New York: Alan Guttmacher Institute, 1999.

Cole, Janet. Obstetrician/gynecologist, former Head of Termination of Pregnancy Services. Gynaecological Oncology Unit, Groote Schuur Hospital. Interview April 18, 2000. Cape Town, South Africa.

Cruywagen, Tersia. Owner, Reproductive Choices. Interview May 19, 2000. Johannesburg, South Africa.

Gho Aspilcueta, Daniel, Obstetrician/gynecologist, CEO/President, Instituto Peruano de Paternidad Responsable (INPPARES). Interview November 12, 2003. Lima, Peru.

Guerrero, Rossina. Psychologist, Programa de Derechos Sexuales y Ciudadanía en Salud, Centro de la Mujer Peruana Flora Tristán. Interview October 31, 2003. Lima, Peru.

Gutiérrez Ramos, Miguel, Obstetrician/gynecologist. Medical Director of Pathfinder International, President-Elect of la Sociedad Peruana de Obstetricia y Ginecología. Interview November 12, 2003. Lima, Peru.

Kyeyune, Joy Kyazike. Vice President, Association of Uganda Women Medical Doctors, Project Manager, Adolescent Friendly Reproductive Health Services Project. Interview April 3, 2002. Kampala, Uganda.

Olea Mauleon, Cecilia. Programa de Derechos Sexuales y Ciudadanía en Salud, Centro de la Mujer Peruana Flora Tristán. Interview November 13, 2003. Lima, Peru.

Owomuhangi, Nestor. Associate Programme Officer of RH Programme, UNFPA. Interview March 7, 2002. Kampala, Uganda.

Petchesky, Rosalind P. "Cross-country Comparisons and Political Visions." In *Negotiating Reproductive Rights: Women's Perspectives Across Countries and Cultures,* ed. Rosalind P. Petchesky and Karen Judd, 295–323. London: Zed Books, 1998.

Qteit, Salwa Bitar. Senior Project Management Specialist, Office of Population and Family Health, United States Agency for International Development (USAID). Interview April 15, 2004. Amman, Jordan.

Quintanilla Zapata, Tammy. Lawyer, Movimiento El Pozo. Interview November 10, 2003. Lima, Peru.

Roberts, Dorothy. *Killing the Black Body: Race, Reproduction, and the Meaning of Liberty.* New York: Vintage Books, 1997.

Silliman, Jael, Marlene Gerber Fried, Loretta Ross, and Elena R. Gutierrez. *Undivided Rights: Women of Color Organize for Reproductive Justice.* Cambridge, MA: South End Press, 2004.

Vargas Vasquez, Trixsi. Coordinadora de Consejeria. Apoyo a Programas de Poblacion (APROPO). Interview November 11, 2003. Lima, Peru.

Index

Abbaro, Seifeldin, 170–71, 173, 181, 187
Abdel-Mohsen, Ayman, 174
abortion. *See also under individual*
    countries
    abortion-related death, 24, 32, 41,
      54–56, 118–19, 121, 153, 201
    consent laws (*see* consent
      laws—abortion)
    illegal, 2, 13, 24, 26, 31–32, 51, 54,
      56, 76–81, 98–99, 104, 118–19,
      134, 179–80, 195
    legalization of, 6, 8, 10, 198 (*see also*
      abortion *under individual countries*)
    mandatory waiting periods, 123–24,
      136
    medically induced, 28, 79, 101, 119,
      137, 155, 179
    other legal restrictions, 100, 120–24,
      136–37
    "partial-birth," 124, 136–37
    postabortion care, 6, 9, 32, 56, 61,
      77–79, 88, 154
    selective, 104–6, 154–56, 160
    taboo/stigma, 2, 55, 81, 98, 103–4, 154
Abu Ra'ad, Basem, 182
AbuZaid, Kholoud, 189–90, 192, 194
access to health services. *See under*
    individual countries
Adams, Abbie, 121–22, 124–25, 130–31
adolescent/teenage reproductive health.
    See under individual countries
Al-Masarweh, Issa, 185, 187
Al-Omari, Nouf, 172, 178, 180
Al-Zu'bi, Zuhair J., 174, 178–80, 185, 199
antiabortion policies, 136–37

antibiotics, 8, 21, 46, 57, 79, 198
Atergire, Jane, 45, 55
Atkins, Rachel, 116, 126, 137

Bernhart, Michael, 175–76, 182, 185
birth control pill
    access to, 51–52, 82
    discontinuation of, 149, 176
    lack of promotion of, 72, 82, 151–52
    misconceptions about, 72, 152, 155,
      175
    promotion of, 140, 177
    rate of use, 20–22, 51, 97, 116, 152
Bishara, Asma, 172, 178, 192
Bitar, Nisreen Haddadin, 179, 185–86,
    189, 192
Bormann, Sita Michael, 143–44, 161
Bush, George W., 9, 75–76, 88, 122, 124,
    136–37, 163

Camp, Brittany, 123
Chávez, Susana, 71–72, 74–75, 80, 84–85
Clinton, William J., 9
Cole, Janet, 16, 19–20, 23, 28–29, 31, 34,
    36, 203
colonialism, 12, 14, 43, 75, 90, 139, 153,
    165
condoms
    access to, 21, 51, 76, 85, 97, 176
    lack of promotion of, 151, 163
    misconceptions about, 114, 116
    promotion of, 58, 64, 72, 97, 159
    rate of use, 35, 42, 51, 59, 97, 116,
      140, 152, 159, 175

sterilization
abuses, 3, 5, 10, 13–15, 30, 67, 81–84, 87, 91, 110–13, 117, 130, 163, 199
consent laws (see consent laws—sterilization)
prevalence of, 22, 97, 175
rights to, 37, 84, 112, 120, 135
tubal ligation, 52, 132, 140, 159, 175, 185
vasectomy, 13–15, 22, 52, 97, 159, 175
structural adjustment programs, 4, 7

teenage pregnancy. See adolescent/teenage reproductive health under individual countries
Tint, Khin San, 31
Toledo, Alejandro, 75–76, 87
tubal ligation. See under sterilization

Uganda
abortion, 40, 46, 51, 54–58, 61, 66
access to health services and family planning, 41, 43, 44–52, 54, 58, 66
adolescent/teenage reproductive health, 42–43, 47, 51, 54, 59–61
contraception, 40–42, 46, 49–54, 56–57, 60, 63, 66
cultural views on fertility and sexuality, 41–42, 50, 52, 54
fertility, 40–41, 50, 60
gender equality, 47, 61, 63–65
health care system, 43–49, 60–61, 63, 66
HIV/AIDS, 40, 45, 57–61, 66
human rights, 62, 66
International Conference on Population and Development (ICPD), 60–62, 65–66
international influences on reproductive rights, 40, 43, 52, 60–64, 66
men's involvement in family planning, 41, 48–52, 63–66
non-governmental organizations (NGOs), 42–43, 52, 61, 63–64
obstacles for health care workers, 46, 57, 63
safe motherhood, 40–41, 44, 50, 58–63
sex education, 42–43, 54, 61, 63, 66

Ugaz, José Carlos, 75, 79, 81
United Nations Population Fund (UNFPA), 4, 9, 49, 54, 57, 59, 62–63, 133, 143, 147, 152, 162–63, 170–71, 173, 186–87, 202
United States Agency for International Development (USAID), 4, 8–9, 57, 61–62, 87–88, 133–34, 144, 158–59, 162–63, 173, 186, 193
United States of America
abortion history, 118–20
abortion today, 109–10, 112–13, 117–18, 120–25
access to health services, 109–10, 112, 115–16, 120, 123, 128–29, 131, 136, 138
adolescent/teenage reproductive health, 113–15, 119, 122, 129–30, 136–38
antiabortion violence, 125–29
contraception, 109–11, 113–20, 30, 132–33, 138
fertility, 109, 134
health insurance, 110, 115, 117, 131, 136 (see also United States of America—Medicaid)
HIV/AIDS and STIs, 113–14, 129–32
International Conference on Population and Development (ICPD), 133–34
mainstream reproductive rights movement, 134–36
Medicaid, 115, 117–18, 120–21, 124–25, 131
men's involvement in family planning, 122–23, 137–38
minority women's health, 109–13, 115–16, 121, 130–33, 135–36
National Association for the Advancement of Colored People (NAACP), 110, 136, 138
opposition to reproductive rights, 135–37
racism and reproductive health, 110–13, 135
sex education, 109, 113–15, 117, 119–20, 129, 137–38
United States Department of Health, Education, and Welfare, 3, 112
United States Supreme Court, 123, 128

DISCARDED